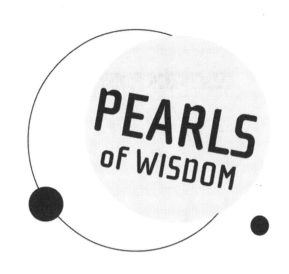

PEARLS of WISDOM

Ophthalmology
BOARD REVIEW

Second Edition

Richard R. Tamesis, M.D.

D1523068

McGraw-Hill
Medical Publishing Division

New York Chicago San Francisco Lisbon London
Madrid Mexico City Milan New Delhi
San Juan Seoul Singapore
Sydney Toronto

Ophthalmology Board Review, Second Edition

1 2 3 4 5 6 7 8 9 0   CUS/CUS   0 9 8 7 6 5

ISBN 0-07-146439-5

The editors were Catherine A. Johnson and Marsha Loeb.
The production supervisor was Phil Galea.
The cover designer was Handel Low.
Von Hoffmann Graphics was printer and binder.

This book is printed on acid-free paper.

Cataloging-in-Publication data for this title is on file at the Library of Congress.

DEDICATION

To Dr. Michael Griffith, who first suggested this project to me. I hope this makes a difference in your review for the board exams.

To Drs. Jack and Milagros Arroyo, Benjamin Cabrera, Victor Caparas, Cesar Espiritu, and Alnette Tan for their friendship and support.

Special thanks to Christine A. Cork, whose tireless dedication, hard work, and sunny optimism was always a source of inspiration.

And to my father, Dr. Jesus V. Tamesis, who first got me interested in ophthalmology. This is for you.

Richard

EDITOR IN CHIEF

Richard R. Tamesis, M.D.
Assistant Professor
Department of Ophthalmology
University of Nebraska Medical Center
Omaha, NE

FIRST EDITION CONTRIBUTORS:

Katherine L. Bergwerk, M.D.
Fellow in Comprehensive
Ophthalmology
Jules Stein Eye Institute
Department of Ophthalmology
UCLA School of Medicine
Los Angeles, CA

Brian A. Bonanni, M.D.
Clinical Associate
Department of Ophthalmology
Duke University
Durham, NC

Jon M. Braverman, M.D.
Assistant Professor
University of Colorado School of
Medicine
Director
Denver Health Medical Center
Denver, CO

Paul W. Brazis, M.D.
Consultant
Department of Ophthalmology and
Neurology
Mayo School of Medicine
Mayo Clinic
Jacksonville, FL

Willie Y.W. Chen, M.D.
Department of Ophthalmology and
Visual Sciences
University of Louisville
Louisville, KY

Thomas W. Hejkal, M.D., Ph.D.
Associate Professor
Department of Ophthalmology
University of Nebraska Medical Center
Omaha, NE

Cameron G. Javid, M.D.
Department of Ophthalmology
Tulane University
New Orleans, LA

Mark Juzych, M.D.
Department of Ophthalmology
Wayne State University
Detroit, MI

James W. Karesh, M.D.
Zanvyl Krieger Chairman
The Krieger Eye Institute
The Sinai Hospital of Baltimore
Associate Professor
The Wilmer Eye Institute
The Johns Hopkins Medical
Institutions
Baltimore, MD

Albert S. Khouri, M.D.
Opthalmology Service
Consulting Clinics Riyadh
Riyadh, Saudi Arabia

Ali M. Khorrami, M.D., Ph.D.
Assistant Professor
Health Science Center of Syracuse
State University of New York
Syracuse, NY

Andrew G. Lee, M.D.
Assistant Professor
Ophthalmology, Neurology and
Neurosurgery
Baylor College of Medicine
Residency Training Director
Cullen Eye Institute
Consultant
Neuro-Ophthalmology
Division of Neurosurgery
M.D. Anderson Cancer Center
The University of Texas
Houston, TX

Donald P. Maxwell, M.D.
Department of Ophthalmology
Tulane University
New Orleans, LA

Kevin M. Miller, M.D.
Associate Professor of Clinical
Ophthalmology
Jules Stein Eye Institute
Department of Ophthalmology
UCLA School of Medicine
Los Angeles, CA

Brian Mulrooney, M.D.
Director
Oculoplastic Services
University of Kansas
Kansas City, KS

Sumit K. Nanda, M.D.
Clinical Associate Professor
Dean A. McGee Eye Institute
University of Oklahoma
Oklahoma City, OK

Scott E. Olitsky, M.D.
Associate Professor
Residency Program Director
Department of Ophthalmology
State University of New York at
Buffalo and the Children's Hospital of
Buffalo
Buffalo, NY

Tony Realini, M.D.
Assistant Professor
Jones Eye Institute
University of Arkansas for Medical
Sciences
Little Rock, AR

Nelson R. Sabates, M.D.
Associate Clinical Professor
Director, Residency Training Program
Director, Retina Service
Department of Ophthalmology
University of Missouri-Kansas City
Kansas City, MO

Carla J. Siegfried, M.D.
Assistant Professor
Department of Ophthalmology and
Visual Sciences
Washington University School of
Medicine
St. Louis, MO

Michael J. Taravella, M.D.
Department of Ophthalmology
University of Colorado Health
Sciences Center
Denver, CO

Menno Ter Riet, M.D.
Department of Anesthesia
Veterans Affairs Medical Center
Miami, FLs

Kristen C. Zeller, M.D.
Department of Ophthalmology
Naval Medical Center
Portsmouth, VA

INTRODUCTION

Congratulations! *Ophthalmology Board Review: Pearls of Wisdom* will help you pass ophthalmology and improve your board scores. This unique format differs from all other review and test preparation texts. Let us begin, then, with a few words on purpose, format, and use.

The primary intent of this book is to serve as a rapid review of ophthalmology principles and serve as a study aid to improve performance on ophthalmology written and practical examinations. With this goal in mind, the text is written in a rapid-fire, question/answer format. The student receives immediate gratification with a correct answer. Questions themselves often contain a "pearl" reinforced in association with the question/answer.

Additional hooks are often attached to the answer in various forms, including mnemonics, evoked visual imagery, repetition and humor. Additional information not requested in the question may be included in the answer. The same information is often sought in several different questions. Emphasis has been placed on evoking both trivia and key facts that are easily overlooked, are quickly forgotten, and yet somehow always seem to appear on ophthalmology exams.

Many questions have answers without explanations. This is done to enhance ease of reading and rate of learning. Explanations often occur in a later question/answer. It may happen that upon reading an answer the reader may think - "Hmm, why is that?" or, "Are you sure?" If this happens to you, GO CHECK! Truly assimilating these disparate facts into a framework of knowledge absolutely requires further reading in the surrounding concepts. Information learned, as a response to seeking an answer to a particular question is much better retained than that passively read. Take advantage of this. Use this book with your ophthalmology text handy and open, or, if you are reviewing on train, plane, or camelback, mark questions for further investigation.

Ophthalmology Board Review risks accuracy by aggressively pruning complex concepts down to the simplest kernel. The dynamic knowledge base and clinical practice of medicine is not like that! This text is designed to maximize your score on a test. Refer to your mentors for direction on current practice.

Ophthalmology Board Review is designed to be used, not just read. It is an interactive text. Use a 3x5 card and cover the answers; attempt all questions. A study method we strongly recommend is oral, group study, preferably over an extended meal or pitchers. The mechanics of this method are simple and no one ever appears stupid. One person holds the book, with answers covered, and reads the question. Each person, including the reader, says "Check!" when he or she has an answer in mind. After everyone has "checked" in, someone states his or her answer. If this answer is correct, on to the next one. If not, another person states his or her answer, or the answer can be read. Usually, the person who "checks" in first gets the first shot at stating the answer. If this person is being a smarty-pants answer-hog, then others can take turns. Try it--it's almost fun!

Ophthalmology Board Review is also designed to be re-used several times to allow, dare we use the word, memorization. I suggest putting a check mark every time a question is missed. A hollow bullet has been arbitrarily provided. If you fill the bullets on re-uses of this book, forget this question! You will get it wrong on the exam! Another suggestion is to place a check mark when the question is answered correctly once; skip all questions with check marks thereafter. Utilize whatever scheme of using the bullets you prefer.

We welcome your comments, suggestions, and criticism. Great effort has been made to verify these questions and answers. There will be answers we have provided that are at variance with the answer you would prefer. Most often this is attributable to the variance between original sources (previously discussed). Please make us aware of any errata you find. We hope to make continuous improvements in future editions and would greatly appreciate any input with regard to format, organization, content, presentation, or about specific questions. Please write to Richard R. Tamesis, M.D. at rtamesis@unmc.edu. We look forward to hearing from you.

Study hard and good luck!

R.R.T.

TABLE OF CONTENTS

FUNDAMENTALS OF OPHTHALMOLOGY

○ **What is the volume of the adult orbit?**

Slightly less than 30 cc or one ounce.

○ **What are the average dimensions of the orbital entrance?**

35 mm in height and 45 mm in width.

○ **Where does the maximum width of the bony orbit occur?**

1 cm behind the anterior orbital margin.

○ **What is the depth range of the adult orbit?**

40-45 mm.

○ **Name the seven bones that make up the orbit.**

Frontal, sphenoid, ethmoid, lacrimal, maxilla, palatine, zygoma.

○ **What bones form the orbital roof?**

Frontal (orbital plate) and lesser wing of sphenoid— (*Front-less*).

○ **What bones form the lateral orbital wall?**

Greater wing of sphenoid and zygoma— (*Great-Z*).

○ **What bones form the orbital floor?**

Palatine, maxilla, and zygoma (orbital plate)— (*PaM-Z*).

○ **What bones form the medial orbital wall?**

Ethmoid (orbital plate), lacrimal, maxilla (frontal process) and lesser wing of sphenoid— (*ELMS*).

"2-2-3-4, all have sphenoid except the floor"— order is roof, lateral, floor, medial.

○ **What bone forms the anterior lacrimal crest?**

Lacrimal.

○   **What bone forms the posterior lacrimal crest?**

Maxilla.

○   **What structure lies 4 mm behind the superior orbital margin medially and of what is it composed?**

The trochlea is composed of hyaline cartilage.

○   **Which bone makes up the largest portion of the medial wall?**

Ethmoid.

○   **What is another name for the ethmoid bone in the medial wall?**

Lamina papyracea.

○   **The nasolacrimal canal extends into what part of the nose?**

Inferior meatus.

○   **What muscle arises from the orbital floor just lateral to the opening of the nasolacrimal canal?**

Inferior oblique.

○   **Name clinical features of a blowout fracture.**

Diplopia, enophthalmos, hypesthesia of the intraorbital nerve, positive forced ductions, fluid level in maxillary sinus, periorbital crepitus.

○   **Which wall of the orbit is thickest and strongest?**

Lateral wall.

○   **What four structures attach to the lateral orbital tubercle?**

Check ligament of the lateral rectus.
Suspensory ligament of the eyeball (Lockwood's ligament).
Lateral palpebral ligament.
Levator aponeurosis.

○   **What structures pass through the optic foramen?**

Optic nerve, ophthalmic artery, sympathetic fibers from the carotid plexus.

○   **What bone does the optic foramen pass through?**

Lesser wing of the sphenoid.

○   **What travels through the supraorbital foramen?**

Blood vessels and the supraorbital nerve (branch of V_1).

○ **What travels through the zygomatic foramen?**

Zygomaticofacial and zygomaticotemporal branches of the zygomatic nerve and the zygomatic artery.

○ **The infraorbital nerve is a branch of which division of CN V?**

V_2— maxillary.

○ **What passes through the superior part of the superior orbital fissure?**

Lacrimal and frontal branches of CN V and the trochlear nerve (*LFT*).

○ **What divides the inferior and superior parts of the superior orbital fissure?**

Origin of the lateral rectus muscle.

○ **What passes through the inferior division of the superior orbital fissure?**

Superior and inferior divisions of CN III, nasociliary branch of CN V, CN VI, superior ophthalmic vein, and the sympathetic nerve plexus.

○ **What passes through the inferior orbital fissure?**

Maxillary and pterygoid parts of CN V, a nerve from the pterygopalitine ganglion and the inferior ophthalmic vein.

○ **Where do the axons of the optic nerve originate?**

Ganglion cell layer of the retina.

○ **How many axons comprise the optic nerve?**

1-1.2 million.

○ **What is the length of the optic nerve?**

35-55 mm, averages 40 mm.

○ **Name the four parts of the optic nerve and their respective lengths.**

Intraocular	1 mm
Intraorbital	25 mm
Intracanalicular	4-10 m
Intracranial	10 mm

○ **What are the dimensions of the optic nerve head?**

1.5 mm horizontally by 1.75 mm vertically.

○   **When do the optic nerve axons become myelinated?**

Normally, after they pass posterior to the lamina cribosa.

○   **Because the optic nerve is developmentally part of the brain, what type of cells surround its fibers?**

Glial cells.

○   **What arises from the Annulus of Zinn?**

The rectus muscles.

○   **Which muscles originate partially from the sheath of the optic nerve and why is this clinically important?**

The superior rectus and medial rectus partially originate from the sheath of the optic nerve, and this may explain why patients with retrobulbar neuritis complain of pain with EOMs.

○   **Why is it clinically important that the dural sheath of the optic nerve is fused to the periosteum in the canal?**

Blunt trauma, especially to the brow, may be transmitted to the optic canal and cause a shearing of the dura and periosteum, compromising blood flow and causing ischemia.

○   **What is the blood supply of the surface of the optic nerve head?**

Central retinal artery or small cilioretinal arteries.

○   **What is the blood supply of the prelaminar region and the lamina cribrosa?**

Branches of the posterior ciliary arteries.

○   **Discuss the watershed zone formed by the terminal posterior ciliary arteries.**

When perfusion pressure drops, the area of the optic nerve contained within the watershed zone is prone to ischemic damage— e.g. anterior ischemic optic neuropathy.

○   **What is the blood supply of the intraorbital part of the optic nerve?**

Intraneural branches of the central retinal artery and pial branches from the peripapillary choroid, the central retinal artery and ophthalmic artery.

○   **What is the blood supply of the intracanalicular part of the optic nerve?**

Ophthalmic artery.

○   **What is the blood supply of the intracranial part of the optic nerve?**

Branches of the internal carotid and ophthalmic arteries.

○   **The superior division of CN III innervates what muscles?**

Superior rectus and levator palpebrae superioris.

○   **The inferior division of CN III innervates what muscles?**

Medial rectus, inferior rectus, and inferior oblique.

○   **What else is carried on CN III, from where does it arise, and what does it innervate?**

Parasympathetics that arise from the ciliary ganglion innervate the pupillary sphincter and ciliary body.

○   **How does a complete paralysis of CN III present?**

Ptosis (levator), inability to move the eye up or in (eye looks down and out), mydriasis (pupillary sphincter).

○   **What is unique about the location of the cell bodies of the part of CN III that innervates the levator?**

They are found in a *single* midline nucleus.

○   **What CN has the longest intracranial course and how long is it?**

CN IV— 75mm

○   **Which superior oblique does the right trochlear nucleus control?**

The right trochlear nucleus controls the left superior oblique.

○   **The motor portion of CN V innervates what structures?**

The muscles of mastication.

○   **Name the three sensory divisions of CN V and the three divisions of CN V_1.**

V_1— ophthalmic (lacrimal, frontal, and nasociliary)
V_2— maxillary
V_3— mandibular

○   **What, other than the lateral rectus muscle, does CN VI innervate?**

Nothing.

○   **Where is the ciliary ganglion located?**

Within the muscle cone, 1 cm in front of the annulus of Zinn, between the optic nerve and the lateral rectus.

O   **Discuss the three roots of the ciliary ganglion.**

Long (sensory) root— arises from the nasociliary branch of CN V and contains sensory fibers from the cornea, iris and ciliary body.

Short (motor) root— arises from the inferior division of CN III, synapses in the ganglion, and carries parasympathetics to the iris sphincter and ciliary muscle.

Sympathetic root— arises from the plexus around the internal carotid artery and innervates blood vessels of the eye and dilator fibers of the iris.

O   **What three ganglions are represented in the short ciliary nerves?**

Ciliary, superior cervical and trigeminal ganglions.

O   **Which muscle does not originate from the orbital apex and from which bone does it originate?**

The inferior oblique originates from the orbital plate of the maxilla.

O   **What is the Spiral of Tillaux?**

It is the shape formed by the insertions of the rectus muscles— 5.5, 6.5, 6.9, and 7.7 mm from the limbus (medial, inferior, lateral, superior). Remember that a suture placed through or under the superior rectus insertion that inadvertently penetrates the sclera could create a hole in the retina.

O   **What is the blood supply of the lateral rectus muscle and why is it unique?**

A single branch of the lacrimal artery supplies the lateral rectus, making it the only extraocular muscle supplied by only one vessel.

O   **Which muscles receive blood supply from the infraorbital artery?**

Inferior oblique and inferior rectus.

O   **What are the names of the two groups of fibers that make up eye muscles and what are their differences?**

1. Fibrillenstruktur— fast or twitch movement, individual neuromuscular junctions, acetylcholine receptor (-).

2. Felderstruktur— slow or tonic movement, multiple neuromuscular junctions, acetylcholine receptor (+).

O   **What are the dimensions of the normal adult palpebral fissure?**

27-30 mm in width by 8-11 mm in height.

O   **How far can a normal levator muscle raise the upper eyelid?**

15 mm.

❍   **How much can the frontalis muscle add to levator function?**

2 mm.

❍   **What is the antagonist muscle of the levator?**

Orbicularis oculi.

❍   **Name the muscle responsible and the clinical feature of the palpebral fissure change that occurs with each of the following conditions: Thyroid disease, Horner syndrome, facial palsy, third nerve palsy.**

Thyroid disease Müller's retraction
Horner syndromeMüller's ptosis
Facial palsy Orbicularis oculi lagophthalmos
Third nerve palsy Levator ptosis

❍   **What is special about the skin of the eyelid?**

It is the thinnest in the body and has no subcutaneous fat.

❍   **Where does the levator aponeurosis form its firmest attachments?**

On the anterior surface of the superior tarsus, 3 mm superior to the lid margin.

❍   **What is the name for the most superficial portion of the orbicularis oculi?**

Gray line— also known as the muscle of Riolan.

❍   **Where are the eyelashes and meibomian gland orifices found on the lid margin in relation to the gray line?**

Eyelashes arise anterior to the gray line.
Meibomian gland orifices open posterior to the gray line.

❍   **Name the respective secretions and locations of the secretory structures found in the eyelid and adenexa.**

Moll	apocrine	lid (*Molly is a sweaty ape*)
Lacrimal	eccrine	superior lateral orbit and lid
Krause and Wolfring	eccrine	plica, caruncle and lid
Meibomian	holocrine	tarsus
Zeis	holocrine	hair follicles, caruncle, and lid
Goblet cells	holocrine	conjunctiva, plica and caruncle

❍   **Describe the anatomic and functional components of the orbicularis oculi muscle.**

Orbital voluntary action
Palpebral voluntary and involuntary actions (blinking)
↳Preseptal
↳Pretarsal

○   **What is the orbital septum an extension of?**

The periosteum of the roof and floor of the orbi

○   **What is found just posterior to the orbital septum?**

Orbital fa

○   **What is an important distinction between orbital and preseptal cellulitis?**

Pain with and restriction of EOMs is associated with orbital, but not preseptal cellulitis.

○   **What happens to the levator muscle when it reaches Whitnall's ligament?**

It turns from a horizontal to a vertical direction and divides anteriorly into the levator aponeurosis and posteriorly into Müller's muscle.

○   **What forms Whitnall's ligament?**

A condensation of tissue surrounding the superior rectus and levator muscles.

○   **What is the tarsus composed of?**

Dense connective tissue, not cartilage.

○   **What are the dimensions of the upper and lower tarsal plates?**

Upper   29 x 1 x 11 mm
Lower   29 x 1 x 4 mm

○   **What is the name for misdirection of the orientation of the eyelids?**

Trichiasis.

○   **What is the name for aberrant growth of eyelashes through the meibomian gland orifices?**

Distichiasis.

○   **What type of muscle is Müller's muscle and how is it innervated?**

Smooth muscle that is sympathetically innervated.

○   **What type of epithelium covers the conjunctiva?**

Nonkeratinized squamous epithelium.

O   **What types of blood cells can be found in the substantia propria of the conjunctiva?**

Lymphocytes, macrophages, mast cells, and plasma cells.

O   **Where are goblet cells most concentrated in the conjunctiva?**

Inferior and medial conjunctiva, plica semilunaris and caruncle.

O   **Where in the conjunctiva can we find no goblet cells?**

In the limbal region.

O   **What structure is fused with the conjunctiva for ~2 mm posterior to the limbus?**

Tenon's capsule.

O   **What two main arteries supply the eyelids?**

External carotid via the facial artery system.
Internal carotid via branches of the ophthalmic artery.

O   **What are the two portions of the venous drainage of the eyelids and into what structures do they drain?**

Pretarsal drains into the internal and external jugular veins.
Posttarsal drains into the cavernous sinus.

O   **Where are lymphatics found in the orbit and to what nodes do they drain?**

Lymphatics are found in the conjunctiva paralleling vessels.
They drain into the preauricular and submandibular lymph nodes.

O   **What is the name for the vestigial structure in the eyelids that is analogous to the nictitating membrane of lower animals?**

Plica semilunaris.

O   **What divides the lacrimal gland into two parts?**

The lateral expansion of the levator aponeurosis.

O   **Why do we biopsy the orbital portion of the lacrimal gland when biopsy is needed?**

To avoid sacrificing the excretory ducts that pass through the palpebral portion.

O   **Where do the excretory ducts of the lacrimal gland empty?**

In the superior fornix approximately 5 mm above the superior border of the tarsus.

O   **When we measure basal tear secretion, what glands are we testing?**

The accessory lacrimal glands of Krause and Wolfring are tested.
The lacrimal gland is responsible for reflex tearing and its contribution is removed from this test by using topical anesthetic.

O   **In what percent of the population do the two canaliculi join to form a common canaliculus?**

90% — the other 10% have two openings into their lacrimal sac.

O   **What percent of full term neonates are born with a closed nasolacrimal duct?**

30% — most resolve spontaneously within 6 months.

O   **What structures penetrate Tenon's capsule?**

Optic nerve Posterior ciliary nerves
Posterior ciliary vessels Vortex veins

O   **The fusion of the sheaths of the inferior rectus muscle, the inferior tarsal muscle, and the check ligaments of the medial and lateral rectus muscles form what structure?**

The suspensory ligament of the globe or Lockwood's ligament.

O   **What is the range of normal for AP diameter in the adult eye?**

21-26 mm.

O   **What is the normal AP diameter of the eye at birth?**

16mm.

O   **When does the eye normally reach its maximum size?**

During puberty.

O   **What are the horizontal and vertical measurements of the adult cornea, anteriorly?**

Horizontal 12 mm
Vertical   11 mm

If viewed from behind, the normal cornea is spherical.

O   **Where is the sclera the thinnest? How thin is it? Why is this clinically important?**

The sclera is thinnest at the insertions of the rectus muscles, where it is only 0.3 mm thick. Inadvertent globe penetration can occur during strabismus surgery or the placement of bridle sutures.

❍ **Where is the sclera the thickest? How thick is it?**

The sclera is 1 mm thick at the posterior pole.

❍ **Where does the inferior oblique insert?**

The medial border inserts at the fovea and the lateral border inserts more anteriorly.

❍ **Describe the position of insertion of the superior oblique.**

Posterior to the equator and temporal to the vertical meridian.

❍ **What is the anatomic relationship between the superior oblique and superior rectus?**

The superior oblique lies beneath the superior rectus.

❍ **What is the function of the vortex veins? How many are there?**

The vortex veins drain the choroid, ciliary body and iris. There is 4-7 per eye.

❍ **How far are the ampullae of the vortex veins from the ora? What does the circle of veins represent?**

They lie 8-9 mm posterior to the ora. The circle of ampullae forms the equator of the fundus.

❍ **How many of each of the following structures are normally found per eye: Short posterior ciliary arteries? Short posterior ciliary nerves? Long ciliary arteries? Long ciliary nerves?**

Short posterior ciliary arteries	~20
Short posterior ciliary nerves	~10
Long ciliary arteries	4
Long ciliary nerves	4

❍ **From where do the ciliary arteries arise?**

Ophthalmic artery.

❍ **What are the layers of the tear film and what structures make them?**

Superficial oily layer	Zeis and Moll
Middle aqueous layer	Krause and Wolfring
Deep mucous layer	Goblet cells

❍ **What is the main refractive part of the eye? What is its strength?**

The cornea, tear film and aqueous form a lens with a power of approximately 43 diopters in air.

○   **What is the central thickness of a normal cornea? Peripheral thickness?**

Central— 0.52 mm; Peripheral— 1.0 mm.

○   **Where is the cornea normally steepest?**

Centrally.

○   **From what embryonic tissue is the corneal epithelium derived?**

Surface ectoderm.

○   **What connects the basal cell layer of the corneal epithelium to its basement membrane?**

Hemidesmosomes.

○   **What makes the corneal surface naturally irregular and what corrects this?**

Microplicae and microvilli give the corneal surface a natural irregularity. This surface is made smooth by the precorneal tear film.

○   **Where are the corneal epithelial stem cells located?**

At the limbus.

○   **How thick is Bowman's layer and why is it called a layer and not a membrane?**

Bowman's layer is 8-14 microns thick. It is acellular and composed of random collagen fibrils.

○   **What happens to Bowman's layer after injury?**

A scar forms because Bowman's is not replaced.

○   **What composes 90% of the corneal thickness? What is it made up of?**

The corneal stroma accounts for 90% of the corneal thickness. It is composed of fibroblasts (keratocytes), ground substance and collagen lamellae.

○   **What is the macroperiodicity of corneal collagen fibrils?**

640 angstroms.

○   **What is corneal ground substance composed of and what synthesizes it?**

It is composed of mucoprotein and glycoprotein and is synthesized by the keratocytes.

○   **What is the basement membrane of the corneal endothelium called? What special stain identifies it?**

Descemet's membrane is the basement membrane of the corneal epithelium. It is PAS-positive.

○   **Describe the two zones of Descemet's membrane.**

The anterior banded zone is created *in utero*.
The posterior nonbanded zone is laid down by the corneal endothelium throughout life.

○   **What is the name for peripheral excrescences of Descemet's membrane? What about central ones?**

Peripheral— Hassall-Henle warts (common); Central— guttata.

○   **From which embryonic tissue is the corneal endothelium derived?**

Neural crest.

○   **How many cell layers make up the corneal endothelium?**

One.

○   **What do adjacent corneal epithelial cells share that endothelial cells lack?**

Desmosomes.

○   **What happens to corneal endothelial cells with age?**

Their numbers decline and they lose mitochondria. Corneal endothelial cells normally do not undergo mitosis.

○   **Where do traumatic scleral ruptures most frequently occur?**

They occur most commonly at the supranasal limbus, but also occur frequently anywhere along limbus, at the rectus insertions and at the equator.

○   **How are the sclera and cornea similar? How are they different?**

Both made up of collagen and are essentially avascular. The sclera is opaque and white due to random collagen orientation and greater water content, while the cornea is clear because its collagen fibrils are arranged in an orderly fashion and its stroma is relatively dry.

○   **What path does extraocular extension of choroidal melanoma take?**

Scleral emissaria allow passage of cells out of the globe.

○   **Name the structures of the anterior chamber angle from anterior to posterior.**

1. Schwalbe's line.
2. Trabecular meshwork.
3. Scleral spur.
4. Ciliary body.
5. Peripheral iris.

○ **Name the structures included in the limbus.**

1. Conjunctiva.
2. Tenon's capsule.
3. Episclera.
4. Corneoscleral stroma.
5. Aqueous outflow apparatus.

○ **Where, anatomically, does the cornea end and the sclera begin?**

At a plane connecting the terminations of Descemet's and Bowman's that extends posteriorly to Schlemm's canal.

○ **What is the cross sectional shape of the trabecular meshwork? What forms its corners?**

It is approximately triangular in cross section.
Apex— Schwalbe's line.
Base— scleral spur and ciliary body.

○ **What are the three parts of the trabecular meshwork and name the part that is responsible for most of the resistance to aqueous outflow?**

Uveal, corneoscleral, and juxtacanalicular.
The juxtacanalicular meshwork causes the greatest resistance to aqueous outflow.

○ **What area of the trabecular meshwork is most pigmented?**

Inferior chamber angle.

○ **What type of endothelium lines the canal of Schlemm?**

Nonfenestrated monolayer of endothelial cells connected by tight junctions.

○ **Where is the thinnest part of the iris located?**

At its junction to the ciliary body— the iris root.

○ **What are posterior synechia?**

Adhesions of the posterior iris surface to the anterior lens capsule.

○ **What are peripheral anterior synechia (PAS)?**

Adhesions of the anterior peripheral iris to the posterior peripheral cornea.

❍   **What structure lies where the gonioscopic slit beam converges to a point?**

Schwalbe's line.

❍   **What is the normal adult AP diameter of the lens up to about age 40? Equatorial diameter?**

AP— 4-5 mm; Equatorial— 9-10 mm.

❍   **What occurs during accommodation?**

The ciliary muscle contracts, decreasing zonular tension, increasing AP lens diameter, and increasing the refractive power of the lens. The pupil also constricts due to stimulation of the pupillary sphincter muscle. Both of these muscles are innervated by parasympathetic fibers.

❍   **What nourishes the lens after regression of the hyaloid vascular system?**

Aqueous and vitreous.

❍   **What is responsible for the innervation of the lens?**

Nothing— the lens lacks innervation.

❍   **What is the PAS-positive basement membrane of the lens epithelial cells?**

Lens capsule.

❍   **Where is the lens capsule thickest? Thinnest?**

Thickest— midway between the anterior pole and the equator.
Thinnest— posterior pole.

❍   **Where can you find dividing lens epithelial cells?**

Beneath the anterior and equatorial lens capsule— not under the posterior capsule
This is why extracapsular cataract extraction has the potential to leave a clear posterior capsule.

❍   **What causes posterior capsular opacification after cataract extraction?**

Migration and proliferation of lens epithelial cells across the posterior capsule.

❍   **What forms the lens sutures?**

Anterior sutures— interdigitations of apical lens fiber cell processes.
Posterior sutures— interdigitations of basal cell processes.

❍   **Where do the zonules originate? Where do they insert?**

They originate from the basal laminae of the nonpigmented epithelium of the pars plana and pars plicata of the ciliary body in the valleys of the ciliary processes and insert on the lens capsule, anterior and posterior to the equator.

O   **What makes up the uveal tract?**

Iris, ciliary body, and choroid.

O   **Where is the uveal tract firmly attached to the sclera?**

Scleral spur, exit points of the vortex veins, and the optic nerve.

O   **Where is the pigmentation located that is responsible for iris color?**

Anterior border layer of the deep stroma.

O   **What forms the bulk of the iris stroma?**

Blood vessels.

O   **What is the posterior pigmented layer of the iris continuous with?**

The nonpigmented epithelium of the ciliary body and the neurosensory retina.

O   **Describe physiologic ectropion.**

The normal continuation of the posterior pigmented layer of the iris around the pupillary border and onto the anterior iris surface for a short distance.

O   **What causes the dilator muscle of the iris to contract?**

Alpha$_2$ adrenergic sympathetic stimulation.

O   **Describe the sympathetic innervation to the iris dilator muscle.**

First-order neuron— originates in the ipsilateral posterolateral hypothalamus, travels through the brainstem and synapses in the intermediolateral gray matter of the spinal cord at C_8 and T_2.

Second-order neuron— leaves the spinal cord, crosses over the pulmonary apex, through the stellate ganglion (no synapse) and synapses in the superior cervical ganglion.

Third-order neuron— exits the superior cervical ganglion, unites with the internal carotid plexus, travels through the cavernous sinus, joins V_1 to enter the orbit, and innervates the dilator muscle of the iris.

O   **The nerve to what muscle carries the post-ganglionic parasympathetic fibers to the iris sphincter?**

The nerve to the inferior oblique from the inferior division of CN III.

○   **In what nucleus do the parasympathetic fibers originate?**

Edinger-Westphal subnucleus.

○   **Where does the ciliary body attach to the sclera?**

Its base attaches to the scleral spur.

○   **What are the two functions of the ciliary body?**

Aqueous humor formation and accommodation.

○   **Where is the pars plana located in relation to the corneal limbus?**

The pars plana is 3-4 mm posterior to the surgical limbus.

○   **What in the ciliary body is responsible for maintaining the blood-aqueous border?**

The zonulae occludentes along the apical border of the nonpigmented epithelium.

○   **How thick is the choroid?**

0.25 mm

○   **Describe the unique features of choroidal blood flow?**

The blood flow of the choroid is high compared to other tissues. Venous blood has only 2-3% less O_2 than arterial blood.

○   **Is Bruch's membrane PAS-positive? Is it a true membrane?**

Yes, it is PAS-positive.
No, it is not a true membrane.

○   **What are the five layers of Bruch's membrane?**

Basal lamina of the RPE.
Inner collagenous layer.
Middle elastic layer.
Outer collagenous layer.
Basal lamina of the choriocapillaris.

○   **Is Bruch's membrane permeable to fluorescein?**

Yes.

○   **What is a potential complication of a break in Bruch's membrane?**

Subretinal choroidal neovascular membranes.

O   **What forms the outer blood-retina barrier?**

Zonulae occludentes and zonulae adherentes of the RPE.

O   **What forms the inner blood-retina barrier?**

Endothelium of the retinal blood vessels.

O   **How are foveal RPE cells different from extrafoveal RPE cells?**

Foveal RPE cells are taller and have more melanosomes than their extrafoveal
counterparts. This is one of the reasons that choroidal flush is relatively dim under the
fovea during IVFA.

O   **What is the location of drusen?**

Between basement membrane of the RPE and inner collagenous layer of Bruch's
membrane.

O   **Where is 90% of cones found in the retina?**

Almost all of the photoreceptors in the fovea are cones, but 90% of the total cones are
found outside the fovea.

O   **A cilioretinal artery contributes to some portion of macular circulation in what
percent of people?**

15% of people have cilioretinal arteries that contribute to their *macular* circulation, but a
cilioretinal artery may contribute to any part of the retina. They are found in 30% of eyes
and 50% of individuals.

O   **What do arterioles and venules in the retina share at their crossings?**

They share a common basement membrane. This is the reason why AV nicking and
venous occlusions at AV crossings.

O   **What forms the external limiting membrane of the retina?**

Attachment sites of adjacent photoreceptors and Muller cells.

O   **Axons of what cells form the nerve fiber layer of the retina?**

Ganglion cells.

O   **What forms the internal limiting membrane of the retina? What can happen if
a break forms in the ILM?**

Foot processes of Muller cells.
A break in the ILM is necessary for epiretinal membrane formation.

❍   **Are the external and internal limiting membranes of the retina true membranes?**

No.

❍   **Where is the retina the thickest? How thick? The thinnest? How thin?**

Thickest	Papillomacular bundle	0.23 mm
Thinnest	Foveola	0.10 mm
	Ora serrata	0.11 mm

❍   **Define the macula histologically and clinically.**

Histologically, it is the area where there is more than one layer of ganglion cell nuclei. Clinically, it is commonly thought of as the area of retina between the arcades.

❍   **What are the two major pigments found in the macula lutea (small yellow spot)?**

Zeaxanthin and lutein.

❍   **We already discussed one reason for decreased choroidal fluorescence under the fovea— name another.**

Xanthophyll pigment found in the macula.

❍   **What is the size of the fovea?**

1.5 mm = 1500 microns ≅ 1 disc diameter.

❍   **What is the foveola and what is found there?**

It is the central depression in the fovea and is also known as the umbo. Only photoreceptors, glial cells and Müller cells are found there.

❍   **What is the name for the cysts found in paraffin sections of the peripheral retina at the ora serrata?**

Blessig-Iwanoff cysts.

❍   **What is the weight, volume and make-up the vitreous?**

Weight	4.0 g
Volume	4.0 ml
Composition	99% water

Hyaluronic acid is responsible for the increased viscosity of the vitreous compared to water.

❍   **How wide is the vitreous base and where does it attach?**

It is 6mm wide.   It extends 2 mm anterior and 4 mm posterior to the ora serrata.

❍   **What forms Cloquet's Canal?**

Regression of the hyaloid vasculature before birth.

❍   **Which cranial nerve has the distinction of having the fewest number of fibers, being the only one to completely decussate, and being the only motor nerve to exit the brainstem dorsally?**

CN IV.

❍   **An aneurysm of the anterior communicating artery could effect which cranial nerve?**

Optic nerve.

❍   **Where is a common place for the occurrence of aneurysms that affect CN III?**

At the junction of the posterior communicating and internal carotid arteries.

❍   **Macular fibers from which quadrant cross anteriorly in the chiasm and bulge into the contralateral optic nerve? What is this bulge called?**

Fibers from the inferonasal macula form Wilbrand's anterior knee.

❍   **What artery most frequently supplies the visual cortex?**

The posterior cerebral artery.

❍   **What structures are found within the cavernous sinus?**

Internal carotid artery.
The sympathetic plexus surrounding the internal carotid artery.
Cranial nerves III, IV, V_1, V_2, and VI.

❍   **What three growth factors that mediate the process of induction in a developing embryo have been identified?**

Fibroblast growth factor   FGF
Insulin-like growth factor-I   IGF-I
Transforming growth factor-beta   TGF-ß

❍   **What is meant by the term induction?**

This term is used to describe the process where one tissue directs the development of another tissue.

❍   **What is the name for the master genes that control the activity of other genes?**

Homeobox genes.
These genes are found in all plants and animals and are conserved evolutionarily.

❍   How many base pairs compose homeobox genes?

180 base pairs.

❍   What is the name for the 60 amino acids encoded by a homeobox gene?

Homeodomain.

❍   How does the homeodomain regulate gene expression?

These proteins bind to specific DNA sequences on other genes, causing either activation or repression. The homeodomain acts as a set of transcription factors.

❍   A mutation in the Pax-6 homeobox gene can produce what ocular abnormalities?

Peter's anomaly or aniridia.

❍   If the Pax-2 homeobox gene contains a mutation, what ocular abnormality can result?

Optic nerve coloboma.

❍   What is the name for the group of anomalies resulting from defects in the migration or terminal differentiation of neural crest cells?

Neurocristopathies.

❍   What ocular structures are derived from mesoderm?

1. Extraocular muscles.
2. Schlemm's canal.
3. Vascular endothelium.
4. Sclera, temporally.

❍   What ocular and orbital structures are derived from neural crest?

1. Cartilage
2. Corneal endothelium
3. Choroidal stroma
4. Corneal stroma
5. Ciliary body stroma
6. Iris stroma
7. Ciliary ganglions
8. Meninges of the optic nerve
9. Ciliary muscles
10. Orbital bones

11. Connective tissue of the extraocular muscles
12. Sclera, other than temporally
13. Trabecular meshwork
14. Connective tissue of the orbit

○   **What ocular structures are derived from neuroectoderm?**

1. Ciliary epithelium
2. Neurosensory retina
3. Iris posterior pigmented epithelium
4. Optic nerve
5. Iris dilator muscle
6. Retinal pigment epithelium
7. Iris sphincter muscle
8. Vitreous

○   **What ocular structures are derived from surface ectoderm?**

1. Cilia
2. Glands
3. Conjunctival epithelium
4. Lacrimal drainage system
5. Corneal epithelium
6. Lens
7. Eyelids
8. Vitreous

○   **On what day of gestation do the optic pits first appear?**

Day 22 or 23.

○   **On what day of gestation does the optic vesicle evaginate?**

Day 25.

○   **On what day of gestation is the lens placode induced by the optic vesicle?**

Day 27 or 28.

○   **On what day of gestation does the embryonic fissure close?**

Day 33.

○   **Where along the embryonic fissure does closure begin?**

Closure begins inferiorly midway between the optic nerve and iris and proceeds anteriorly and posteriorly simultaneously.

○   **Complete fusion of the embryonic fissure encloses what artery within the globe?**

Hyaloid artery.

○ **When does the retina complete its development?**

Remodeling of foveal elements is not complete until approximately 4 years of age.

○ **What is the name for the inner plexiform layer of the retina prior to its maturation?**

Transient nerve fiber layer of Chievitz.

○ **How many optic nerve axons are present at 16 weeks gestation?**

3.7 million.

By 33 weeks, however, attrition has decreased the number of optic nerve axons to the adult total of around 1.1 million.

○ **Primary lens fibers form what part of the lens?**

The embryonic nucleus.

○ **By what day of gestation have the primary lens fibers filled the lens vesicle?**

Day 45.

○ **During which month of gestation do the eyelid folds meet and fuse together?**

Third month.

○ **During which month of gestation do the eyelids begin to separate?**

Fifth month.

○ **During which month of gestation does the hyaloid vascular system begin to regress?**

Fourth month.

○ **During which month of gestation is the regression of the hyaloid vascular system complete?**

Eighth month.

○ **During which month of gestation is the anterior chamber angle completed?**

Eighth month.

○ **During which month of gestation do the retinal vessels reach the temporal periphery?**

Ninth month.

O   **What remains of the primary vitreous in a normal adult?**

Cloquet's canal is the only normal remnant of the primary vitreous.
Bergmeister's papilla and Mittendorf's dot are two other common remnants.

O   **What structure does the secondary vitreous become?**

The main vitreous body.

O   **The tertiary vitreous is involved in the development of what structure?**

The zonular apparatus.

O   **At what age is the adult 68° angle of ocular alignment reached?**

At about 3 years of age the globes reach their adult orientation.
At birth the angle is 71°.

O   **What is the name for a substance or factor that causes or increases the incidence of physical anomalies in a developing embryo?**

Teratogen.

O   **Name some classes of nongenetic teratogens.**

1. Developmental failures
2. Nutritional deficiencies
3. Drugs
4. Radiation
5. Maternal infections
6. Toxins

O   **During which trimester can teratogens cause major orbital and ocular structural abnormalities?**

First trimester.

O   **Exposure of the fetus to alcohol during certain critical periods can cause what ocular abnormalities?**

1. Anterior lenticonus
2. Microphakia
3. Colobomas
4. Microphthalmos

O   **What is the name for total absence of ocular tissues?**

Anophthalmos.

The diagnosis of this very rare condition can only be confirmed histologically.

○   **Which type of anophthalmos is lethal and why?**

Secondary anophthalmos is lethal because it is caused by complete suppression of the development of the forebrain.

○   **What is the name given to a small, but otherwise normal globe?**

Nanophthalmos.

○   **How can nanophthalmos be inherited?**

Autosomal dominant or autosomal recessive.

○   **What is the name for a small malformed globe?**

Microphthalmos.
Most cases of clinical anophthalmos are actually severe cases of microphthalmos.

○   **Name two genetic aneuploidy (abnormal number of chromosomes) conditions that can result in microphthalmos.**

Trisomy 13 (Patau syndrome).
Trisomy 18 (Edwards syndrome).

○   **What is the name for a single midline eye?**

Cyclopia.

○   **Where is the proboscis (primitive nose) located in true cyclopia?**

Above the midline ocular structure.

○   **Is cyclopia compatible with life?**

No, cyclopia is a lethal condition.

○   **What is the name for two incomplete globes joined at the midline?**

Synophthalmia.

○   **Is synophthalmia compatible with life?**

No, like cyclopia, synophthalmia is also lethal.

○   **What is the name for the condition caused when the optic vesicles remain in an embryonic state?**

Cystic eye.

❍   **What is the name for the condition that occurs when faulty closure of the embryonic fissure causes a remnant of the optic vesicle to be displaced outside the globe?**

Cystic coloboma.

❍   **What is the name for a cystic abnormality found in the orbit that contains elements from all primitive germ layers?**

Orbital teratoma.

❍   **What is the name for a mass of cerebral tissue protruding through an orbital suture?**

Encephalocele.

❍   **What is the name for the condition caused by failure of the eyelid folds to form, leaving a single layer of skin lying over a usually malformed eye?**

Cryptophthalmos.

❍   **In cryptophthalmos, where can the eyebrows be found if they are present at all?**

Usually the eyebrows are completely absent, but if present, they will be small and displaced far temporally.

❍   **What causes the risk of a trisomy to increase?**

Increasing maternal age.

❍   **What is the name given to the meiotic abnormality that leads to monosomy or trisomy?**

Nondisjunction.

❍   **What is the only sex chromosome aneuploidy that is known to have characteristic ocular findings?**

Turner syndrome (45,X).

EXTERNAL DISEASE AND CORNEA

❍ **Describe the technique for performing a gram stain.**

1. Crystal violet x 1 minute, rinse with tap water.
2. Gram's iodine x 1 minute, rinse.
3. Tilt and decolorize slide.
4. Safranin solution x 1 minute, rinse, dry.
5. Examine with oil-immersion.

❍ **What are Hassall-Henle bodies?**

Peripheral excrescences of Descemet's membrane toward to anterior chamber.

❍ **What is the best slit lamp technique to see Hassall-Henle bodies?**

Specular reflection.

❍ **When are Hassall-Henle bodies pathologic?**

When they are found centrally (corneal guttata).

❍ **Tiny dot and comma shaped opacities in the deep corneal stroma composed of lipofuscin are known as what?**

Corneal farinata.

❍ **What substance is deposited in band keratopathy and in what layer?**

Calcium hydroxyapatite in Bowman's layer.

❍ **Why should thyroid function tests be requested for in superior limbic keratoconjunctivitis?**

SLK is associated with thyroid dysfunction in about half of all cases.

❍ **What is the definitive treatment for SLK?**

Surgical resection of the superior bulbar conjunctiva.

❍ **What is the average corneal endothelial cell count of a person between the ages of 40 and 90?**

2400 cells/mm^2 (range 1500-3500).

❍   **What is defined as increased variability of corneal endothelial cell shape and size?**

Shape – pleomorphism.
Size – polymegethism.

❍   **What method of indirect illumination with the slit lamp uses total internal reflection in the cornea to highlight areas of reduced light transmission?**

Sclerotic scatter.

❍   **Describe techniques of qualitative and quantitative corneal esthesiometry.**

Qualitative -   use a wisp of cotton from a common CTA.
Quantitative - an esthesiometer uses a filament that increases with rigidity as it is
                shortened to test sensation.

❍   **What cranial nerve is tested by corneal esthesiometry?**

Trigeminal nerve.

❍   **What assumption in keratometry makes it useless in evaluating irregular astigmatism, and what is a better tool for this?**

Keratometry assumes that the cornea is a spherocylindrical surface with two perpendicularly opposed curvatures that lie 3mm apart on the central cornea. Computerized videokeratoscopy is better at evaluating irregular astigmatism.

❍   **What substances in our tears act to control the conjunctival flora and reduce bacterial adherence?**

Lactoferrin, lysozyme, beta-lysin, and secretory IgA.

❍   **What is stained by Rose bengal?**

Devitalized cells and cells that have lost their mucin surface.

❍   **The bulbar conjunctiva vessels are terminal branches of which artery?**

Ophthalmic artery.

❍   **What is an anterior embryotoxon?**

This is arcus juvenilis characterized by a white ring in the anterior peripheral cornea present either at birth or up to middle age.

❍   **What is the difference between trichiasis and distichiasis?**

Trichiasis is a misdirection of the lashes, while distichiasis is the presence of accessory lashes arising from the meibomian gland orifices.

○ **What is the difference between madarosis and poliosis?**

Madarosis is patchy or diffuse loss of lashes - poliosis is patches of whiting in the lashes.

○ **What is the difference between papillae and follicles?**

Papillae have a vascular core, while follicles are collections of lymphocytes with a germinal center.

○ **Why do giant papilla form?**

After prolonged conjunctival inflammation the anchoring septae weaken and papillae become confluent.

○ **What is the difference between membranes and pseudomembranes?**

Membranes cause bleeding when stripped - pseudomembranes do not cause bleeding. They are both formed from fibrinous exudate.

○ **To what nodes do the lymphatics from the eye drain?**

Preauricular and Submandibular.

○ **What is the difference between punctate epithelial erosions (PEE) and punctate epithelial keratopathy (PEK)?**

PEE are depressions, while PEK are raised areas on the corneal epithelium.

○ **What are corneal epithelial filaments?**

Strands of mucous and degenerated epithelial cells attached to the cornea at one end that is pulled in the direction of movement of the upper eyelid.

○ **What is the radius of curvature of the anterior cornea?**

7.5 mm.

○ **What is a focal lymphocytic nodule lying on the limbus representing a cell-mediated hypersensitivity reaction to staph?**

Phlyctenule.

○ **What syndrome is characterized by granulomatous conjunctivitis with an enlarged preauricular node?**

Oculoglandular syndrome.

○ **What pathogens can stimulate the alternate complement pathway?**

Gram negative bacteria contain endotoxins, which activate this pathway.

❍ **Where are the accessory lacrimal glands located?**

The glands of Wolfring are located in the tarsus, while the glands of Krause are in the conjunctival fornices.

❍ **What is the difference between micropannus and macropannus?**

Micropannus is <1 mm
Macropannus is >1 mm

❍ **What cells are found in suppurative stromal keratitis? Nonsuppurative?**

Suppurative - neutrophils; Nonsuppurative – monocytes.

❍ **What is the name for a circular pattern of nonsuppurative stromal keratitis?**

Wessely ring.

❍ **Can xanthelasma occur despite the presence of normal serum cholesterol?**

While xanthelasma occurs in patients with hypercholesterolemia, it is most common in female patients with normal serum cholesterol levels.

❍ **What ocular structure forms the mucous layer of tears?**

Goblet cells.

❍ **What arthropods cause collarettes to form during extensive infestation?**

Demodex folliculorum and *Demodex brevis*.

❍ **What is ophthalmia nodosa?**

A focal conjunctival granuloma caused by insect and arachnid hairs.

❍ **What causes the blue coloration of the sclera after an episode of scleritis?**

Thinning of the sclera allows the color of the uvea to come through.

❍ **What are Hudson-Stahli lines?**

They are horizontal lines in the corneal epithelium and are associated with old age.

❍ **What are Haab's striae?**

They are splits in Descemet's membrane and occur in congenital glaucoma.

❍ **What are the differences between pedunculated and sessile papillomas with respect to location, corneal involvement, spontaneous resolution and papillomavirus strains?**

Pedunculated - inferior tarsal or fornix conjunctivitis, occasional punctate epithelial erosions, common spontaneous resolution, strains 6 and 11.

Sessile - limbus may spread onto cornea, uncommon spontaneous resolution, strain 16 (18 rarely).

❍   **What are the different treatment choices when dealing with chalazia?**

Hot compresses, intralesional steroids, surgical incision and drainage.

❍   **What are the most common causes of blepharitis?**

Staph aureus infection, seborrhea and meibomian gland dysfunction.

❍   **Where do the sensory afferents of the cornea run through to connect to the ciliary ganglion?**

They pass through the long ciliary nerves.

❍   **What is the only bacteria causing conjunctivitis that commonly produce preauricular lymphadenopathy and conjunctival membranes?**

Gonococci.

❍   **What percentage of patients with gonococcal conjunctivitis will also have concurrent chlamydial venereal disease?**

30%.

❍   **Poliosis is associated with which type of blepharitis?**

Staphylococcal blepharitis.

❍   **What external eye disease is associated with tuberculosis?**

Phlyctenular keratoconjunctivitis has been associated with tuberculosis.

❍   **What is the leading cause of preventable blindness worldwide?**

Trachoma - spread by the common housefly and other household fomites.

❍   **What connective tissue disorder is characterized by sicca and anti-SSA and anti-SSB autoantibodies?**

Sjögren's syndrome

❍   **There are many tests to evaluate for dry eye syndrome/aqueous tear deficiency (ATD). Describe a few.**

1. Inspection of the tear meniscus (normal is 1.0 mm).
2. Tear Breakup Time (normal greater than 10 seconds).

3. Basic Secretion Test (with anesthesia)<5 mm highly suggestive, 5-10 mm equivocal at 5 min.).
4. Schirmer I ((without anesthesia) >10 mm at 5 min is normal).
5. Schirmer II ((BST with nasal stimulation) > 15 mm after 5 min is normal).
6. Tear film osmolarity (increased in dry eye/aqueous tear deficiency).

O   **What is Mikulicz's syndrome?**

Systemic diseases such as leukemia, lymphoma, or sarcoidosis are causing an enlargement of the lacrimal and/or salivary glands and aqueous tear deficiency.

O   **What do the deposits of Schnyder's crystalline corneal dystrophy consist of?**

Cholesterol and neutral fats in the corneal stroma, which stain positive with, oil red O or Sudan red.

O   **Conjunctival autografts (patch grafts) have been found to be useful in the treatment of a variety of surface abnormalities. List some of these.**

1. Primary or recurrent pterygium.
2. Cicatricial strabismus.
3. Repair after conjunctival excisional surgery (neoplasms).
4. Fornix reconstruction.

O   **What are the clinical signs of keratoconjunctivitis sicca(KCS)?**

1. Conjunctival and corneal staining with rose bengal.
2. Decreased tear lake.
3. Mucous debris in tear film.
4. Decreased tear breakup time.

O   **Vitamin A deficiency results in changes in mucosal surfaces, including the conjunctiva. What two classic signs of this disease may be clinically apparent in the conjunctiva?**

1. Bitot's spots- triangular, grey, foamy, tangles of keratin and bacteria (usually *Corynebacterium xerosis*).
2.   Xerosis- metaplasia of the conjunctival epithelium leads to a stratified squamous type with loss of goblet cells.

O   **What forms the oily layer of tears?**

Meibomian glands.

O   **What is the histopathological difference between herpes zoster iritis and herpes simplex iritis?**

Herpes zoster iritis is a lymphocytic vasculitis, whereas herpes simplex iritis is a diffuse lymphocytic infiltrate of the iris stroma.

❍ **What antibiotic is an effective treatment for both the meibomian gland dysfunction and facial skin complications of acne rosacea?**

Oral doxycycline.

❍ **What is an alternative antibiotic to tetracycline for the treatment of rosacea?**

Oral erythromycin.

❍ **Which has a greater effect in enhancing drug absorption of topical medications through the cornea: increasing water solubility or increasing lipid solubility?**

Increasing lipid solubility increases drug absorption of topical medications by allowing the drug to penetrate the intact, lipid-rich corneal epithelium.

❍ **What is oculodermal melanocytosis (nevus of Ota)?**

It is a congenital nevus of the conjunctiva and uvea with ipsilateral blue nevus of the periocular skin, most frequently in the distribution of the first and second divisions of the trigeminal nerve. Melanocytes in the episclera produce a blue color to the overlying conjunctiva. Ipsilateral iris hyperchromia is common, and melanomas of the uveal tract, optic nerve head, skin and CNS may occur in some patients.

❍ **How often does glaucoma occur in patients with nevus of Ota?**

Glaucoma occurs in 10% of patients on the same side as the skin lesions. Trabecular hyperpigmentation is present.

❍ **A 16-year-old female presents for a routine eye exam and refraction. Best-corrected visual acuity is only 20/30 to 20/40 OU. High "with the rule" astigmatism, about 4 to 5 diopters is present in both eyes. Retinal exam is normal, and there is to cataract. Keratometry readings confirm high "with the rule" astigmatism and are slightly distorted. What are likely findings on slip lamp exam and retinoscopy? What other tests might be helpful in making the diagnosis?**

The most likely diagnosis is keratoconus. The drop in best-corrected acuity is due to irregular astigmatism. Retinoscopy can help confirm the presence of irregular astigmatism. A scissors reflect or teardrop reflex might be seen. Slit lamp exam may reveal central corneal thinning, vertical striae and iron line at the base of the cone and enlarged corneal nerves. Qualitative exam with a placido disc or computerized corneal topography will help confirm the diagnosis.

❍ **What gland is responsible for reflex tearing?**

Main lacrimal gland.

❍ **What glands are responsible for basal tear secretion?**

The accessory lacrimal glands of Krause and Wolfring.

O   **What are the most common organisms causing fungal keratitis in the United States?**

Fusarium and *Aspergillus* are the most common causes of fungal keratitis in the southern U.S. and warmer climates, while *Candida* is more common in the northern U.S. and in colder regions.

O   **What bacterial organisms are the most common causes of central corneal ulcers?**

Pseudomonas, pneumococcus, staphylococcus and *Moraxella lacunata*.

O   **Why do infants with chlamydial neonatal conjunctivitis require systemic erythromycin?**

They can develop a chlamydial pneumonitis.

O   **What stain would you request for on conjunctival scrapings of suspected chlamydial conjunctivitis, and what will this show?**

Giemsa stain to identify intracytoplasmic inclusion bodies.

O   **What is "peculiar substance?"**

It is a PAS-positive material found in Meesman's dystrophy.

O   **What is the pattern of inheritance of Meesman's dystrophy?**

Autosomal dominant.

O   **Why is Reis-Bücklers' dystrophy difficult to cure?**

Recurrence in corneal grafts is very common.

O   **A 30-year old HIV positive male presents with the complaint of irritation in both eyes. Diffuse, grey-white opacities giving the corneal epithelium a granular appearance are present. Minimal conjunctivitis is present. The cornea is otherwise clear and the rest of the ocular exam is normal. What is the most likely diagnosis? What is the easiest test to perform to confirm this diagnosis?**

Microsporidial keratoconjunctivitis caused by an obligate intracellular protozoal parasite; either *Nosema corneum* or *Encephalitozoon hellem*. Gram stain of conjunctival scrapings will often reveal the gram positive spore form. Treatment with topical Amphotericin B and oral itraconazole have been reported to be successful.

O   **A 25-year-old HIV positive male presents with a complaint of bilateral ocular irritation and foreign body sensation. The cornea, anterior chamber, and retinal exam are normal. There is a very mild papillary conjunctivitis. What is the most likely diagnosis?**

Keratoconjunctivitis sicca. Dry eye is a well-known but poorly understood complication of HIV infection.

❍ **What does Alcian blue stain for and what corneal dystrophy is it used to demonstrate in corneal specimens?**

It stains for mucopolysaccharides and is used to stain specimens with macular dystrophy.

❍ **What does the material found in corneas with lattice dystrophy consist of?**

Amyloid.

❍ **Bilateral corneal edema in a newborn with normal intraocular pressures and normal corneal diameters suggests what diagnosis?**

Congenital hereditary endothelial dystrophy. Two forms are recognized; one with an autosomal dominant pattern of inheritance, the other with a recessive pattern of inheritance. Deafness is sometimes an associated finding. Normal intraocular pressure and normal corneal diameter help distinguish this entity from congenital glaucoma.

❍ **What Chlamydial serotypes cause inclusion conjunctivitis?**

Serotypes D to K.

❍ **What chlamydial serotypes cause trachoma?**

Serotypes A to C.

❍ **What is the recommended treatment for gonorrheal infection in an otherwise healthy adult?**

Ceftriaxone 1 gm IM for 5 consecutive days.

❍ **What are the main antibodies found in tears?**

IgA and secretory IgA.

❍ **If taken in high doses taken for long periods of time, what type of deposit can chlorpromazine produce in the cornea?**

It can produce a brownish, powder-like deposit in the deep stroma of the cornea.

❍ **What is Mooren's ulcer?**

It is a peripheral ulcerative keratitis caused by ischemic necrosis from vasculitis of limbal vessels.

❍ **Describe the two varieties of Mooren's ulcer.**

The limited or torpid type is usually unilateral (75%) and seen in an older patient population with equal sex distribution. The second type is usually bilateral (75%), rapidly progressive and typically found in young Nigerian males, which may be an antigen-antibody reaction to helminthic toxins.

○   **Which member of the herpes virus family does not produce a keratitis?**

CMV.

○   **What is Artl's line?**

It consists of subconjunctival scarring along the upper tarsal plate and is seen in trachoma.

○   **What are Cogan's patches?**

Dellen anterior to horizontal rectus insertions in the elderly.

○   **What is an easy way to distinguish episcleritis from scleritis?**

Topical phenylephrine will blanch the inflamed episcleral vessels, but not the scleral ones.

○   **What is the most common cause of the 29% of deaths that occur within five years of the onset of necrotizing scleritis?**

Complications of systemic vasculitis.

○   **Patients with long-standing rheumatoid arthritis can develop a necrotizing scleritis without signs of inflammation known as what?**

Scleromalacia perforans.

○   **What is the definition of giant papillae?**

Papillae ≥1 mm.

○   **What are Haab's striae?**

They are horizontal curvilinear lines representing healed breaks in Descemet's membrane and occur in eyes with congenital glaucoma.

○   **What are Vogt's striae?**

They are vertical stress lines in the corneal stroma which disappear with external pressure and are an early sign of keratoconus.

○   **What is Munson's sign?**

It is a late sign of keratoconus and characterized by indentation of the lower eyelid by the cornea in downgaze.

○ **What are Tranta's dots?**

Tranta's dots are white spots composed of eosinophils at the limbus of patients with the limbal form of vernal conjunctivitis and may also occur in atopic keratoconjunctivitis and soft contact lens wear.

○ **What is a Bitot's spot?**

It is a foamy white lesion found at the limbus found in association with vitamin A deficiency.

○ **What are Herbert's pits?**

They are regressed limbal follicles leaving behind depressed scars and are found in trachoma.

○ **What is the inheritance pattern of Reiss-Bücklers' dystrophy?**

Autosomal dominant.

○ **What are the causes of interstitial keratitis?**

1. Viral: herpes simplex, herpes zoster, mumps.
2. Bacterial: syphilis, tuberculosis, leprosy, Lyme disease, brucellosis.
3. Parasitic: acanthamoeba, trypanosomiasis, onchocerciasis, leishmaniasis, filariasis.
4. Cogan's syndrome.

○ **What type of hypersensitivity reaction occurs in phlyctenules?**

Type IV hypersensitivity to microbial proteins, eg. Staphylococcal and tuberculin.

○ **What is Cogan's syndrome?**

It is a bilateral interstitial keratitis associated with bilateral deafness, tinnitus and vertigo. Early diagnosis and treatment with systemic steroids may prevent permanent deafness.

○ **What systemic disease may be associated with Cogan's syndrome?**

Polyarteritis nodosa.

○ **What other disease besides Cogan's syndrome can cause interstitial keratitis associated with deafness?**

4% of patients with syphilitic interstitial keratitis eventually become deaf months or years after the acute episode.

○ **What are some causes of enlarged corneal nerves?**

1. Keratoconus.
2. Multiple endocrine adenomatosis (MEA).
3. Congenital ichthyosis.
4. Idiopathic.
5. Refsum's disease.
6. Neurofibromatosis.
7. Leprosy.
8. Posterior polymorphous dystrophy.
9. Fuch's endothelial dystrophy.
10. Reiss-Bückler's dystrophy.

❍   **Beading of corneal nerves or a string of pearls appearing to the corneal nerves suggests what systemic problem?**

Leprosy. Lid skin may be thickened and lashes can be absent. In addition, the iris may show characteristic creamy white "pearl" lesions.

❍   **What is Ferry's line?**

It is an iron deposit in the cornea near a filtering bleb.

❍   **A 39-year-old nurse presents with a history of non-healing corneal abrasion that is associated with pain, redness and dense ring infiltrate. She was treated previously with two weeks of intense fortified antibiotics. Cultures performed prior to starting her topical antibiotics were negative for bacteria and fungus. What is the most likely diagnosis?**

Anesthetic abuse; more common in health care personnel that have access to proparacaine and tetracaine. Suspect the diagnosis in non-healing corneal ulcers or abrasions which are culture negative. Dense white ring infiltrates, corneal edema, and even a hypopyon are possible findings.

❍   **What malignancies are associated with multiple endocrine adenomatosis type IIb (Sipple-Gorlin syndrome)?**

Medullary thyroid carcinoma, pheochromocytoma and mucosal neuromas.

❍   **A 30-year-old male presents for a routine eye exam and refraction. Slit lamp exam reveals arc shaped superior corneal thinning with blood vessels extending from the limbus across the area of thinning. Lipid deposition is present at the central edge of the thinned cornea. The epithelium over the are of thinning is intact. The opposite eye appears normal on slit lamp exam. What is the diagnosis?**

Terrien's marginal degeneration. Note that this is often bilateral but can be present unilaterally.

❍   **What would the refraction of the case above most likely show?**

High "against the rule" astigmatism in the opposite axis of the thinning.

❍ **What are the ocular features of Ehlers-Danlos syndrome?**

1. Anterior segment: keratoconus, keratoglobus, blue sclera, lens subluxation.
2. Posterior segment: high myopia and retinal detachment.

❍ **What is Ehlers-Danlos syndrome?**

It is a dominantly inherited collagen disorder caused by a deficiency in hydroxylysine. Its main systemic features are:

1. Hyperelastic skin that bruises easily and heals slowly.
2. Joint hypermobility.
3. Cardiovascular disease.
4. Daphragmatic hernia.
5. Diverticuli of the respiratory and GI tracts.

❍ **What are the ocular features of osteogenesis imperfecta?**

1. Blue sclera.
2. Keratoconus.
3. Megalocornea.

❍ **What mucopolysaccharidoses are associated with corneal clouding?**

Hurler's, Scheie's, Morquio's and Maroteaux-Lamy's but not in Hunter's and Sanfilippo's

❍ **What is the primary antibiotic of choice for an identified Gram-positive keratitis?**

Fortified cephalosporins, eg. Cefazolin

❍ **What is the significance of the presence of hypopyon in association with bacterial keratitis?**

Unless there has been ocular perforation, the presence of hypopyon is almost always a reactive phenomenon and does not signify endophthalmitis.

❍ **Is an intraocular tap and systemic antibiotics indicated in patients with bacterial keratitis and reactive hypopyon?**

No. An intraocular tap may be hazardous in patients with this condition, since it runs the risk of introducing the organisms into the eye.

❍ **What are the systemic causes of scleritis?**

1. Rheumatoid arthritis.
2. Collagen vascular disorders: Wegener's granulomatosis, polyarteritis nodosa, systemic lupus erythematosus.
3. Relapsing polychondritis.

4. Herpes zoster.
5. Porphyria.

❍ **What viruses usually cause acute hemorrhagic conjunctivitis?**

Enterovirus 70 and coxsackie A24, although adenovirus type 11 and 37 have also been implicated.

❍ **What are some causes of corneal verticillata?**

1. Drugs: amiodarone, anti-malarials, indomethacin, tamoxifen, chlorpromazine, meperidine, amodiaquine.
2. Fabry's disease.

❍ **What is Fabry's disease?**

It is a disorder caused by a deficiency in the enzyme alpha-galactosidase. Patients develop angiokeratomas, cardiovascular and renal lesions and episodes of severe pain in the fingers and toes.

❍ **What other anterior segment findings are found in Fabry's disease?**

Spoke-like lens opacities.

❍ **What does the material in granular dystrophy consist of, and what is the best stain for it?**

The granular material is composed of hyalin and stains bright red with Masson's trichrome stain.

❍ **What is Salzmann's nodular degeneration?**

It is the late sequela of a keratitis and may not appear until years after the active disease. It presents as midperipheral, smooth, bluish gray nodules on the cornea.

❍ **What is the appearance of Salzmann's nodules histopathologically?**

Localized replacement of Bowman's layer by hyaline and fibrillar material

❍ **A middle-aged man presents with a peripheral ulcerative keratitis and a positive hepatitis B surface antigen (HbsAg) lab result. What systemic disease may this patient possibly have?**

Polyarteritis nodosa

❍ **What are the ocular features of polyarteritis nodosa?**

1. Anterior segment: peripheral ulcerative keratitis, necrotizing scleritis, secondary Sjögren's syndrome.

2. Posterior segment: retinal artery occlusion, cotton wool spots, choroidal vasculitis, anterior ischemic optic neuropathy.

❍   **What is Stocker's line?**

It is an iron deposit on the cornea in front of a pterygium.

❍   **What are some systemic associations of peripheral ulcerative keratitis?**

1. Rheumatoid arthritis.
2. Wegener's granulomatosis.
3. Polyarteritis nodosa.
4. Relapsing polychondritis.
5. Systemic lupus erythematosus.

❍   **What is a Tzanck prep?**

This is a Giemsa stain of corneal scrapings of HSV epithelial infection, revealing multinucleated giant cells.

❍   **Do patients with central cloudy corneas of François complain of decreased vision?**

No. Central cloudy cornea of François is bilateral, hereditary, deep, central shagreen that has no effect on vision.

❍   **What is the name for the noninflammatory, slowly progressive thinning of the peripheral cornea that begins superiorly and has an associated vascular pannus?**

Terrien's marginal degeneration.

❍   **What type of astigmatism may develop from Terrien's marginal degeneration?**

"Against-the-rule" astigmatism.

❍   **Thinning in the lucid area posterior to corneal arcus is know as what?**

Furrow degeneration.

❍   **What percent of patients with map-dot-fingerprint will have corneal erosions?**

10%.

❍   **What percent of patients with corneal erosions will have map-dot-fingerprint?**

50%.

❍   **A 3 day old infant is noted to have progressive corneal edema with vertical posterior striae. What is the most likely cause of this ocular condition?**

Birth trauma (forceps delivery) with rupture of Descemet's membrane and endothelium.

❍   **What are some systemic disorders associated with keratoconus?**

1. Atopic dermatitis.
2. Down's syndrome.
3. Marfan's syndrome.
4. Ehlers-Danlos syndrome.
5. Osteogenesis imperfecta.
6. Mitral valve prolapse.

❍   **What type of hypersensitivity reaction may be invoked in ocular rosacea?**

Type IV hypersensitivity.

❍   **What stains can be used to identify fungi?**

1. Gomori Metamine silver stain.
2. Periodic acid-Schiff.
3. Giemsa stain.

❍   **What is blood agar used to culture for?**

It is used primarily for isolation of aerobic bacteria and will allow the growth of saprophytic fungi at room temperature.

❍   **Which anti-Epstein-Barr virus antibody does not peak during the first 6 to 8 weeks of infection with EBV?**

EBNA (Epstein-Barr nuclear antigen).

❍   **Which anti-EBV antibodies remain detectable for life after infection with EBV?**

EBNA and VCA-IgG.

❍   **What are other ocular disorders associated with keratoconus?**

1. Vernal and atopic keratoconjunctivitis.
2. Leber's congenital amaurosis.
3. Retinitis pigmentosa.
4. Aniridia.
5. Ectopia lentis.

❍   **What do the deposits in spheroidal degeneration represent, and what are they caused by?**

Spheroidal degeneration is characterized by golden brown spherules in the superficial corneal stroma. They are proteinaceous material resulting from the combined effects of genetic predisposition, aging, actinic exposure, and environmental trauma.

❍   **What are the causes of corneal clouding in infants?**

1. Corneal edema (birth trauma, glaucoma).
2. Infectious keratitis (rubella, intersitial, gonococcal).
3. Metabolic abnormalities (mucopolysaccharidoses, mucolipidoses).
4. Dystrophies (endothelial and stromal).
5. Sclerocornea.

❍   **What is the appropriate management of malignant melanoma of the conjunctiva?**

Excision using a no-touch technique with care to include 3-4 mm of normal adjacent conjunctiva and double freeze-thaw applications to the surrounding conjunctiva.

❍   **What is a Kayser-Fleischer ring?**

It consists of copper deposits in Descemet's membrane and is found in Wilson's disease.

❍   **What species is responsible for lice infection of the lids (ocular pediculosis)?**

Phthirus pubis (crab louse).

❍   **What is the Ziehl-Neelsen stain used to stain for?**

Mycobacteria and Nocardia.

❍   **What culture medium is used to grow mycobacteria?**

Löwenstein-Jensen.

❍   **What are the causes of band keratopathy?**

1. Juvenile rheumatoid arthritis.
2. Hereditary band keratopathy.
3. Chronic iridocyclitis in adults.
4. Hypercalcemia and hyperphosphatemia.
5. Chronic mercurial exposure.
6. Congenital ichthyosis.
7. Silicone oil in anterior chamber.
8. Phthisis bulbi.
9. Idiopathic in elderly.

❍   **How do you remove band keratopathy?**

Apply 0. 5 mol/L to 0.25 mol/L disodium EDTA solution topically to soften the calcium, then scrape the deposit off. The eye is then patched or a bandage contact lens is applied to allow the epithelium to heal.

❍   **What are the anterior segment features of Marfan's syndrome?**

1. Bilateral upward lens subluxation.
2. Microspherophakia.
3. Blue sclerae.
4. Keratoconus.
5. Angle anomalies.
6. Hypoplastic dilator pupillae.

○   **How does *Onchocerca volvulus* cause blindness?**

It produces a sclerosing keratitis.

○   **What is the vector of *Onchocerca volvulus*?**

Black fly.

○   **What are Henderson-Patterson bodies?**

They are intracytoplasmic inclusion bodies in the hyperplastic epithelium in umbilicated, nodular lesions caused by molluscum contagiosum. The bodies are small and eosinophilic deep inside the lesion but basophilic and larger near the surface.

○   **What type of polymorphonuclear leukocytes are usually present in the conjunctival epithelium of patients with vernal conjunctivitis?**

Eosinophils.

○   **What is the most appropriate surgical management of squamous cell carcinoma of the conjunctiva?**

Wide no-touch surgical excision with supplementary cryoablation.

○   **A patient with decompensated Fuch's dystrophy presents with a well-circumscribed, chalky white infiltrate with overlying ulceration associated with pain, photophobia and tearing for the past 4 days. What is the most likely organism in this case?**

Staphylococcus aureus.

○   **What stains can be used to identify the presence of amyloid deposits in the cornea, and what type of reaction do they exhibit?**

1. Dichroism with Congo Red stain.
2. Metachromasia with crystal violet stain.
3. Fluorescence with thioflavin T.

○   **An alcoholic elderly patient who lives in the streets presents with a nonperforated corneal ulcer for the past week and a half and maceration of the skin at the lateral canthus. What will the gram stain of the corneal scraping likely show?**

Large gram negative diplobacilli of *Moraxella lacunata*.

❍ **If Acanthamoeba keratitis is suspected, what type of culture media should be used?**

Nonnutrient agar with heat-killed E. coli overlay.

❍ **What culture media should be used for the growth of fungi?**

Sabouraud's agar.

❍ **What condition associated with HLA-DR3 is characterized by recurrent episodes of tearing, foreign body sensation, photophobia, decreased vision, and multiple small corneal epithelial lesions?**

Thygeson's superficial punctate keratitis.

❍ **What infectious diseases can cause interstitial keratitis (IK)?**

1. Syphilis.
2. Tuberculosis.
3. Leprosy.
4. *B. burgdorferi.*
5. Rubeola.
6. EBV.
7. *C. trachomatis.*
8. *Onchocerca volvulus.*

❍ **A 44-year-old woman presents with intense eye irritation associated with hypertropic conjunctiva at the superior limbus with adjacent filamentary keratitis. What is your diagnosis?**

Superior limbic keratoconjunctivitis.

❍ **What systemic disease may be associated with superior limbic keratoconjunctivitis (SLK)?**

Thyroid disease in 50% of patients with SLK.

❍ **What is the treatment for SLK?**

In mild cases artificial tears and ointment may be sufficient. In more severe cases, 0.5 to 1% silver nitrate (in wax ampoules, *not* cautery sticks) applied to the superior bulbar and tarsal conjunctiva for 10-20 seconds. Thermal cautery, pressure patching, or bandage contact lenses may be employed. Conjunctival resection may be necessary.

❍ **This is usually a seasonal recurring, bilateral inflammation of the conjunctiva, which occurs most commonly in male children and young adults.**

Vernal keratoconjunctivitis.

❍ **What type of ulcer is associated with vernal?**

Shield ulcer.

O   **What is used as prophylaxis against seasonal recurrences of vernal?**

4% Cromolyn sodium qid started at least one month prior to usual onset of symptoms.

O   **What type of keratoconjunctivitis may be associated with shield-shaped anterior subcapsular or posterior subcapsular lens opacities?**

Atopic keratoconjunctivitis.

O   **What is a congenital syndrome associated with aqueous tear deficiency (ATD)?**

Riley-Day (familial dysautonomia) or Shy-Drager (idiopathic autonomic dysfunction).

O   **What is the most common cause of dacryocystitis in adults? In children?**

Pneumococcus and *Haemophilus influenza* respectively.

O   **What is the diagnostic value of Wright's stain in regards to conjunctivitis?**

It is a cytologic stain that highlights eosinophils and their granules - found in hay fever conjunctivitis.

O   **What is a classic slit lamp finding of staphylococcal blepharitis?**

Collarettes.

O   **What should always be on the differential of ocular surface inflammation in patients that have been using topical medication?**

Medicamentosa - toxic reaction that can occur after long-term use of topical medication.

O   **How do the dermoids of epidermal nevus syndrome differ from those of Goldenhar's syndrome?**

They tend to be bilateral and more extensive.

O   **What is the treatment for gonococcal conjunctivitis?**

Ceftriaxone 1gm IM once (or IV). Copious irrigation with normal saline should be instituted. Since concurrent chlamydial infection has been reported in a third of patients, supplemental oral antibiotics should be given to treat chlamydia (tetracycline, doxycycline, minocycline, erythromycin, or azithromycin).

O   **What organisms are most commonly associated with phlyctenulosis?**

Chronic infection with *Staphylococcus aureus* is the most common cause of phlyctenulosis. Tuberculin antigen was most commonly linked to phlyctenulosis in the past.

❍ **What is the classic slit lamp finding of *Demodex* infection?**

Sleeving of eyelash bases.

❍ **How is *Trichinella spiralis* contracted?**

Ingestion of raw or half-cooked pork.

❍ **What is the treatment for *Trichinella* infections?**

Thiabendazole.

❍ **What are Schaumann bodies?**

They are nonspecific intra-giant cell deposits commonly seen in sarcoid.

❍ **What does scurf on eyelashes indicate?**

Seborrhea.

❍ **What can be seen histopathologically at Descemet's membrane in corneas with deep stromal involvement by herpes simplex?**

There is a granulomatous reaction to Descemet's membrane.

❍ **What type of staining pattern will likely be seen in a patient wearing rigid gas-permeable lenses who complains of a scratchy sensation after 6 to 8 hours of wearing time?**

3 and 9 o'clock staining, which occurs in up to 80% of RGP-wearing patients.

❍ **What is Sattler's veil?**

This is central epithelial edema resulting from hypoxic stress, which may occur with either rigid or soft contact lenses, and is best seen with sclerotic scatter or retroillumination. This is usually associated with a tight lens fit. Patients will complain of hazy vision or blur after removing their contact lenses that usually dissipates after about an hour.

❍ **What organism commonly causes infectious crystalline keratopathy and in what clinical setting is it usually seen?**

Streptococcus viridans usually causes infectious crystalline keratopathy. It most often occurs in the setting of a compromised host, such as a post-corneal graft patient on long-standing corticosteroid treatment.

❍ **What antibiotic would be appropriate for a streptococcal infection of the cornea?**

Fortified cephalosporin or vancomycin.

❍   **What is the recurrence rate of herpes simplex in the corneal graft following penetrating keratoplasty for herpetic corneal ulcers?**

Approximately 20%.

❍   **What is a Fleischer ring?**

It is iron deposition at the basal epithelium and is diagnostic of keratoconus.

❍   **Which disease produces greater corneal anesthesia in keratitis of comparable severity, herpes simplex or herpes zoster?**

Herpes zoster, which can markedly diminish corneal sensation even in the mildest cases of keratitis, produces greater corneal anesthesia than herpes simplex.

❍   **How does pellucid marginal degeneration differ from keratoconus?**

In pellucid marginal degeneration, the thinnest area is not at the apex of the cone but in a crescentic distribution near the inferior limbus.

❍   **What is the appropriate management for acute corneal hydrops in a patient with keratoconus?**

Cycloplegics are used to manage the mild iritis that may be present, and topical hypertonic saline drops and ointment may help to reduce the swelling of the corneal stroma and epithelium.

❍   **What stain is used to identify the trophozoites and cysts of *Acanthamoeba* in corneal sections?**

Calcofluor white stain.

❍   **What does immunofluorescent staining of conjunctival specimens from patients with ocular cicatricial pemphigoid (OCP) demonstrate?**

C3, IgG, IgM, and IgA are localized to the basement membrane.

❍   **What is the treatment for ocular cicatricial pemphigoid?**

Systemic corticosteroids, diaminodiphenylsulfone (Dapsone), cyclophosphamide (Cytoxan), and azathioprine (Imuran) are all currently being tried. Epilation/cryotherapy for trichiasis, mucosal grafting for fornix reconstruction, and topical corticosteroids for acute exacerbations are adjunctive measures.

❍   **What is the difference between pemphigus vulgaris and ocular cicatricial pemphigoid with regards to the conjunctival changes produced?**

Pemphigus vulgaris forms intraepithelial bullae, a mild, self-limiting conjunctivitis, and no scar formation nor involvement of the substantia propria or dermis. OCP produces subepithelial fibrosis, subconjunctival scarring, and fornix foreshortening and symblepharon formation.

○ **A 75-year-old female with history of open angle glaucoma presents with a pigmented lesion in the inferior fornix of the left eye. A biopsy is performed to rule out melanoma but comes back negative for melanin. What might this represent?**

Adrenochrome deposit from the use of epinephrine compounds for her glaucoma.

○ **What is a pyogenic granuloma?**

They are composed of granulation tissue and proliferating vascular endothelial cells in reaction to an inciting event such as strabismus surgery, inflammation (chalazion), chemical burns, limbal surgery, or foreign bodies. They are rapidly developing lesions - onset is typically days to weeks.

○ **What is thioglycolate broth used to culture for?**

Anaerobic bacteria.

○ **How thick is the central cornea?**

0.5 mm.

○ **What are Krukenberg's spindles?**

They are melanin deposits oriented vertically on the endothelium and are found in pigment dispersion syndrome or pigmentary glaucoma.

○ **In what age group does ligneous conjunctivitis usually affect?**

Ligneous conjunctivitis is an idiopathic chronic conjunctivitis that usually affects children.

○ **What part of the conjunctiva is usually affected by ligneous conjunctivitis?**

A fibrinous exudate first develops usually in the upper palpebral conjunctiva, which is then infiltrated by granulation tissue, although the bulbar conjunctiva can also be involved.

○ **In what other extraocular locations can ligneous conjunctivitis manifest?**

Nasopharynx, buccal mucosa, middle ear, tympanic membrane, vagina, and cervix.

○ **What is the most dangerous complication of herpes zoster keratitis?**

Neuroparalytic epithelial breakdown and diffuse stromal edema and infiltration, which can result in chronic trophic ulceration, corneal melting and perforation.

❍   **How would you treat herpes zoster neuroparalytic keratitis that has resulted in a trophic ulcer?**

This may respond to soft contact lens wear or to cyanoacrylate gluing in advanced cases. Neovascularization is a sign of healing and should be allowed to take place. These eyes are poor surgical risks for keratoplasty.

❍   **A patient with herpes zoster keratitis is fitted with a therapeutic bandage contact lens. Two days later, he presents with hypopyon. There is no corneal infiltrate seen. How would you manage this case?**

An infection is probably unlikely if the hypopyon follows the application of a bandage lens by only 2 or 3 days and if a stromal infiltrate is absent or of long duration. Sterile uveitis and hypopyon has been associated with lens fit too steeply and may be related to anterior segment ischemia. This complication can be managed by cycloplegia and lens removal.

❍   **What are the main indications for use of a Gunderson conjunctival flap?**

1. Chronic sterile ulcerations, eg. Herpes simplex, herpes zoster, chemical and thermal burns, sicca, neurotrophic ulcers.
2. Bullous keratopathy.
3. Closed but unstable corneal wounds.
4. Eyes being prepared for a prosthetic shell.

❍   **What topical medications can produce a cicatrizing conjunctivitis?**

Timolol, pilocarpine, echothiophate iodide and idoxuridine.

❍   **What is the importance of Hutchinson's sign?**

In patients with HZO, vesicles and itching at the tip of the nose indicates involvement of the nasociliary branch of the trigeminal nerve, which also supplies the cornea and other intraocular structures.

❍   **Where does most of the glucose for corneal epithelium comes from?**

Aqueous humor.

❍   **What type of collagen do Descemet's membrane and Bowman's membrane consist of?**

Descemet's membrane consists of type IV collagen while Bowman's membrane is made of type I collagen.

❍   **How far do myelinated nerve fibers extend into the normal cornea?**

Myelination ends within 2 mm of the limbus.

❍   **What percentage of patients with Terrien's marginal degeneration are male?**

75%.

❍   **What type of astigmatism is usually associated with Terrien's marginal degeneration?**

"Against-the-rule" astigmatism.

❍   **A 58-year-old patient presents with bilateral interstitial keratitis and hearing problems. Serologic tests for syphilis are negative. What is the probable diagnosis and how could deafness be prevented?**

Cogan's syndrome, which is a bilateral non-luetic interstitial keratitis associated with bilateral deafness. Early systemic steroid administration will prevent deafness.

❍   **What percentage of patients with syphilitic interstitial keratitis will become deaf?**

4% of patients with syphilitic interstitial keratitis will become deaf, which may occur months or years after the acute episode.

❍   **What are Leber cells?**

Leber cells are macrophages that have phagocytosed debris and are found in the conjunctival stroma in patients with trachoma.

❍   **What is the definition of microcornea?**

Corneal diameter ≤10 mm.

❍   **What type of astigmatism is produced by keratoconus?**

Irregular astigmatism.

❍   **What sign is seen on retinoscopy of an eye with keratoconus?**

Scissoring reflex.

❍   **What is Rizzuti's sign?**

It is a conical reflection on the nasal cornea when a light is shown from the temporal side in an eye with keratoconus.

❍   **What are causes of decreased corneal reflexes?**

1. Keratitis (herpes simplex, herpes zoster, leprosy).
2. Corneal dystrophies (lattice, Reiss-Bückler's, Schnyder's).
3. Diabetes, especially juvenile onset.
4. Cerebello-pontine angle tumors, eg. Acoustic neuroma.
5. Cavernous sinus and superior orbital lesions.
6. Intracranial aneurysms.

7. Iatrogenic (cataract and corneal surgery, prolonged contact lens wear, surgical section of the trigeminal nerve).
8. Riley-Day syndrome.

O   **What systemic diseases are associated with lattice dystrophy types 1 and 2?**

Lattice dystrophy type 1 is not associated with any systemic disease, but type 2 is associated with systemic amyloidosis (Meretoja syndrome).

O   **What is the relative risk of ulcerative keratitis among users of extended-wear contact lenses and daily wear soft contact lenses who wore them overnight as compared to users of such lenses who did not?**

Users of extended wear contact lenses who wore them overnight had a 10 to 15 times greater risk of microbial keratitis as users of daily wear lenses who did not. Users of daily wear soft contact lenses who sometime wore them overnight had 9 times the risk of the users of such lenses who did not.

O   **What are corneal filaments composed of?**

Mucus and desquamated epithelial cells.

O   **What is the definition of megalocornea in a child age 1 year?**

>12 mm horizontally.

O   **What medications appear to be useful in treating *Acanthamoeba* keratitis?**

1. Neomycin-polymyxin B-gramicidin.
2. Neomycin.
3. Natamycin 5% topical suspension.
4. Miconazole 1% topical solution.
5. Propamidine isethionate 0.1% drops (Brolene).
6. Dibromopropamidine 0.15% ointment.

O   **What are the eosinophilic intranuclear inclusion bodies of HSV epithelial infection called?**

Lipschütz bodies.

O   **Which anti-viral agent may produce preauricular lymphadenopathy as a hypersensitivity reaction?**

Idoxuridine.

O   **Which anti-viral medications inhibit DNA synthesis by acting as thymidine analogs?**

Trifluridine and idoxuridine.

❍ **How does acyclovir inhibit HSV DNA synthesis?**

Acyclovir, activated only by herpes virus-induced thymidine kinase, irreversibly binds to viral DNA polymerase and acts as a viral DNA chain terminator.

❍ **What abnormality of the eye is normally the cause of iron deposition?**

Abnormalities of tear pooling.

❍ **Deep stromal deposition of gold is seen in what condition?**

Chrysiasis.

❍ **This syndrome is characterized by hyperkeratotic lesions of the palms, soles, and elbows, and nonstaining corneal pseudodendrites.**

Richner-Hanhart syndrome (tyrosinemia type II).

❍ **Endothelial cells that ultrastructurally behave like epithelium and form contractile membranes are found in what syndrome?**

ICE syndrome (iridocorneal endothelial syndrome).

❍ **What is the distinctive corneal change seen in sphingolipidoses?**

Corneal verticillata.

❍ **What is the most common corneal lipid deposition condition?**

Arcus senilis.

❍ **Asymmetric arcus should lead to what kind of work-up?**

Carotid artery work-up is indicated.

❍ **A photophobic very short person with polychromatic conjunctival and corneal crystals and photophobia probably has what disease?**

Cystinosis.

❍ **What topical medication could be used to reduce the density of crystals in the previously mentioned shot person?**

Cysteamine drops.

❍ **Which bacterial conjunctivitis can produce preauricular lymphadenopathy?**

Gonococcal conjunctivitis.

❍ **What type of blepharoconjunctivitis does *Moraxella lacunata* produce?**

Angular blepharoconjunctivitis.

O   **How do you treat *C. diphtheriae* conjunctivitis?**

Use systemic antibiotics to treat the conjunctivitis and diphtheria antitoxin to prevent systemic effects of the exotoxin.

O   **What topical eye medications are recommended by the Centers for Disease Control (CDC) for the prevention of ophthalmia neonatorum?**

Erythromycin 0.5% ophthalmic ointment, tetracycline 1% ophthalmic ointment or silver nitrate 1% aqueous solutions are used within 1 hour of delivery on neonates.

O   **What is an important difference between neonatal and adult inclusion conjunctivitis in terms of conjunctival response?**

A follicular response is rarely seen in neonatal inclusion conjunctivitis.

O   **What is the most common anterior segment infection in HIV patients?**

Herpes zoster ophthalmicus is probably the most common infection in the anterior segment. The keratitis and uveitis may be unusually severe and have a protracted course.

O   **What is a Khodadoust line?**

It is a line of keratic precipitates on the endothelial surface of a corneal graft at the margin of the graft and the host occurring during corneal endothelial graft rejection.

O   **What is the cause of corneal graft failure in the immediate postoperative period?**

In the immediate postoperative period, graft failure is often due to a defect in the donor material itself and is never due to immunologic rejection.

O   **When does corneal graft rejection occur after a corneal transplant?**

The term corneal graft rejection is used to define an immunologically mediated process in which the graft, having been clear for several weeks to months, suddenly develops graft rejection with inflammatory signs.

O   **How long can topical steroids be used to reduce posttraumatic iritis and inflammation following an alkali burn?**

1% prednisolone or 0.1% dexamethasone applied topically several times a day for the first 10 days is safe and effective in reducing posttraumatic iritis and inflammation. However, if after 10 days corneal reepithelialization has not occurred, the steroid dosage must be tapered rapidly and discontinued within 1 to 2 days to avoid accelerating stromal ulceration.

O   **What HLA type is found more frequently in ocular pemphigoid?**

HLA-B12.

○   **A young male presents with extensive molluscum contagiosum in upper and lower eyelids bilaterally. What other serological test would you obtain?**

An HIV test is necessary in this case.

○   **Name 3 indication for amniotic membrane transplantation.**

Steven-Johnson syndrome, chemical burn, persistent cornea epithelial defects.

○   **What is the most common indication for limbal transplantation?**

Chemical injury may result in the complete loss of corneal epithelium and stem cells.

○   **What kind of allergic eye diseases is 4% Cromolyn sodium approved for?**

Vernal conjunctivitis and atopic keratoconjunctivitis but not seasonal or hay-fever allergic conjunctivitis.

○   **What is Maxwell Lyon sign?**

In vernal conjunctivitis, the mucus production becomes thicker and tenacious. The ropy strands have mucous discharge and an elastic quality described as the Maxwell Lyon sign.

○   **Describe the distribution of papillary hypertrophy in atopic keratoconjunctivitis (AKC), vernal conjunctivitis (VKC) and giant papillary conjunctivitis (GPC).**

In AKC, the papillary hypertrophy is often prominent in inferior palpebral conjunctiva. In contrast, VC and GPC tend to have papillae in the superior tarsus.

○   **What is the major difference between allergic conjunctivitis versus toxic conjunctivitis?**

Papillary reactions are both seen in allergic and toxic conjunctivitis, but a follicular component may be present in toxic conjunctivitis. In addition, the hyperemia and chemosis may occur less diffusely and relatively spare the superior aspect of bulbar conjunctiva.

○   **What are some of the infectious causes of Parinaud's oculoglandular syndrome?**

1. Cat-scratch disease (*Bartonella henselae*).
2. Tularemia (*Francisella tularensis*).
3. Sporotrichosis (*Sporotrichum schenckii*).
4. Lymphogranuloma venereum (serotypes L1, L2, L3).
5. Syphilis.
6. Tuberculosis.

○   **What is Paton's sign?**

Multiple, short, comma-shaped conjunctival capillary segments found near the limbus in SS disease and SC disease of sickle cell anemia.

○   **What enzyme screening test is required prior to treating cicatricial pemphigoid with dapsone?**

Make sure the patient is not glucose-6-phosphate dehydrogenase-deficient.

○   **What viruses are more likely to cause pedunculated papilloma?**

Human papilloma virus (HPV) type 6 and 11.

○   **What is the most common ocular finding in Graft-Versus-Host disease (GVHD)?**

The most common ocular manifestation is keratoconjunctivitis sicca (KCS).

○   **What is the maximum size of corneal perforation that can be sealed with tissue glue?**

2 mm.

○   **What are the ocular manifestations reported in dermatitis herpetiformis?**

Chronic or recurrent cicatrizing conjunctivitis producing subepithelial fibrosis and symblepharon

○   **How early after birth can you detect a clinical follicular response in conjunctiva?**

A follicular response is not seen prior to 6-8 weeks of life.

○   **Where is the most common place to find conjunctival intraepithelial neoplasia?**

95% of lesions occur at limbal region, within the interpalpebral fissure.

○   **What are the histological findings that can differentiate mucoepidermoid carcinoma from squamous cell carcinoma?**

Histologically, both conjunctival mucoepidermoid carcinoma and squamous cell carcinoma consist of squamous cells. However, squamous cell carcinoma does not have goblet cells while mucoepidermoid carcinoma does.

○   **What is the differential diagnosis when you see a patient with a smooth "fish-flesh" mass in the inferior conjunctiva?**

Amyloidosis, lymphoma and benign reactive lymphoid hyperplasia.

○ **Where do ocular dermoids and dermolipomas commonly occur?**

Dermoids most commonly involve the inferotemporal limbal corneal and epibulbar region. Dermolipomas arise near the insertion of lateral rectus muscle and may extend upward to the superior fornix.

○ **What is the treatment for molluscum contagiosum?**

Treatment includes excision, curetting, or cryotherapy of the lesions.

○ **What is floppy eyelid syndrome?**

Often associated with obesity, floppy eyelid syndrome results from extreme laxity of the upper lid. It is proposed that eversion of the lid occurs during sleep which allows contact of the conjunctiva with the pillow or bedding. The patient develops chronic papillary conjunctivitis as a result of repeated trauma.

○ **What is the treatment for floppy eyelid syndrome?**

Treatment consists of taping the lid closed and wearing a shield. Horizontal lid shortening procedures may also be performed.

○ **What is the most common causative agent in hyperacute conjunctivitis?**

Neisseria gonorrhea (or, less often, *N.meningitidis*)

○ **What are the histological findings of pingueculas?**

Normal, atrophic, or hyperkeratotic conjunctival epithelium. The substantia propria shows basophilic degeneration.

○ **When does keratoconus usually progress, and when does it usually stabilize?**

Progression during adolescence and stabilization when patient is fully-grown.

○ **What is a very early retinoscopic sign of keratoconus?**

Scissoring of the red reflex.

○ **What is the mainstay of treatment used in keratoconus that is not at the stage for penetrating keratoplasty?**

Glasses and RGP contact lenses.

○ **What will a rupture of Descemet's membrane cause in a keratoconus patient?**

Acute corneal hydrops.

○ **Does this usually heal or is surgery immediately indicated?**

This usually heals is 6-12 weeks, and surgery is not immediately indicated.

O   **Which abnormal layer of the cornea is responsible for the initiation of keratoconus?**

Bowman's layer becomes fibrillated and fragmented.

O   **What disease may be associated with a pinguecula that is brownish in hue?**

Gaucher's disease.

O   **What metabolites accumulate in the mucopolysaccharidosis syndromes?**

Heparin, dermatin and keratin sulfates

O   **A 50-year-old male born in Halifax county, North Carolina presents with elevated translucent-white limbal lesions which have dilated vessels. On questioning his father and grandfather have similar lesions. The patient also has leukoplakic oral lesions. What is your diagnosis?**

Benign hereditary intraepithelial dyskeratosis.

O   **What factors are associated with the development of conjunctival intraepithelial neoplasia (CIN)?**

1. Actinic exposure.
2. Heavy cigarette smoking.
3. Exposure to petroleum products.
4. Light hair and ocular pigmentation.
5. Xeroderma pigmentosa.
6. HIV infection.
7. Soft contact lens wear.

O   **In what percentage of patients does primary acquired melanosis (PAM) of the conjunctiva progress to malignant melanoma?**

30%.

O   **What does the "rule of thirds" when speaking of conjunctival melanoma state?**

1/3 arise from nevi (mortality 20%), 1/3 arise from PAM (mortality 40%), and 1/3 arise de novo (mortality 40%).

O   **What is the most important prognostic indicator in conjunctival melanoma?**

Thickness. A positive relationship between thickness and mortality has been found.

O   **Where do conjunctival melanomas most commonly metastasize to?**

Conjunctival melanomas share with cutaneous melanomas the ability to invade lymphatics and metastasize, most commonly the preauricular and intraparotid nodes.

❍ **What are the causes of membranous conjunctivitis?**

1. Alkaline chemicals.
2. *Corynebacterium diphtheriae.*
3. Pneumococcus.
4. Gonococcus.
5. Adenovirus.
6. Stevens-Johnson.
7. OCP (ocular cicatricial pemphigoid).
8. Herpes simplex virus.
9. Ligneous conjunctivitis.
10. Neonatal inclusion conjunctivitis.
11. Vernal and atopic conjunctivitis.
12. Staphylococcus.
13. Beta-hemolytic streptococci.

❍ **Angular blepharitis is most commonly caused by which organisms?**

Moraxella lacunata and staphylococcus.

❍ **A 25-year-old male is referred from a family practitioner with chronic conjunctivitis which initially responded to sulfacetamide drops. Symptoms return when the patient was taken off drops after two weeks. Slit lamp exam reveals a fine micropannus, punctate keratopathy, and follicular conjunctivitis in the right eye with minimal signs in the left. What is the diagnosis?**

Chlamydia inclusion conjunctivitis; initially suppressed but not eradicated by sulfacetamide drops.

❍ **How does neonatal inclusion conjunctivitis differ from the adult version?**

Caused by the same serotypes of C. trachomatis (D-K), the neonatal form is more likely to be associated with conjunctival membranes. Intracytoplasmic inclusions are seen in greater numbers on Giemsa staining. There tends to be no follicular response, there is a greater discharge, and the infection is more likely to respond to topical medications (erythromycin or sulfacetamide).

❍ **What are the three most common bacteria isolated from the normal eyelid?**

Staphylococcus aureus, *Propionibacterium acnes*, and *Corynebacterium species.*

❍ **What are causes of acute follicular conjunctivitis?**

1. Adenoviral infections.
2. Herpes simplex.
3. Inclusion (chlamydial).
4. Newcastle disease (poultry handlers or veterinarians).
5. Enterovirus.
6. Cat-scratch fever.

○   **A patient with a diagnosis of dry eye presents with a worsening of symptoms over the last several weeks. Examination does not reveal any signs of infection of allergy. Her Schirmer's test is dramatically decreased from previous baseline studies. What is the most likely cause?**

The patient may have been placed on a new medication such as antidepressant, diuretic or antihistamine.

○   **A patient with a diagnosis of dry eye presents with worsening symptoms over the last several weeks. She has not started on any new systemic medications and recently increased the dosing frequency of her current eye drops, an over the counter artificial tear preparation, from four times a day to every hour. What is the most likely cause and what would be seen on slit lamp exam?**

This patient most likely has medicamentosa from using drops containing preservatives such as benzlyalkonium chloride. Slip lamp exam would reveal diffuse punctate epithelial keratopathy and inflamed conjunctiva. Treatment would consist of discontinuing her current drops and starting on preservative free teardrops. Punctal occlusion could also be considered.

○   **A 30-year-old female patient presents with unilateral follicular conjunctivitis, diffuse punctate epithelial keratopathy, and a palpable small preauricular lymph node. What is the differential diagnosis?**

The differential diagnosis would include herpes simplex, adenovirus and chlamydia keratoconjunctivitis. Other causes include cat-scratch fever (Parinaud oculoglandular syndrome) and herpes zoster. Some topical medications such as carbachol and timolol can cause a toxic follicular response.

○   **Would topical steroid drops be helpful in this patient?**

Although topical steroid drops would make the patient more comfortable and less photophobic in the case of adenoviral keratoconjunctivitis, the differential diagnosis includes herpes simplex, which would be made worse by the use of this therapy. Especially since the infection is unilateral, this possibility must be kept in mind.

○   **What corneal dystrophies usually do not recur following corneal transplantation?**

Only Fuch's and posterior polymorphous dystrophy does not usually recur.

○   **Epithelial vesicles that appear as tiny bubble-like blebs on retroillumination in the intrapalpebral area of the corneal surface are found in this anterior corneal dystrophy.**

Meesman's dystrophy.

○   **Which stromal dystrophy is caused by an abnormal synthesis of keratin sulfate?**

Macular dystrophy.

○   **Which stromal dystrophy is associated with hyperlipoproteinemia or elevated serum cholesterol in up to 50% of cases?**

Central crystalline dystrophy of Schnyder.

○   **What are the different causes of symblepharon?**

1. Ocular cicatricial pemphigoid.
2. Steven-Johnson syndrome.
3. Old chemical or radiation injury.
4. Atopic keratoconjunctivitis.
5. Ocular rosacea is a less common cause.
6. Topical drops associated with conjunctival scarring include idoxuridine (IDU), pilocarpine, timolol, epinephrine, and echothiophate iodide.

○   **What three corneal dystrophies map to chromosome 5q?**

Avellino, Lattice type 1, and granular corneal dystrophies are autosomal dominant stromal dystrophies that have been mapped to chromosome 5.

○   **A 45-year-old female patient notes pain, photophobia, and slightly decreased vision in one eye on awakening. This is the third episode in an many months. Describe the corneal lesions that might be associated with this problem.**

This patient has recurrent corneal erosions. She may have a localized area of microcysts in any area of repeated breakdown. This is most likely to occur if the patient has a history of corneal abrasions. Map line, dots and fingerprint lesions are all characteristic of epithelial basement membrane dystrophy and may be present in one or both eyes. Synthesis of a thickened, reduplicated, abnormal basement membrane is responsible for the appearance and the poor adhesion of the overlying epithelium.

○   **What type of treatments might be appropriate for recurrent corneal erosions?**

Treatment would consist of a trial of hypertonic saline drops and ointment at bedtime. A bandage contact lens could also be tried. Unresponsive cases might require superficial keratectomy or anterior corneal stromal puncture.

○   **Which of the following alkalies penetrate the eye quickest: ammonia, lye, caustic potash (KOH), magnesium hydroxide, or lime (calcium hydroxide)?**

Penetration of alkali is cation dependent and is most rapid with ammonia. Magnesium hydroxide is important because it is found in many fireworks. Eye injuries occurring with fire works can be a combination of mechanical, chemical and thermal trauma. The other agents noted are listed in order of most rapid to least rapid penetration.

○   **What is the total power of the cornea in air?**

The cornea has a power in air of approximately - 45 D. This is because the posterior surface is more curved than the anterior surface. The refractive effect of the posterior surface is neutralized by aqueous. A favorite board question.

○   **What ocular finding could help distinguish the peripheral corneal ulceration associated with Mooren's ulcer and a similar corneal problem in a patient with Wegner's granulomatis?**

Associated scleritis would most likely be seen in the patient with Wegner's granulomatosis and not in a patient with Mooren's ulcer.

○   **What percentage of patients with recurrent HSV eye disease will have stromal involvement?**

<15%.

○   **What complication of HSV disease can lead to nonhealing trophic epithelial defects?**

Corneal anesthesia.

○   **What percentage of adults will experience zoster infection?**

20%.

○   **What percentage of patients with HZO will have ocular involvement?**

70%.

○   **What is the leading risk factor for the development of fungal keratitis?**

Trauma caused by plant or vegetable material.

○   **The most important symptom differentiating episcleritis from scleritis is what?**

Pain. The ocular pain occurring in scleritis is often described as a deep, boring, and pain whereas patients with episcleritis generally have only mild discomfort or irritation.

○   **What is the recommended treatment for trachoma?**

Topical and oral tetracycline or erythromycin.

○   **What is the proposed cause of subepithelial infiltrates associated with EKC (adenoviral)?**

Immune response to viral antigens deposited in the superficial corneal stroma.

○   **Where does herpesvirus reside while in a latent nonpathologic state prior to reactivation in the eye?**

Trigeminal ganglion.

❍   **What is the difference between a dendrite and a pseudodendrite?**

Dendrites have terminal bulbs, while pseudodendrites do not.

❍   **What is the most commonly associated ocular finding in patients with sclerocornea?**

Cornea plana.

❍   **What is nonprogressive corneal enlargement that is not the result of congenital glaucoma?**

Megalocornea.

❍   **How is megalocornea inherited, and is it unilateral or bilateral?**

X-linked recessive and bilateral.

❍   **What is an eye that is small but otherwise normal and an eye that is small and malformed?**

Nanophthalmos and microphthalmos, respectively.

❍   **What is the name for a cornea that is less than 43 diopters?**

Cornea plana.

❍   **What is thought to be the main cause of pingueculae?**

Ultraviolet light exposure (actinic damage).

❍   **What layer of the cornea is invaded and destroyed by pterygia?**

Bowman's layer.

❍   **What type of astigmatism is associated with pterygia?**

"Against-the-rule."

❍   **What is the recurrence rates after simple resection of a pterygium and if a conjunctival autograft is used?**

Simple resection - 40%. Resection with conjunctival autograft - 5%.

❍   **Histopathologically, what are common conjunctival concretions?**

Epithelial inclusion cysts filled with epithelial debris and keratin.

○   **In what layer of the cornea do you find the lipid that causes arcus senilis?**

Corneal stroma.

○   **Arcus in patients under 40 is an indicator of what and a prognosticator of what?**

Indicates hyperlipoproteinemia and prognosticates coronary artery disease.

○   **Which stromal dystrophy has mild stromal haze composed of polygonal gray areas that clears peripherally?**

Central cloudy dystrophy of Francois - aka posterior crocodile shagreen.

○   **This is a rare, dominant, stationary dystrophy that presents at birth with central corneal clouding that is often confused with congenital glaucoma.**

Congenital hereditary stromal dystrophy (CHSD).

○   **Why is it important to note corneal gutatta in pre-operative patients?**

Progression to corneal decompensation and edema may be accelerated after intraocular surgery. As many as 1/3 of corneal endothelial cells may be lost during uncomplicated cataract extraction.

○   **In what group of patients is Fuch's endothelial dystrophy most common?**

Postmenopausal women.

○   **At what time of day are the symptoms of Fuch's dystrophy the worst and why?**

Morning - decreased corneal surface evaporation while asleep.

○   **Which corneal dystrophy can show endothelial bands with scalloped edges composed of large endothelial cells that stain positive for keratin?**

Posterior polymorphous dystrophy (PPMD).

GLAUCOMA

○ **How many axons are present in a typical optic nerve?**

1 to 1.2 million axons.

○ **What is the best method for examining of the optic nerve head?**

A slit lamp examination with a posterior pole lens gives the best magnification and stereoscopic view.

○ **Name the two cell types found within the ganglion cell layer and their functions.**

M cells (magnocellular) have large diameter axons, synapse in the magnocellular layer of the lateral geniculate body, and are sensitive to changes in dim illumination. P cells (parvocellular) comprise the majority of the ganglion cells, have small diameter axons, synapse in the parvocellular layers of the lateral geniculate body, and are used in color and fine detail.

○ **Name the four layers of the optic nerve and their respective vascular supply.**

Nerve fiber layer	central retinal artery.
Prelaminar layer	short posterior ciliary arteries.
Laminar layer	short posterior ciliary arteries.
Retrolaminar layer	branches of the meningeal arteries and central retinal artery.

○ **How do the short posterior ciliary arteries in the optic nerve differ from those of the choriocapillaris?**

The short posterior ciliary arteries in the optic nerve resemble retinal capillaries. They are surrounded by pericytes, have tight junctions, and lack fenestrations.

○ **Why does glaucomatous cupping occur earlier in children than in adults?**

The scleral ring surrounding the optic nerve expands with increased IOP in children and infants.

○ **What supplies essential nutrients and removes waste from the lens, cornea, and trabecular meshwork?**

The aqueous humor acts as a substitute blood for these avascular tissues.

❍   **What percentage of plasma proteins is filtered out by the blood-aqueous barrier in the formation of aqueous humor?**

More than 99% of plasma proteins are absent from aqueous. Normal aqueous has a protein content of about 0.02g/100 ml, while plasma contains about 7g/100 ml.

❍   **How far away is the optic nerve head from fixation in the visual field?**

10-15°.

❍   **What retinal layer is most damaged by glaucoma?**

Nerve fiber layer.

❍   **Patient's with which type of glaucoma are most likely to have splinter hemorrhages of the optic disc?**

Normal-tension glaucoma.

❍   **What photographic technique best demonstrates early nerve fiber layer thinning?**

High contrast black-and-white photography.

❍   **What is the initial medical management for ciliary-block (malignant) glaucoma?**

Atropine and corticosteroids as well as aqueous suppressants to control IOP as needed.

❍   **How does the Schiøtz tonometer work?**

The IOP is determined by measuring the indention of the cornea by a known weight on a linear scale on the instrument. This value is then converted using a table to IOP in mmHg.

❍   **When should digital palpation be used to measure IOP and how accurate is it?**

IOP estimation by digital palpation should be reserved for uncooperative patients only, because it is only useful in detecting large differences in IOP between two eyes.

❍   **Why is it important to clean tonometers between uses?**

Many viruses, including those causing AIDS, EKC and hepatitis, can be recovered from the tears of infected individuals.

❍   **What type of inheritance pattern is seen in juvenile-onset glaucoma?**

Juvenile-onset glaucoma has been shown to follow an autosomal dominant inheritance pattern by large pedigree studies, and a genetic marker has been identified on chromosome 1q.

❍ **What is the first assessment that should be made when evaluating an automated visual field?**

Noting the percentage of fixation losses, false positives, false negatives, and fluctuations should first assess the quality of the test.

❍ **What is the average fluctuation seen between points on an automated visual field in normal and abnormal subjects.**

The average fluctuation should be less than 2 dB in a normal field, less than 3 dB in cases of early damage, and less than 4 dB in cases of moderate damage.

❍ **How is adult-onset primary open angle glaucoma thought to be inherited?**

It most closely follows an autosomal recessive pattern.

❍ **What is Sampaolesi's line?**

Pigment deposited anterior to Schwalbe's line, which is seen in pseudoexfoliation syndrome and pigmentary dispersion syndrome.

❍ **What type of artifact will be produced if a patient quits responding midway through a Humphrey visual field test?**

A cloverleaf-shaped field is a common artifact seen in automated visual field testing.

❍ **What effect is seen if a patient's spectacle correction is not used during automated perimetry?**

Generalized depression of visual sensitivity.

❍ **What effect does a media opacity, such as a cataract, has on the results of automated perimetry?**

Media opacities cause a generalized depression of the visual field with a normal pattern standard deviation. Miotic pupils can cause similar artifacts.

❍ **The goal of serial visual field testing is to detect progression of glaucomatous damage. What is mandatory for this type of interpretation?**

An accurate baseline field.

❍ **What is the mechanism of action for the antimetabolites 5-fluorouracil and mitomycin C to increase the success rate of glaucoma filtering surgery?**

Both of these medications inhibit the proliferation of fibroblasts and mitomycin C also affects the proliferation of vascular endothelial cells. 5-FU is a fluorinated pyrimidine inhibitor of thymidylate synthase and is an S-phase specific agent. Mitomycin C is a cell cycle nonspecific alkylating agent.

O   **A diurnal fluctuation of greater than 10 mmHg suggests what diagnosis?**

Glaucoma.

O   **What antioxidant is found at levels 10 to 50 times higher in aqueous than plasma?**

Ascorbic acid (vitamin C).

O   **What enzyme found in the aqueous provides essential antibacterial activity?**

Lysozyme.

O   **Low-tension glaucoma patients have been divided into what two groups by some authorities. What are they?**

1. The senile sclerotic group has a characteristic shallow, pale sloping of the optic nerve rim.
2. The focal ischemic group suffers deep, focal notching in the optic nerve rim.

O   **How do the typical visual field defects of low-tension glaucoma patients differ from those of high-tension glaucoma patients?**

They are usually more dense, focal, and closer to fixation.

O   **Does low-tension glaucoma seem to have any race predilection?**

Yes, it seems to have a higher prevalence among Japanese patients.

O   **What test should be used clinically to rule out POAG before making a diagnosis of low-tension glaucoma?**

Diurnal IOP measurement.

O   **What in a patient's medical history could explain the optic neuropathy and visual field loss that would otherwise be labeled normal-tension glaucoma?**

History of hemorrhagic shock, myocardial infarction, anemia, syphilis, or vasculitis

O   **What growth modulatory factor shows increased levels in the aqueous when any ocular neovascularization is present?**

Vascular endothelial growth factor (VEGF).

O   **How do you perform the dark room prone test?**

This test is done in patients with suspiciously narrow angles. IOP is first measured, and then the patient is seated for 30-60 minutes in a darkened room with the head down on a cushioned table. The IOP is again measured in the darkened room. A rise of 6-8 mm Hg or greater or a significant asymmetric rise in IOP accompanied by gonioscopic confirmation of further angle closure is a positive test, and a laser iridotomy is performed. Placing the patient in a brightly-lit room for 5 minutes after this test and observing a significant lowering of IOP is further confirmation of a positive test.

❍ **Why do some glaucoma experts advocate the use of calcium channel blockers in low-tension glaucoma patients?**

Calcium channel blockers may increase perfusion to the optic nerve.

❍ **What oral osmotic agent should be used to lower the IOP of a diabetic patient with an attack of acute angle closure glaucoma?**

Isosorbide.

❍ **What neurological complication can result from use of osmotic agents such as mannitol and urea?**

Brain shrinkage with traction on vessels and subsequent subarachnoid hemorrhage.

❍ **Which part of the ciliary body is responsible for active secretion of aqueous?**

Nonpigmented ciliary epithelium.

❍ **What are the partial pressures of oxygen and carbon dioxide in the aqueous?**

Oxygen: 55 mm Hg
Carbon dioxide: 40-60 mmHg

❍ **What is the normal pH of aqueous humor?**

Normal range is 7.5-7.6.

❍ **What is the most prevalent type of adrenergic receptors in the ciliary epithelium?**

Beta$_2$ receptors.

❍ **A patient presents for exam one day following a trabeculectomy. She is comfortable, the anterior chamber is shallow and the IOP is 2. The bleb is flat and no choroidals are present. What test will make the diagnosis apparent?**

Seidel testing. This patient has the classic findings of a wound leak with a low IOP, shallow AC and a flattened filtering bleb.

❍ **What does the fibrillar material deposited in the anterior chamber of the eye in pseudoexfoliation syndrome resembles histochemically?**

Amyloid.

❍   **Which is the only form of primary angle closure glaucoma that is not totally caused by a pupillary block mechanism?**

Plateau iris.

❍   **Is there a difference in the success rate between limbus-based and fornix-based conjunctival flaps?**

No. A fornix-based flap is easier to dissect and close but there is an increased risk of leakage at the limbus, especially with the use of adjunctive antimetabolites.

❍   **What method is most commonly used to measure the rate of aqueous formation?**

Fluorophotometry.

❍   **What is the mean IOP of the population in general?**

The mean IOP is approximately 16 mmHg and there is a standard deviation of 3 mmHg. The distribution is skewed toward the higher values, and this is more apparent in people over 40.

❍   **Why does the pattern of deposits on the anterior lens capsule in pseudoexfoliation syndrome resembles a target?**

The iris rubs off the material during normal pupillary size changes, leaving a clear zone between areas of central and peripheral deposition.

❍   **Why is a relatively shallow anterior chamber a common finding in patients with pseudoexfoliation syndrome?**

Forward movement of the lens-iris diaphragm sometimes occurs secondary to the zonular weakness that accompanies the disorder.

❍   **What is the mechanism of action of latanoprost?**

Latanoprost is a prostaglandin $F_{2\alpha}$ prodrug, which lowers IOP by increasing uveoscleral outflow of aqueous.

❍   **Acutely, how would the IOP change with a 4 mmHg rise in episcleral venous pressure?**

The IOP would also rise 4 mmHg. There is a 1:1 change in IOP with acute changes in episcleral venous pressure. This does not hold true for chronic conditions.

❍   **What is the approximate turnover time of aqueous humor?**

About 1% of the aqueous is replaced every minute, so turnover time is approximately 100 minutes.

❍ **What happens to outflow facility as a person ages?**

Outflow facility decreases as age increases.

❍ **What are two complications of cataract surgery seen frequently in patients with pseudoexfoliation syndrome?**

Zonular dehiscence and vitreous loss.

❍ **What region of the world has the highest prevalence of pseudoexfoliation syndrome?**

Pseudoexfoliation syndrome is responsible for up to 50% of open-angle glaucoma in Scandinavian countries.

❍ **When may releasable sutures be removed from a trabeculectomy?**

Releasable sutures usually are pulled at any time between 1 and 21 days. This time may be extended with the use of adjunctive antimetabolite therapy and an effect may be seen up to one year postoperatively according to some reports.

❍ **What causes the iris transillumination defects seen in pigment dispersion syndrome?**

It is thought that zonular contact with the iris pigment epithelium is responsible for the release of pigment.

❍ **What type of drug is brimonidine?**

It is a selective alpha$_2$ adrenergic agonist.

❍ **How does alcohol use affect IOP?**

Consumption of alcohol decreases IOP for a short time.

❍ **How does the risk of developing glaucoma change over time in an eye with angle recession?**

The risk of developing glaucoma drops off substantially after a few years.

❍ **What is the treatment of choice for angle recession glaucoma?**

Aqueous suppressants.

❍ **How many times more common is glaucoma among blacks as compared to whites?**

The prevalence of glaucoma is 3 to 6 times higher in blacks than in whites.

❍ **In what way is glaucoma associated with cyclodialysis clefts?**

An abrupt increase in IOP may occur as the cleft closes. When a cleft is open, hypotony is more likely because of increased uveoscleral outflow.

O   **What type of eyes is associated with anatomically narrow angles?**

Small, hyperopic eyes, e.g. nanophthalmos.

O   **Why has some experts advocated laser peripheral iridotomy (LPI) for patients with pigmentary glaucoma?**

To relieve the posterior bowing commonly seen in the peripheral iris of these patients and subsequently decrease contact between the iris pigment epithelium and zonules, LPI has been advocated by some, but its efficacy has not yet been established.

O   **What physiologic mechanisms are responsible for aqueous humor production, and which mechanism produces most of the aqueous?**

Diffusion, ultrafiltration, and active secretion produce aqueous. It is widely believed that most of the aqueous is produced by active secretion, which involves a Na-K ATPase active transport pump.

O   **Compare the concentrations of sodium, potassium, magnesium, calcium, and lactate in plasma and aqueous.**

The concentration of sodium, potassium and magnesium in aqueous is similar to plasma, while calcium is about half that found in plasma. Lactate concentrations in aqueous is higher than in plasma.

O   **What happens to IOP as a patient lies down?**

IOP is usually higher when lying down as compared to sitting upright.

O   **How does phacolytic glaucoma occur?**

It occurs when denatured lens proteins from a hypermature cataract leak through an intact lens capsule, causing an inflammatory reaction in the anterior chamber. Macrophages engorged with lens proteins, fill the anterior chamber and clog the trabecular meshwork, causing a rise in intraocular pressure.

O   **What effect does cannabis has on IOP?**

Cannabis use decreases IOP, although it has no established clinical use in this regard.

O   **Does caffeine affect IOP?**

Yes, caffeine sometimes causes a transient rise in IOP.

O   **What is the difference between choroidal detachments and retinal detachments with regards to their anterior extent on B-scan ultrasonography?**

Choroidal detachments can extend to the scleral spur, while retinal detachments end at the ora serrata.

○ **What types of glaucoma are nanophthalmic eyes prone to?**

Angle closure glaucoma.

○ **What group of patients is at increased risk for developing glaucoma following a hyphema?**

Patients with any of the sickle cell hemoglobinopathies are at increased risk because sickled red blood cells are more likely to clog the trabecular meshwork.

○ **What medication should be avoided in sickle cell patients with a hyphema?**

Carbonic anhydrase inhibitors are thought to increase sickling in the anterior chamber.

○ **Name two conditions that can produce elevated episcleral venous pressure and dilated episcleral vessels.**

Sturge-Weber syndrome and arteriovenous fistulas.

○ **An infant with congenital glaucoma has cloudy corneas. What is the surgical treatment of choice?**

Trabeculotomy, since this does not require a clear cornea to be performed.

○ **What position must the patient be in when you perform Koeppe gonioscopy?**

The patient must be supine.

○ **When is Koeppe gonioscopy most commonly used?**

During examinations under anesthesia and when performing goniotomy.

○ **What are the lenses changes following an attack of angle closure glaucoma called?**

Glaukomflecken.

○ **What is the explanation for the increased risk of choroidal and exudative detachments when performing surgery on nanophthalmic eyes?**

Nanophthalmic eyes are small with thick sclera, which impedes vortex vein drainage.

○ **Describe the normal diurnal variation of IOP.**

Over a 24-hour period, IOP varies between 2-6 mmHg in the normal population.

○ **What is the difference between a cyclodialysis and an angle recession?**

A cyclodialysis is a separation of the ciliary body from the scleral spur, while an angle recession is a separation of the longitudinal and circular muscles of the ciliary body.

○ **Two weeks after filtering surgery, a glaucoma patient presents with an IOP of 40 mm Hg, a low lying bleb and a deep anterior chamber. What is the cause for the high pressure in this patient?**

Gonioscopy will probably show blockage of the sclerostomy. YAG laser therapy may reopen it.

○ **Which miotic agent has both indirect and direct cholinergic activity?**

Carbachol, which is an acetylcholine analog and a competitive inhibitor for acetylcholinesterase.

○ **What are the major risk factors for spikes in intraocular pressure after argon laser trabeculoplasty?**

Posterior laser burns, dense trabecular pigment, and poor outflow facility.

○ **What phacomatoses are associated with congenital glaucoma?**

Sturge-Weber syndrome and neurofibromatosis type 1 (NF-1).

○ **What angle structure is the peripheral termination of Descemet's membrane?**

Schwalbe's line.

○ **What portion of the trabecular meshwork is adjacent to Schlemm's canal?**

The trabecular meshwork has three portions: uveal, corneoscleral and juxtacanalicular. The juxtacanalicular meshwork lies adjacent to Schlemm's canal.

○ **A diabetic patient presents with acutely elevated IOP following a vitreous hemorrhage. She appears to have a small hypopyon. What is the name for this secondary glaucoma and what is the pseudohypopyon composed of?**

Ghost cell glaucoma may present with a pseudohypopyon that is actually composed of degenerated red blood cells or erythroclast. These decomposing cells can mechanically block aqueous outflow.

○ **What is the most likely cause for a shallow anterior chamber with a low intraocular pressure and a flat bleb in the immediate postoperative period following a trabeculectomy for primary open angle glaucoma?**

Bleb leak.

○ **What is the main advantage of using dipivefrin over topical epinephrine?**

Dipivefrin is a prodrug of epinephrine that must first enter the cornea to be activated by esterases within the stroma; hence systemic side effects are reduced.

○   **Name three techniques that the patient can do to improve the absorption of ocular medications.**

1. Digital nasolacrimal compression.
2. Close the eyes for 5 minutes after instillation of drops.
3. Wait 10 minutes in between the administration of different drops.

○   **How can systemic sulfonamides produce glaucoma?**

Systemic sulfonamides can cause idiosyncratic choroidal detachments and precipitate angle closure glaucoma.

○   **Is a posterior embryotoxon typically associated with primary infantile glaucoma?**

A prominent, anteriorly displaced Schwalbe's line or posterior embryotoxon can be seen in Axenfeld-Rieger syndrome but is not typically seen in primary infantile glaucoma.

○   **What is the most common reason for long-term visual loss in primary infantile glaucoma?**

Amblyopia.

○   **A glaucoma patient taking betaxolol, pilocarpine, acetazolamide, and dipivefrin is scheduled to undergo cataract surgery. Which of his medications should be discontinued temporarily?**

Pilocarpine and adrenergic agonists such as dipivefrin can weaken the blood-aqueous barrier and worsen inflammation. They should therefore be discontinued prior to surgery if possible.

○   **A patient with open angle glaucoma is started on carteolol eye drops to his right eye. What can you expect to see occur in the left eye after two weeks of therapy?**

There will often be a reduction of intraocular pressure in the contralateral eye with unilateral use of a topical beta-blocker, although less than in the treated eye.

○   **What are the main sources of blood supply to the anterior optic nerve?**

Posterior ciliary arteries via the peripapillary choroid or the short posterior ciliary arteries.

○   **What are the most common causative organisms in a late bleb-associated endophthalmitis?**

H. influenzae and *S. pneumoniae*.

○   **What risks factors can be associated with chronic primary angle-closure glaucoma?**

Hyperopia, cataract progression, advancing age, and pseudoexfoliation syndrome.

○   **How many optic nerve axons must be lost before kinetic perimetry will show a visual field defect?**

50% of the axons in the optic nerve.

○   **Why should gonioscopy be performed in patients with narrows angles and chronic angle-closure glaucoma after starting miotic therapy?**

Miotic therapy can increase relative pupillary block by allowing forward movement of the lens against a constricted pupil, thereby exacerbating chronic angle-closure and precipitating an acute attack of angle-closure glaucoma. Gonioscopy must be performed in these patients to determine if worsening of angle closure is occurring.

○   **What are Haab's striae?**

They are breaks in Descemet's membrane in eyes with enlarged corneas resulting from congenital glaucoma. Irregular astigmatism is often present.

○   **Two days after a trabeculectomy, a 72-year-old patient presents with an IOP of 45 mm Hg, shallow anterior chamber, patent iridectomy and no choroidal detachment on B-scan. How would you manage this patient, and is miotic therapy indicated?**

This patient has malignant glaucoma and should be started on beta-blockers, carbonic anhydrase inhibitors to reduce the IOP and topical cycloplegic therapy to relieve the pupillary block by tightening the zonules and posteriorly displacing the lens. Miotic therapy will exacerbate the block and increase inflammation. Vitrectomy is indicated if medical therapy is not successful.

○   **In what types of patients are peripupillary iris transillumination defects and radial peripheral iris transillumination iris defects more commonly found in?**

Peripupillary iris transillumination defects may be present in pseudoexfoliation syndrome, while radial peripheral iris transillumination defects are more commonly found in pigmentary dispersion syndrome.

○   **A 45-year-old Filipino patient presents with an acute attack of angle closure glaucoma despite having patent laser iridotomies done previously. The slit lamp examination shows the anterior chamber to be deep centrally and the iris plane to be flat. What is the most likely diagnosis?**

Plateau iris syndrome.

○   **What procedure is indicated in a patient with plateau iris syndrome in which the angle remains appositionally closed or occludable after laser iridotomy?**

Laser peripheral iridoplasty. The anterior positioning of the ciliary processes causes the iris root to remain in contact with the angle structures.

○ **Identification of gonioscopic landmarks is simplest in which portion of the angle?**

The inferior angle is usually wider and more pigmented.

○ **Describe the gonioscopic findings seen in angle closure.**

The trabecular meshwork is not visible because the peripheral iris obstructs it.

○ **Describe the gonioscopic findings in plateau iris configuration.**

The peripheral anterior chamber appears closed with a flat iris plane while the central anterior chamber is deep, resulting from an anterior position of the ciliary processes and an abnormal configuration of the peripheral iris.

○ **What does pressure on a Goldmann indirect gonioscopy lens does to the angle? What about a Zeiss lens?**

The angle is falsely narrowed when pressure is applied to a Goldmann lens. Pressure applied to a Zeiss lens will falsely open the angle.

○ **How can pressure applied to the central cornea with a Zeiss lens (indentation gonioscopy) is used clinically?**

This technique can be used to distinguish peripheral anterior synechia (PAS) from iridocorneal touch.

○ **What visual field abnormality would most likely be seen in a patient with a progressive nuclear sclerotic cataract in the absence of other abnormalities?**

Progressive nuclear sclerotic cataracts are more likely to cause a generalized depression of the central visual field and an even depression of thresholds rather than focal defects or scotomas. The pattern standard deviation will probably remain the same.

○ **What type of glaucoma medication is apraclonidine?**

It is an $alpha_2$-adrenergic agonist.

○ **What is the pathogenesis of angle closure glaucoma secondary to neovascularization of the iris?**

Contraction of myofibroblasts that accompany the new vessels lead to PAS and closure of the angle.

○ **During gonioscopy you note a prominent scleral spur, abnormally wide ciliary body band, and torn iris processes in the temporal angle of a patient's right eye.**

What are your diagnosis and what history should you try to obtain from the patient?

Angle recession is the diagnosis and you should ask about a history of trauma to the right eye.

❍   **What is the desired tissue response of an argon laser trabeculoplasty?**

Blanching of the trabecular meshwork. Minimal bubble formation may also be noted with correct laser treatment.

❍   **In patients with increased pigmentation of the trabecular meshwork, should the power be increased or decreased?**

Decreased. As pigmentation increases, the current of laser energy absorbed increases. Laser power settings may require adjustment as pigmentation varies in differing quadrants.

❍   **What effect does thymoxamine has on the pupil and outflow facility?**

Thymoxamine causes miosis but has no effect on outflow facility.

❍   **What are some causes of a depressed ring of peripheral points in a central 30° visual field program?**

Lens rim artifact, ptosis, and retinal disorders, eg. Chorioretinal scars, retinitis pigmentosa.

❍   **What term is used to describe low pressure after filtration surgery associated with choroidal folds decreased visual acuity and retinal pigment epithelial changes?**

Hypotony maculopathy.

❍   **What does the pattern standard deviation in an automated perimetry signify?**

It highlights localized visual field defects rather than diffuse generalized visual field depression.

❍   **Filtering blebs in the inferior quadrants or in the intercanthal region increase the risk of what serious complication?**

Endophthalmitis.

❍   **What finding on slit lamp examination is important to differentiate a bleb infection from endophthalmitis?**

Cells in the vitreous cavity indicating involvement of the posterior segment.

❍   **What optic nerve findings will be suggestive of glaucomatous optic nerve damage in a patient with elevated intraocular pressure?**

1. Cup-to-disc ration asymmetry greater than 0.2.
2. Notch formation in the optic nerve rim, even in patients with 0.4 cups.

❍   **What is the mechanism for angle closure glaucoma following extensive panretinal photocoagulation?**

Swelling and anterior rotation of the ciliary body, which does not respond to laser iridectomy.

❍   **What procedure should be considered in patients at risk for development of intraoperative and postoperative choroidal hemorrhage (e.g. Sturge-Weber syndrome)?**

Prophylactic sclerotomies.

❍   **How does carbonic anhydrase inhibitors (CAIs) lower intraocular pressure?**

They suppress aqueous humor production by an indirect inhibition of sodium transport in the nonpigmented ciliary epithelium.

❍   **Do patients taking CAIs develop a metabolic alkalosis or acidosis?**

Carbonic anhydrase inhibitors can produce a metabolic acidosis because of alkaline diuresis and loss of sodium, potassium and bicarbonate in the kidneys.

❍   **What serious CAI-induced side effect can occur in patients already taking glucocorticosteroid, thiazide diuretics or digitalis?**

Hypokalemia-induced cardiac arrhythmias.

❍   **What are the risk factors for failure of goniotomy?**

Glaucoma diagnosis at birth, other ocular abnormalities, corneal diameter > 14 mm or age > 2 years.

❍   **What are the most serious hematologic side effects of carbonic anhydrase inhibitors?**

Thrombocytopenia and aplastic anemia, which is idiosyncratic.

❍   **What is the most common reason for discontinuation of a Simmons shell used to tamponade a bleb leak?**

Patient discomfort.

❍   **What is the most serious complication of laser peripheral iridotomy?**

Elevation of IOP. Treatment with topical apraclonidine significantly decreases both the frequency and magnitude of the rise in IOP. IOP should always be measured 1-2 hours after the procedure.

○   **What is the treatment for patients with angle closure glaucoma following panretinal photocoagulation for diabetic retinopathy?**

Topical cycloplegics and corticosteroid therapy may cause posterior rotation of the ciliary body and open the angle. Laser iridoplasty is performed if the angle closure fails to respond to medical therapy.

○   **An elderly patient develops sudden, severe eye pain 36 hours after filtering surgery while going to the restroom. What diagnosis is most likely?**

Suprachoroidal hemorrhage.

○   **What procedure must be performed to distinguish pupillary block from plateau iris configuration?**

Peripheral iridotomy or iridectomy.

○   **Can topical betaxolol (Betoptic) be safely used in a patient with congestive heart failure?**

No. Both nonselective and beta-1 selective beta-blockers, such as betaxolol, can worsen congestive heart failure.

○   **What beta-blockers can be combined with dipivefrin to produce a greater additive effect than dipivefrin alone?**

A greater additive effect of dipivefrin with betaxolol can be seen over dipivefrin with nonselective beta-blockers, such as timolol and levobunolol.

○   **What side effects can epinephrine and possibly dipivefrin is associated with in aphakic eyes?**

Cystoid macular edema.

○   **In what conditions is blood in Schlemm's canal commonly seen?**

Hypotony, Sturge-Weber syndrome, carotid-cavernous sinus fistulas.

○   **What transient side effect can apraclonidine produce in eyelids?**

Transient lid retraction.

○   **With regards to corticosteroid responsiveness, what percentage of offspring of POAG patients is high responder?**

25%.

○   **What percentage of the general population are high steroid responders?**

5%.

O   **What percentage of patients with established POAG are high steroid responders?**

90%.

O   **Would laser iridotomy be useful in treating a patient with elevated IOP and ICE syndrome?**

No. The mechanism of glaucoma in eyes with ICE syndrome is through angle closure, but there is no pupillary block present.

O   **What is the most likely cause for severe blurring of vision in a young, highly myopic patient following a single application of a drop of pilocarpine?**

Increased myopia.

O   **Can miotics are used in a glaucoma patient who has aniridia and open angles?**

Yes. The effect of miotic agents is mediated through the ciliary muscle and not the pupillary sphincter.

O   **What conditions can produce glaucomatous visual field-like defects?**

Optic nerve drusen, retinal vascular occlusive disease and ischemic optic neuropathy.

O   **Can cataract extraction resolve or prevent glaucoma in a patient with pseudoexfoliation syndrome?**

No. The pseudoexfoliative material will continue to be produced by nonpigmented ciliary epithelium and other ocular tissues. This can be found on the anterior chamber angle, iris, corneal endothelium, and lens capsule in pseudophakic and aphakic eyes.

O   **What is the difference between Rieger's anomaly and Rieger's syndrome?**

Both conditions have posterior embryotoxon and iris anomalies (corectopia, stromal hypoplasia, pseudopolycoria, and ectropion uveae). When dental anomalies (hypodontia and microdontia) and facial anomalies (maxillary hypoplasia, telecanthus, hypertelorism, broad nasal bridge) are present, the condition is called Rieger's syndrome.

O   **What is a posterior embryotoxon?**

Anteriorly displaced Schwalbe's line.

O   **If a patient has a posterior embryotoxon and no other abnormality, what is this condition called?**

Axenfeld's anomaly.

O   **What is the inheritance pattern of Rieger's anomaly?**

Autosomal dominant.

O	**How often does glaucoma develop in eyes with Rieger's anomaly?**

50%, usually during childhood or early adulthood.

O	**A patient reports worsening ptosis and diplopia with use of topical beta-blockers. What is the most likely explanation for this?**

The patient may have myasthenia gravis, which can be exacerbated by topical beta-blockers.

O	**What are the main causes of a shallow anterior chamber following filtering surgery?**

1.	Wound leak.
2.	Excessive filtration.
3.	Pupillary block.
4.	Malignant glaucoma.

O	**What complications can result from excising the block too far posteriorly during a trabeculectomy?**

Excising the block too posteriorly can result in vitreous loss and an inadvertent cyclodialysis cleft. Hemorrhage can also occur if the major arterial circle to the iris is cut.

O	**What type of aniridia is associated with neuroblastoma or Wilms' tumor?**

Sporadic, nonfamilial aniridia.

O	**Is the episcleral venous pressure increased or decreased in Sturge-Webber syndrome?**

Increased.

O	**What is the normal rate of aqueous flow?**

2 to 3 µL/min.

O	**What type of medication is dapiprazole and what is it used for?**

It is an alpha-adrenergic antagonist used to reverse sympathomimetic-induced pupillary dilation.

O	**A patient has bilaterally narrow angles and IOPs of 28 mm Hg OU. The IOP does not decrease after thymoxamine administration. What does this indicate, and how will it affect your management?**

Patients with mixed mechanism glaucoma have open angle glaucoma with partial angle closure secondary to pupillary block. Thymoxamine, an alpha-adrenergic antagonist, causes miosis and lessens pupillary block without affecting outflow facilityand is useful in determining whether partial angle closure due to pupillary block is present. In this case where thymoxamine-induced miosis fails to lower IOP, partial angle closure is not present, and iridotomy may not be helpful in lowering IOP.

○ **A glaucoma patient taking echothiophate drops requires abdominal surgery. What complication should the anesthesiologist be alert for in this patient if general anesthesia is used?**

Echothiophate decreases serum pseudocholinesterase activity and accentuates the effect of succinylcholine, resulting in prolonged respiratory paralysis after general anesthesia.

○ **An 80-year-old patient presents with normal intraocular pressures, rubeosis iridis with synechial angle closure, midperipheral retinal hemorrhages and poor vision in his left eye. What is the most likely diagnosis?**

Ocular ischemic syndrome.

○ **Where in the angle is resistance to aqueous outflow greatest?**

Juxtacanalicular meshwork.

○ **A 60-year-old patient presents to your clinic with headache, right eye pain and redness. She has a history of sudden loss of vision in her right eye 4 months ago. The IOP in her affected eye is 42 mm Hg. The gonioscopic examination reveals angle neovascularization. What is the procedure of choice for treating this patient?**

Panretinal photocoagulation

○ **What are the mechanisms by which uveal melanomas can produce glaucoma?**

1. Direct invasion of the anterior chamber angle by tumor.
2. Angle closure from forward displacement of the lens-iris diaphragm.
3. Clogging of the trabecular meshwork with pigment or macrophages filled with pigment from necrotic tumor.
4. Iris neovascularization.

○ **Which parts of the optic disk neuroretinal rim is most affected early in normal tension glaucoma?**

Temporal and inferotemporal neuroretinal rim.

○ **When does epithelial downgrowth occur?**

It occurs when the ocular surface epithelium enters the eye through a surgical or traumatic wound and forms a sheet of nonkeratinizing squamous epithelium that grows over the anterior chamber angle, iris and ciliary body.

○ **What is the mean value for outflow facility in the normal eye?**

0.28 µL/min/mm Hg.

O   **What is nanophthalmos?**

It is a rare disease characterized by a small eye, high hypermetropia, weak but thick sclera, and a tendency to angle closure glaucoma.

O   **Why should eye surgery in a nanophthalmic eye be avoided where possible?**

Any surgery, but especially intraocular surgery and even laser trabeculoplasty may be complicated by severe uveal effusion.

O   **What is the most common pathophysiologic mechanism behind developmental glaucoma?**

Trabeculodysgenesis.

O   **How much does aqueous humor production decrease when active transport is inhibited by ouabain?**

Aqueous production decreases by 70%, thus 30% is due to ultrafiltration and diffusion.

O   **Which part of the autonomic nervous system is important in aqueous humor production?**

Both parasympathetic and sympathetic impulses are important in the release of aqueous humor.

O   **When is intraocular pressure highest and lowest?**

It is highest in the morning and lowest at midnight.

O   **In what condition is Sampaolesi's line seen?**

Sampaolesi's line, which is a pigment line seen anterior to the trabecular meshwork, is seen in cases of pseudoexfoliation and pigmentary dispersion syndrome.

O   **What procedure is most appropriate for a patient with an attack of angle closure glaucoma and media opacities or a flat chamber which precludes the use of a laser for a peripheral iridotomy?**

Surgical peripheral iridectomy.

O   **What is Posner-Schlossman syndrome?**

It is a unilateral ocular hypertensive cyclitis in a white eye.

O   **What procedure must be performed to distinguish pupillary block from ciliary block glaucoma?**

Peripheral iridotomy or iridectomy.

○ **What are the gonioscopic features of congenital glaucoma?**

The angle is open with a high insertion of the iris root and a membrane (Barkan's membrane) covering the angle.

○ **What are the risk factors for the development of ciliary block (malignant) glaucoma?**

Eyes with chronic angle closure glaucoma, peripheral anterior synechiae, and uncontrolled IOP are at increased risk postoperatively.

○ **What are glaukomflecken?**

Glaukomflecken are anterior, subcapsular lens opacities caused by foci of cortical fiber necrosis.

○ **What is the main advantage of applanation tonometry over Schiøtz tonometry?**

Scleral rigidity does not affect the readings of applanation tonometry.

○ **What principle does applanation tonometry utilize?**

Applanation tonometry uses the Imbert-Fick principle ($P = F/A$, where P = pressure inside a sphere, F = force necessary to flatten its surface, and A = area of flattening).

○ **At what diameter of corneal flattening does the resistance of the cornea to flattening and the force exerted by the tear meniscus pulling the tonometer towards the cornea cancel each other out?**

3.06 mm.

○ **How is IOP measurement with an applanation tonometer affected by corneal edema or scarring?**

Corneal edema produces falsely low readings.
Corneal scars produce falsely high reading.

○ **What happens to the IOP reading if too much or too little fluorescein is used?**

Too much fluoresceinproduces wide mires = falsely high reading.
Too little fluoresceinproduces narrow mires = falsely low reading.

○ **What must you do to obtain accurate applanation tonometry readings in a patient with high corneal astigmatism?**

Two readings taken 90∞ apart can be averaged or the red mark on the tonometer head can be rotated to match the patient's negative corneal axis.

O   **What is the mechanism of action of cyclodestructive procedures?**

These procedures lower pressure by producing necrosis of the secretory cells of the ciliary epithelium and may also damage the vascular supply of the ciliary body.

O   **In what condition are Krukenberg's spindles seen?**

Krukenberg spindles are vertically oriented pigment lines in the shape of a spindle on the corneal endothelium and are a sign of pigment dispersion syndrome.

O   **What is the most common cause of a flat or shallow chamber after filtration surgery?**

Overfiltration.

O   **A patient who recently underwent scleral buckling for retinal detachment develops an acute attack of angle closure glaucoma. What is the mechanism of angle closure in this case, and is peripheral iridectomy indicated?**

Obstruction of venous outflow by the buckle can produce choroidal effusions that cause anterior rotation of the ciliary body and secondary angle closure. Peripheral iridectomy is ineffective because there is no pupillary block present. The buckle may need to be repositioned if medical treatment of the glaucoma is not effective.

O   **What is the cause of the elevated IOP seen in phacolytic glaucoma?**

This is believed to be due to obstruction of the trabecular meshwork by high molecular weight lens protein, although macrophages filled with engulfed lens material can also be seen.

O   **What techniques can be used to open a miotic pupil for cataract surgery?**

Multiple sphincterotomies, sector iridectomy with secondary closure, manual pupil stretching, hooks inserted thru limbal punctures or pupil-expanding rings can be utilized.

O   **Approximately when postoperatively do Tenon's cyst tend to form?**

Tenon's capsule may form a thick-walled cyst within 3-6 weeks after filtering surgery in 10-15% of eyes. Most cases resolve with aqueous suppressants and do not require surgical revision.

O   **What is the incidence of primary open angle glaucoma in the general population aged over 40 years?**

0.5 to 1%.

O   **Which goniolenses are useful for distinguishing appositional angle closure from synechial angle closure using indentation gonioscopy and why?**

Zeiss and Sussman goniolens are better suited for indentation gonioscopy than the Goldmann lens because of their smaller diameters.

❍   **What is the normal range for episcleral venous pressure?**

8 to 12 mm Hg.

❍   **What is the difference between hemolytic glaucoma versus ghost cell glaucoma with regards to the cause of the rise in IOP?**

In hemolytic glaucoma, macrophages filled with hemoglobin from fresh hemorrhage clog the trabecular meshwork. In ghost cell glaucoma, which is seen weeks to months later after a vitreous hemorrhage, degenerated red blood cells from the vitreous enter the anterior chamber and obstruct the trabecular meshwork.

❍   **What is the medical treatment for angle closure glaucoma in a patient with microspherophakia?**

Cycloplegics to relieve pupillary block.

❍   **What is the incidence of POAG among patients with Fuch's dystrophy?**

15%.

❍   **How can iris cysts be prevented when treating POAG with strong miotics such as phospholine iodide?**

Concomitant use of phenylephrine can prevent iris cysts through an unknown mechanism.

❍   **What are the ocular manifestations of aniridia?**

1. External: microcornea, pannus, sclerocornea, epibulbar dermoids, and keratolenticular adhesions.
2. Lenticular: cataract, upward subluxation, and persistent pupillary membrane.
3. Glaucoma in 50%.
4. Posterior segment: foveal hypoplasia, disc hypoplasia, choroidal coloboma.
5. Congenital nystagmus.

❍   **What part of the visual field do paracentral scotomas occur more frequently?**

Upper half of the visual field.

❍   **How much of a reduction in sensitivity in the visual field is produced by loss of half the number of axons?**

This leads to a 5 dB reduction in sensitivity.

❍   **What are the causes of a ring scotoma?**

1. Retinitis pigmentosa.
2. Glaucoma (double arcuate scotoma).
3. Refractive scotoma with aphakic glasses.

○   **What is the earliest visual field change in chronic glaucoma?**

The earliest change is a generalized constriction of all isopters, which is nonspecific. The earliest clinically significant visual field defect is a paracentral scotoma.

○   **What is the treatment for congenital glaucoma?**

Goniotomy, trabeculotomy, trabeculectomy.

○   **A 6-month-old child has an IOP of 18 mm Hg when examined under general anesthesia. Does this rule out the diagnosis of congenital glaucoma?**

No, because general anesthesia may lower IOP. The appearance of the optic disc, the cornea and the corneal diameter are also important in making the diagnosis.

○   **How often is aniridia bilateral?**

98% of cases.

○   **In what conditions is the use of intravenous mannitol to lower IOP contraindicated?**

Pulmonary congestion and edema, heart failure, dehydration and renal disease.

○   **What do high false positive and high false negative error values on a Humphrey visual field indicates?**

A high false positive value suggests a trigger-happy patient, while a high false negative value suggests inattention.

○   **What percentage of total aqueous outflow facility does uveoscleral outflow account for?**

10 to 20%.

○   **A patient who had a complicated cataract surgery has considerable postoperative corneal edema. What tonometers are useful for measuring IOP in this case?**

Pneumotonometer and MacKay-Marg tonometer both applanate a very small area of the cornea and are useful in the presence of corneal edema or corneal scars.

○   **How well does pseudoexfoliation glaucoma respond to treatment?**

Patients with pseudoexfoliation glaucoma are often resistant to medical therapy but are very responsive to laser trabeculoplasty.

❍   **A patient with very narrow angles receives dilating eye drops to his eye. If this patient develops an attack of primary angle closure glaucoma, when is this most likely to occur?**

It generally takes place after full dilation as the pupil constricts to midposition and maximal iris-lens contact occurs.

❍   **How do you break an attack of acute angle closure glaucoma?**

The IOP should first be lowered using topical beta-blockers, carbonic anhydrase inhibitors and/or hyperosmotic agents. The iris may not respond to miotics if the IOP is very elevated. Once the IOP is controlled, a laser iridotomy is performed. The other eye should also be treated with a prophylactic laser iridotomy. If laser iridotomy cannot be performed, a surgical iridectomy is indicated.

❍   **How is the prone-dark provocative test performed?**

The IOP is measured before and after 30 minutes to an hour with the patient lying prone in a totally dark room. Lying prone will move the lens forward, and the dark will dilate the pupils, thereby increasing pupillary block and causing angle closure in susceptible patients.

❍   **What is the most popular flow-restricted or nonresistance tube shunt devices?**

Molteno and Baerveldt tube shunt designs.

❍   **What is the mechanism of acute angle closure glaucoma following a recent CRVO?**

Transudation of serum into the vitreous by the elevated intravascular pressure can cause vitreous swelling and secondary angle closure.

❍   **Why is succinylcholine and ketamine not recommended for use in examining a patient with a possible ruptured globe under anesthesia?**

Both agents can raise IOP and cause further prolapse of intraocular contents through the wound.

❍   **A 38-year-old woman complaining of blurred vision and haloes in her right eye presents with corneal edema in her right eye, minimal corectopia, normal IOP and broad based peripheral anterior synechiae. What is the probable diagnosis?**

Chandler's syndrome, a one of the iridocorneal endothelial syndromes, is characterized by severe corneal changes. Corectopia may be mild to moderate. Stromal atrophy is absent in about 60% of cases. Glaucoma is usually less severe than in Cogan-Reese syndrome and progressive iris atrophy, and the IOP may be normal at presentation.

○ **How do you distinguish between Rieger's anomaly and progressive iris atrophy, both of which are characterized by peripheral anterior synechiae, iris stromal atrophy, hole formation and corectopia?**

Rieger's anomaly, an autosomal dominant trait, is usually bilateral and occurs in childhood or early adulthood. An anteriorly displaced Schwalbe's line (posterior embryotoxon) is present. Progressive iris atrophy, which is one of the iridocorneal endothelial syndromes, typically affects one eye in young to middle-aged woman. The endothelium may have a beaten-metal appearance similar to Fuch's dystrophy. Posterior embryotoxon is not present.

○ **What could Cogan-Reese syndrome be misdiagnosed with?**

Diffuse iris melanoma.

○ **An infant presents with a dense, white central corneal opacity in both eyes with iris adhesions to its margins. The lens cannot be visualized. What is the probable diagnosis?**

Peter's anomaly.

○ **What complications are patients with Sturge-Weber syndrome, who have glaucoma, at high risk for if trabeculectomy is attempted?**

Intraoperative choroidal effusion and expulsive hemorrhage.

○ **What is the most common complication seen following Nd:YAG and argon laser iridotomies?**

Acute glaucoma.

○ **Which laser iridotomy has a greater chance of spontaneous closure, Nd:YAG or argon laser iridotomy?**

Nd:YAG laser iridotomy.

○ **Which of the following drugs is the most potent ocular hypotensive agent among the topical beta, blocking agents: timolol, betaxolol, levobunolol, carteolol and metipranolol?**

Timolol, levobunolol, metipranolol and carteolol are all equivalents to each other in terms of IOP-lowering effect, while betaxolol is less effective as an ocular hypotensive agent when compared to the other topical beta blockers.

○ **What drug when added to betaxolol will produce an ocular hypotensive effect equivalent to timolol and other topical beta-blockers?**

Dipivefrin.

❍ **What is the success rate of a primary trabeculectomy (without antimetabolites) in patients with open angle glaucoma?**

Approximately 80-85%.

❍ **What are the appropriate laser settings when performing argon laser trabeculoplasty?**

50 µm spot size, 0.1 sec duration, initial power setting between 600 to 800 mW and then adjusted to obtain a blanch or small bubble formation.

❍ **Approximately what percentage of eyes of patients with open angle glaucoma respond to initial therapy with argon laser trabeculoplasty?**

According to the Glaucoma Laser Trial, 80% of individuals responded with at least a 20% reduction in intraocular pressure.

❍ **What is the postulated mechanism by which argon laser trabeculoplasty lowers IOP?**

Trabecular outflow is increased due to shrinkage of adjacent tissues and opening of the trabecular channels. In addition, there may be acceleration of the phagocytic activity of the trabecular cells.

❍ **Following argon laser trabeculoplasty, what is the incidence of a postoperative IOP elevation of >10 mmHg?**

Approximately 8%. The use of apraclonidine has decreased this incidence to 2%.

❍ **How do you define threshold in perimetry?**

It is the differential light sensitivity at which a stimulus of given size and duration of presentation is seen 50% of the time. In practical terms, it is the dimmest spot detected during testing.

❍ **What is an isopter?**

It is a line connecting points with the same threshold on a visual field representation.

❍ **What is the most serious idiosyncratic hematologic side effect of carbonic anhydrase inhibitors?**

Aplastic anemia.

❍ **How much of the enzyme carbonic anhydrase must be inhibited in order to reduce aqueous flows significantly?**

99%.

❍   **What carbonic anhydrase inhibitor is available for topical use, and how effective is it in lowering IOP?**

Dorzolamide hydrochloride 2% administered three times a day effectively reduces IOP and avoids the systemic side effects of oral administration of carbonic anhydrase inhibitors. The IOP lowering effect is about 5 mm throughout the day in clinical studies up to 1 year's duration.

❍   **How effective is betaxolol's ability to lower IOP when compared to timolol?**

Betaxolol is about 85% as effective in lowering IOP as timolol. However, the deficit can be made up by its greater additive effect in combined therapy with epinephrine or dipivefrin.

❍   **What is the aim of medical therapy of low-tension glaucoma?**

Medical therapy is aimed at rapidly reducing IOP to the lowest level possible in order to enhance vascular perfusion of the optic nerve, not just at treating on the basis of extent of cupping and field loss.

❍   **What systemic medications have some favorable therapeutic effect on low-tension glaucoma?**

Calcium channel blockers and the anti-serotonin agent nastidrofuryl are vasodilators and may be useful in treating low-tension glaucoma.

❍   **What are the most common causative organisms in filtering bleb-associated endophthalmitis?**

Haemophilus or *Streptococcus* species.

❍   **What laser settings are used to release scleral flap sutures after trabeculectomy?**

Argon laser, 50 micron spot, 0.1 second duration, Power 200-600 mW.

❍   **What are some patient characteristics associated with an increased risk of suprachoroidal hemorrhage?**

Advanced glaucoma, high preoperative IOP, aphakia, vitrectomized eyes systemic vascular disease, and patients with uncontrolled hypertension.

❍   **What two questions did the Ocular Hypertension Treatment Study (OHTS) set out to answer?**

1. Does lowering IOP prevent or delay the onset of glaucoma?
2. What are the risk factors for converting from ocular hypertension (OHT) to glaucoma?

❍   **What was the conclusion of the OHTS study with regards to whether lowering IOP prevents or delays glaucoma?**

In this study, 1500 OHT patients were randomized either to observation or to treatment with IOP-lowering medications. After five years, 9.5% of the control group developed early signs of glaucoma while only 4.4% in the treated group did so. Treating ocular hypertension therefore prevents the onset of glaucoma.

❍   What are the risk factors for converting from OHT to glaucoma identified by the OHTS study?

1. Older age
2. Higher untreated IOP
3. Increased cup-to-disc diameter
4. Decreased central corneal thickness
5. African descent

LENS AND CATARACT

○ **Where is the lens epithelium located?**

Immediately behind the anterior lens capsule is a single layer of epithelial cells. The most mitotic activity occurs in a ring around the anterior lens known as the germinative zone. The newly formed cells migrate to the lens equator where they differentiate into fibers.

○ **What is the lens capsule and its composition?**

It is the basement membrane laid down by the lens epithelium and is composed of type IV collagen.

○ **How thick is the posterior capsule?**

4 microns.

○ **The most common indication for cataract surgery is a patient's desire for improved vision. Name or describe the medical indications for cataract removal.**

1. Phacoantigenic uveitis.
2. Phacolytic glaucoma.
3. Phacomorphic glaucoma.
4. Anterior dislocation of the crystalline lens.
5. Inability to view the posterior segment.

○ **What are the causes of postoperative hypotony?**

1. Wound leak.
2. Inadvertent cyclodialysis.
3. Anterior choroidal effusion with ciliary body detachment.
4. Retinal detachment.

○ **How thick is the anterior capsule?**

14 microns centrally and 21 microns midperipherally.

○ **How much greater is the risk of zonular breaks and vitreous loss when performing cataract extraction with a pupil less than 4.5 mm as compared to a pupil size greater than 4.5 mm?**

There is a 5 times greater risk of vitreous loss when the pupil size is less than 4.5 mm.

○ **How are the Y sutures in the lens arranged?**

The lens sutures are arranged in an Y shape anteriorly and an inverted Y shape posteriorly.

○ **Where in the human lens is glycolysis the primary means of energy production?**

Everywhere except in the anterior epithelial cell layer. Lens fiber cells are devoid of organelles including nuclei, mitochondria, and ribosomes, and lack the machinery for generating energy through oxidative phosphorylation.

○ **What is a lens coloboma due to?**

Faulty closure of the fetal fissure.

○ **Which class of medications, taken orally on a chronic basis, is associated with the deposition of pigment in the anterior lens epithelium in an axial and stellate configuration?**

Phenothiazine.

○ **What circumstances preclude implantation of a plate-haptic intraocular lens?**

1. Tears or discontinuities in the anterior capsulorrhexis.
2. Tears in the posterior capsule other than a small posterior capsulorrhexis.

○ **What is the average speed of sound through the phakic eye?**

1555 m/sec.

○ **What part of the lens undergoes the most change in shape during accommodation?**

Central anterior capsule.

○ **What determines the time it takes for vacuum to build to vacuum limit in a peristaltic machine?**

Aspiration flow rate.

○ **What is the maximum safe dose of 2% lidocaine for local injection in adults?**

15 ml.

○ **What is the maximum safe dose of 0.75% bupivacaine for local injection in adults?**

25 ml.

○ **Describe the incisional funnel.**

The incisional funnel is a theoretical construct. It relates cataract incision length and location to induced corneal astigmatism. The closer is an incision to the center of the cornea or the longer its chord length, the greater is its astigmatic effect. Imaginary lines that connect the ends of incisions of equal astigmatic effect theoretically define a two-dimensional incisional funnel. The wide end of the funnel is 3 to 4 mm behind the limbus in the sclera and the narrow end of the funnel is several millimeters onto the surface of the cornea.

O   **What can be said about the location of intraocular lenses within the eye as the A constant increases?**

The higher the A constant, the more posteriorly the lens will sit inside the eye. Anterior chamber lenses generally have low A constants while lenses with posteriorly-angulated haptics intended for implantation in the capsular bag generally have high A constants.

O   **Explain the difference between hydrodissection and hydrodelineation.**

Hydrodissection is the separation of lens cortex from capsule using balanced salt solution while hydrodelineation is the separation of nucleus from cortex. A distinction between nucleus, epinucleus, and cortex is not readily apparent histologically. So while these terms are useful clinically and surgically, they have no histologic counterpart. Hydrodelineation can be performed in multiple layers of the lens.

O   **When should warfarin therapy be discontinued prior to surgery?**

96 to 115 hours (4 doses).

O   **What is the cause of true exfoliation of the lens?**

Infrared exposure, especially among glass blowers and furnace operators. Peeling and scrolling of the anterior lens capsule clinically recognize it.

O   **What is pseudoexfoliation of the lens?**

This is characterized by deposition of a basement membrane-like material on the lens capsule, iris, conjunctiva, trabecular meshwork and visceral organs.

O   **What is the incidence of anterior subcapsular cataracts in patients with atopic dermatitis?**

10%.

O   **Kelman-style anterior chamber lenses come in different overall lengths (12.5, 13.0, 13.5 mm etc.). How does a surgeon determine the correct lens to implant in an aphakic patient?**

A useful starting place is to measure the horizontal white-to-white distance and add 1 mm. If the lens seems small or large after implantation (this can be determined by intraoperative gonioscopy, if necessary) it can be exchanged.

O   **What factor is primarily responsible for the surge of fluid from an eye after an occlusion break?**

Compliance of the vacuum tubing.

O   **What type of aspiration pump is capable of the fastest vacuum rise?**

Venturi pump.

O   **When does the lens vesicle form during embryonic development?**

The lens vesicle forms at the 16 mm stage of embryonic development.

O   **What is the treatment for capsular contraction syndrome?**

Capsular contraction syndrome is a postoperative contraction of the capsulorhexis opening and has been described in patients with pseudoexfoliation syndrome, retinitis pigmentosa, advanced age and previous uveitis. The treatment consists of multiple radial Nd:YAG laser anterior capsulotomies.

O   **An eye is found to have an axial length of 24.60 D by A-scan ultrasonography. The axial length is accidentally entered into the lens power calculation formula as 26.40 mm. How far off and in what direction will the resulting refractive error be?**

At a normal axial length of 24.60 D, a 1 mm error in axial length measurement corresponds to a 3 D error in calculated lens power. As the error in this example is 1.8 mm, the calculated lens power will be off by 5 to 6 D. The lens will be under-powered and result in a hyperopic refractive error.

O   **What type of lenticonus is present in Lowe's syndrome?**

The most common ocular complications of Lowe's syndrome are congenital cataracts and posterior lenticonus.

O   **What is the most common cause of UGH syndrome?**

The inappropriate sizing of anterior chamber intraocular lenses usually causes uveitis-Glaucoma-Hyphema syndrome.

O   **What is Alport's syndrome?**

It is an autosomal dominant disorder characterized by nephropathy, deafness, anterior lenticonus, and polar cataracts.

O   **What are the most common surgical techniques for reducing corneal astigmatism at the time of cataract removal?**

1. Placing the cataract incision in the meridian of greatest corneal astigmatism.
2. Performing simultaneous astigmatic keratotomy.

❍   **What is the medical treatment of choice in a patient with microspherophakia who develops angle closure glaucoma?**

Cycloplegics will decrease pupillary block by tightening zonular fibers, decreasing the anteroposterior lens diameter and pulling the lens posteriorly in these patients.

❍   **A mentally retarded child presents to you with congenital cataracts, small crystalline lenses that appear disk shaped, and glaucoma. What is the probable diagnosis?**

Lowe's (oculocerebrorenal) syndrome, which consists of microspherophakia, congenital cataract, glaucoma, and aminoaciduria.

❍   **What is a Mittendorf dot?**

It is a remnant of the tunica vasculosa lentis, which is usually located on the inferonasal posterior capsule.

❍   **Which maternal infections are associated with the development of bilateral congenital cataracts?**

1.   Toxoplasmosis.
2.   Rubella.
3.   Cytomegalovirus.
4.   Syphilis.
5.   Varicella.

❍   **During which trimester of pregnancy will a maternal rubella infection produce congenital cataracts in the infant?**

The rubella syndrome occurs if the mother is infected during the first trimester of pregnancy and may result in nuclear or lamellar congenital cataracts, corneal opacity, pigmentary retinopathy, hearing defects, and cardiac defects.

❍   **What postoperative complication can occur if not all lens material is removed during cataract extraction in an infant with rubella syndrome?**

The rubella virus is present in the lens up to three years after birth. Incomplete removal of the lens will result in a viral-induced iridocyclitis.

❍   **What systemic disorder may be associated with "Christmas tree" cataracts?**

Myotonic dystrophy may be associated with multicolored, posterior subcapsular "Christmas tree" cataracts." These are composed of polychromatic iridescent crystals in the lens cortex and are composed of whorls of plasmalemma from the lens fibers.

❍   **Immediately after administering a posterior orbital injection in preparation for cataract surgery, a systemically healthy patient becomes apneic. What probably happened?**

The needle probably penetrated the inferior orbital fissure or the optic nerve sheath and anesthetic reached the patient's brainstem.

○   **A patient gets hit in the eye by a tennis ball. On examination, you note a ring of iris pigment on the anterior lens surface. What is this called?**

Vossius ring.

○   **Where is the anterior surgical limbus located, and what does this histologically correspond to in the cornea?**

The anterior surgical limbus is located superiorly at the insertion of the conjunctiva onto the cornea and corresponds to the end of Bowman's layer.

○   **What does the midsurgical limbus histologically corresponds to, and where is it located?**

It overlies the end of Descemet's membrane or Schwalbe's line and lies approximately 1 mm posterior to the insertion of the conjunctiva onto the cornea.

○   **Where is the posterior surgical limbus located, and what structure does it overlie?**

It is located 2 mm from the anterior surgical limbus and overlies the iris root and scleral spur.

○   **What type of lens changes are produced by Wilson's disease?**

In 20% of cases, copper accumulates in the anterior capsule and underlying cortex in a petaloid configuration.

○   **Assuming a watertight incision, what determines intraocular pressure during phacoemulsification and irrigation-aspiration?**

The height of the irrigation bottle above the eye.

○   **A patient who had cataract surgery with implantation of a posterior chamber IOL in his right eye complains of vertical diplopia when reading through the bifocal segment of his glasses. His distance refraction is –1.00 OD and –4.75 OS and corrects his vision to 20/20 OU. He refuses to wear contact lenses or to have refractive surgery. What can you do to correct this problem?**

Bifocal glasses with slab off grinding of the more minus lens, which, in this case, is the left lens.

○   **What type of glaucoma are patients who have microspherophakia prone to developing?**

Pupillary block glaucoma.

❍ **A patient develops a posterior subcapsular cataract. Which will be more greatly affected by the cataract, his near vision or his distance vision?**

Near vision.

❍ **What type of lens changes can amiodarone produce?**

Anterior capsular opacities.

❍ **What type of lens changes can be associated with atopic dermatitis?**

Posterior subcapsular cataracts.

❍ **What are the known environmental risk factors for the development of posterior subcapsular cataract?**

1. Trauma.
2. Corticosteroid use.
3. Ionizing radiation.
4. Ultraviolet radiation.

❍ **What systemic disorder has been associated with corneal melting several weeks following an uncomplicated cataract extraction?**

Rheumatoid arthritis with keratoconjunctivitis sicca.

❍ **What is the attachment of anterior hyaloid to posterior lens capsule called?**

Wieger's ligament.

❍ **A patient who had previously undergone extracapsular cataract extraction without an intraocular lens implant years ago is observed to have a ring of cortex fused between the anterior and posterior capsule during slit lamp examination. What is this finding called?**

Sommering's ring.

❍ **What factors increase the likelihood of a thermal burn at the cataract incision during phacoemulsification?**

1. Reduced irrigation around the phacoemulsification needle because of incision tightness.
2. Prolonged phacoemulsification time at a high-energy setting.

❍ **What disorder is associated with spontaneous rupture of the lens capsule and absorption of the lens proteins?**

Hallermann-Streiff syndrome, which is characterized by congenital cataract, microcornea, microphthalmia, and a "bird-like" facies.

O   **What syndromes can produce inferior displacement of the lens?**

Homocystinuria and Weill-Marchesani syndrome.

O   **How is capsulorrhexis in infants and children different from that in adults?**

The lens capsule is thinner and more elastic in infants. It tends to radialize more quickly because the sclera is less rigid and the anterior chamber collapses more easily.

O   **What are the risk factors for intraoperative suprachoroidal hemorrhage?**

1. Advanced age.
2. Uncontrolled glaucoma.
3. Systemic hypertension.
4. Myopia.
5. Generalized arteriosclerosis.
6. Recent eye trauma or surgery with active inflammation.
7. Intraoperative Valsalva maneuver.

O   **What is Weill-Marchesani syndrome?**

It is an autosomal recessive disorder characterized by microspherophakia, pupillary block glaucoma, bradycephaly, small stature, small hands with spade-like, stubby fingers, prominent knuckles, and knobby interphalangeal joints. Cutaneous and vascular anomalies are not present.

O   **What is the location of the lens displacement seen in Marfan's syndrome?**

The lens is displaced superiorly and temporally in Marfan's syndrome.

O   **What is the incidence of lens dislocation in Marfan's syndrome?**

60%.

O   **What type of lens anomaly is also associated with Marfan's syndrome?**

Microspherophakia.

O   **How do the zonules of patients with Marfan syndrome and homocystinuria differ?**

The zonules stretch but remain intact in Marfan syndrome, whereas the zonules are brittle and break more easily in homocystinuria.

O   **How many years after birth can live rubella virus be cultured from the human lens in congenitally acquired infection?**

Three years.

❍   **Which of the available intraocular lens materials is associated with the greatest contraction of the anterior capsulorrhexis after cataract surgery?**

Silicone.

❍   **What is the most common postoperative complication following extracapsular cataract extraction?**

Posterior capsule opacification.

❍   **In what metabolic disorder are "oil-droplet" cataracts seen?**

Galactosemia.

❍   **What is the sunset syndrome?**

This is an inferior displacement of the intraocular lens implant within the capsular bag due to zonular dialysis or capsular tears.

❍   **What type of intraocular lenses has the highest rate of lens dislocations?**

Iris-fixated IOLs.

❍   **Why is cardiac monitoring important following retrobulbar anesthesia and the use of a Honan balloon to soften the eye?**

Bradycardia may result because of stimulation of the oculocardiac reflex.

❍   **What is epikeratophakia?**

It is the surface implantation of prelathed donor corneal tissue after removal of the epithelium of the recipient's cornea for the correction of hyperopia and aphakia.

❍   **A patient with a giant retinal tear undergoes successful pars plana vitrectomy, scleral buckle placement, and silicone oil injection. Eight months later, cataract surgery is performed and the patient achieves 20/20 (6/6) unaided acuity with an appropriately powered biconvex PMMA lens. Four months later the silicone oil is removed. What happens to the patient's refractive error?**

The patient becomes moderately myopic.

❍   **What is the enzymatic defect present in homocystinuria?**

In this autosomal recessive disorder, there is an absence of cystathione beta-synthetase resulting in serum elevations of homocysteine.

❍   **What complication can result in patients with homocystinuria who undergo general anesthesia?**

Vascular thrombosis.

❍   **What are the primary advantages of capsulorrhexis over can-opener capsulotomy?**

1. A capsulorrhexis has no radial tears to extend posteriorly if excessive pressure is placed on the lens.
2. A capsulorrhexis will center the intraocular lens as the capsule contracts whereas a can-opener capsulotomy may allow one haptic to migrate into the ciliary sulcus.

❍   **What type of body habitus do patients with homocystinuria have, and what complication are they at risk of developing following cataract surgery?**

These patients are tall and have a marfanoid habitus. They are myopic and at risk for developing a retinal detachment after surgery.

❍   **Several weeks after a long but otherwise uneventful cataract operation, a patient complains of an oval-shaped dark spot above fixation in the operated eye. What is the most likely diagnosis?**

A scotoma caused by retinal phototoxicity from the operating microscope.

❍   **What are the principal advantages of topical or topical-intraocular anesthesia over posterior orbital injection anesthesia?**

1. No injection risks.
2. No need for an eye patch if the incision is stable.
3. Immediate recovery of vision.

❍   **How is O'Brien akinesia performed?**

This involves blocking the proximal trunk of the facial nerve before it divides in front of the ear. Locate the condyloid process of the mandible by placing a finger in front of the tragus and asking the patient to open and close his mouth. Inject 2-3 ml of anesthesia and be careful not to inject it into the joint space.

❍   **What is the effect on corneal astigmatism of a 3.0 to 3.5 mm phacoemulsification incision placed just inside the limbus?**

A reduction of astigmatism of 0.5 D in the meridian of the incision.

❍   **What is the affect of age on astigmatic keratotomy?**

Older patients experience a greater change in astigmatism than younger patients given the same incision do.

❍   **How is Atkinson akinesia performed?**

Atkinson akinesia involves blocking the superior branch of the facial nerve by injecting anesthetic along the inferior aspect of the zygomatic bone and arch along a line drawn down from the lateral canthus to the top of the ear.

❍   **What intraocular lens shape minimizes the change in refractive error that results from replacing vitreous gel with silicone oil or silicone oil with balanced salt solution?**

Positive meniscus shape in which the posterior radius of curvature of the lens equals the distance from the posterior lens surface to the fovea

❍   **How is Nadbath akinesia performed?**

This technique involves anesthesia of the facial nerve as it exits the stylomastoid foramen, which is located by palpating the space between the ramus of the mandible and the mastoid process.

❍   **What complication can result following Nadbath akinesia?**

Difficulty swallowing and speech as well as respiratory arrest can result with inadvertent block of the vagus nerve, the pharyngeal nerve and the spinal accessory nerve.

❍   **Which anesthetic technique has the advantage of sparing the lower face and mouth?**

Atkinson akinesia.

❍   **What is the embryological origin of the lens?**

Surface ectoderm.

❍   **What intraoperative complication are patients with pseudoexfoliation syndrome at risk of developing during cataract surgery?**

These patients have weak zonular support and are at risk of developing a dropped nucleus during cataract surgery.

❍   **What is the name applied to the flecks of brown pigment on the anterior lens capsule that mark the remnant of the anterior aspect of the tunica vasculosa lentis?**

Epicapsular star.

❍   **How often does cystoid macular edema (CME) develop in patients following intracapsular (ICCE) and extracapsular cataract extraction (ECCE)?**

Up to 50% of patients who undergo ICCE and 15% following ECCE will develop angiographically detectable CME within the first 6 weeks after surgery.

❍   **How much error in IOL power results for every millimeter of deviation from the true axial length?**

Approximately 3 diopters.

❍   **The pupil of a patient with pseudoexfoliation syndrome is 4 mm despite repeated use of mydriatics. Will addition of topical flurbiprofen (Ocufen) augment the preoperative pupillary dilation?**

No. Flurbiprofen is a prostaglandin synthetase inhibitor used to prevent intraoperative miosis and maintain mydriasis during surgery. It does not increase preoperative pupillary dilation.

❍   **Which type of congenital cataract is more amblyogenic, nuclear cataracts or posterior polar cataracts?**

Congenital nuclear cataracts are high amblyogenic, while posterior polar cataracts are usually visually insignificant.

❍   **What happens to color discrimination after removal of dense nuclear cataracts?**

It improves, particularly for colors at the short wavelength end of the visible spectrum such as blues and greens.

❍   **In general, how large should congenital lens opacities be before they are considered visually significant?**

3 mm or more.

❍   **What serious complications are associated with retrobulbar and peribulbar anesthetic injections?**

1. Globe perforation.
2. Optic nerve trauma.
3. Retrobulbar hemorrhage.
4. Brainstem anesthesia.

❍   **What is the change in the index of refraction of the aging crystalline lens due to?**

It is due to the increased content of water-insoluble lens proteins.

❍   **What is the average anteroposterior diameter of the crystalline lens at birth and at maturity?**

3.5 mm at birth, 5 mm in adults.

❍   **What intraoperative problems are typically encountered in patients with pseudoexfoliation syndrome?**

1. Poor dilation.
2. Floppy iris.
3. Weak zonules.

○   **Where is the oldest protein in the human lens located?**

The oldest protein is located in the primary lens fiber cells at the center of the lens nucleus.

○   **What is the most common type of congenital or infantile cataract by morphology?**

Lamellar or zonular cataract.

○   **What is the average equatorial length of the lens at birth and at maturity?**

6.4 mm at birth, 9 mm at maturity.

○   **What systemic disease should be considered in the setting of a 35-year-old woman with posterior subcapsular cataracts, thin atrophic skin, moderate obesity, and adult onset diabetes mellitus?**

Cushing's disease.

○   **What type of receptors do epinephrine and phenylephrine stimulate?**

Epinephrine is an alpha and beta-adrenergic agonist, while phenylephrine is an alpha-adrenergic agonist.

○   **What is "second sight"?**

The myopic shift in refraction that often accompanies cataract development, allowing presbyopic individuals who were formerly emmetropic to read without glasses.

○   **A patient who is taking amitriptyline for postherpetic neuralgia from a bout of shingles is scheduled to undergo cataract surgery. Why should phenylephrine not be used to dilate his pupil?**

Tricyclic antidepressants and monoamine oxidase inhibitors can augment the adrenergic effects of phenylephrine and precipitate a hypertensive crisis.

○   **What mechanism is thought to play a role in lens opacification in diabetes?**

Increased intracellular levels of sugar alcohols from increased aldose reductase activity, which leads to increased osmotic pressure and destructive changes in lens fibers and results in loss of lens transparency.

○   **What type of cataracts is associated with trisomy 21?**

Coronary cataracts, which consist of peripheral cortical opacities encircling the nucleus in a radial fashion and punctate, bluish nuclear opacities.

○   **What are Elschnig pearls?**

They are the result of migration of lens epithelial cells from the periphery of the lens through spaces between anterior and posterior capsule following cataract surgery, where they form accumulations of cortical material.

O   **What vascular anomalies may be present in Marfan's syndrome?**

Dilated proxima aortic arch with aortic insufficiency, mitral valve prolapse and aortic dissection.

O   **What is the effect on the postoperative refraction if a biconvex posterior chamber IOL is implanted in the ciliary sulcus rather than in the lens capsular bag?**

The correction will become approximately 0.7 diopters more myopic.

O   **What is the definition of anisometropia?**

A difference of 3 diopters or more in refraction between two eyes.

O   **A patient who had previously undergone a successful scleral buckling procedure for retinal detachment develops a clinically significant cataract in that eye. What is the incidence of a recurrent retinal detachment following uncomplicated ECCE?**

≤3%.

O   **A bilaterally aphakic patient wearing contact lenses elects to have a sutured posterior chamber IOL placed in one eye. What will be the effect of the IOL on image size as compared to the other eye wearing a contact lens?**

Pseudophakia results in about 1 to 2% image magnification while aphakic contact lenses magnify images by about 8 to 12%. Aphakic eyeglasses result in an image magnification of 20 to 35%. In this case, the image in the pseudophakic eye will appear slightly smaller than in the eye wearing the contact lens.

O   **What complications are associated with Nd:YAG capsulotomy?**

1. Transient elevation of intraocular pressure.
2. Lens pits and cracks.
3. Lens decentration or dislocation.
4. Retinal detachment.

O   **Close to the end of a routine, uncomplicated cataract extraction, the anterior chamber suddenly shallows, the red reflex disappears, and iris starts prolapsing through the wound. What is the most likely explanation for these findings?**

Expulsive choroidal hemorrhage. The surgeon should immediately close the wound with sutures and perform posterior sclerotomies to drain the suprachoroidal blood.

O   **What preoperative test is the best predictor of postoperative endothelial function?**

Early morning pachymetry is a better predictor than specular microscopy, since the endothelium is under greatest stress after the eyelids are closed during sleep.

○ **A patient with a prosthetic mitral valve taking coumadin requires cataract surgery. What is the best method of removing the cataract in this case?**

Clear corneal cataract extraction under topical anesthesia. Anticoagulation therapy should not be stopped in patients with prosthetic heart valves or deep vein thrombosis.

○ **When should sutures be cut in order to reduce postoperative corneal astigmatism following cataract surgery?**

Six weeks after surgery and after topical corticosteroids have been tapered.

○ **What complication can occur if the optic nerve sheath is penetrated during retrobulbar anesthesia?**

Respiratory depression can occur if inadvertent subdural injection occurs.

○ **Which procedure causes temporary loss of vision more frequently, retrobulbar or peribulbar anesthesia?**

Retrobulbar anesthesia.

○ **What are the potential complications of Nd:YAG laser capsulotomy?**

Increased IOP, cystoid macular edema, IOL damage, corneal endothelial damage, uveitis, vitreous prolapse, macular holes, retinal tears and retinal detachment.

○ **What is the incidence of retinal detachment following Nd:YAG laser capsulotomy and how soon after the procedure is performed do they most frequently occur?**

The incidence of retinal detachment following Nd:YAG laser has been reported to be about 0.1to 3.6%. The majority of retinal detachments occur within the first year.

○ **A 60-year-old pseudophakic patient reports a sudden decrease in central vision a few days after undergoing an uncomplicated Nd:YAG laser capsulotomy for an opacified posterior capsule, which could not be improved to better than 20/200. The IOL is well centered, the IOP is normal, and no retinal detachment is seen. What is the most likely explanation for the decrease in vision?**

Macular hole formation, which has been reported to occur soon after Nd:YAG laser posterior capsulotomy.

○ **A 35-year-old patient, who had an uncomplicated cataract extraction with implantation of a single piece silicone posterior chamber IOL, returns one month later with a significant posterior capsular opacity, which reduces his vision to 20/50. How soon after surgery can you do a Nd:YAG laser capsulotomy to correct this?**

Three to six months to allow capsular fibrosis around the IOL and to reduce the chance of spontaneous enlargement of the posterior capsulotomy and subsequent dislocation of the IOL.

O   **What medications can you use to pretreat a patient about to undergo a Nd:YAG capsulotomy to prevent a postoperative rise in IOP?**

Timolol 0.5% and apraclonidine or brimonidine eye drops.

O   **What is the cause of the elevated IOP seen in phacolytic glaucoma?**

This is believed to be due to obstruction of the trabecular meshwork by high molecular weight lens protein, although macrophages filled with engulfed lens material can also be seen.

O   **What type of refractive change is associated with a large and rapid increase in blood glucose?**

Increased myopia.

O   **If bilateral congenital cataracts are left untreated, when will nystagmus typically develop?**

3 months after birth.

O   **How often do cataracts occur in children with congenital rubella syndrome?**

Cataracts are present in 20% of patients and are bilateral 75% of the time.

O   **A patient who previously had refractive surgery in both eyes develops a significant cataract in one eye and wishes to have it removed. If the refraction and keratometric measurements prior to refractive surgery are unavailable, what can you do to calculate the true corneal power of the patient?**

First determine the patient's refraction. Next, place a plano hard contact lens of known base curvature on the cornea and refract over it. Subtract the resulting refractive error (with the contact lens in place) from the initial refraction to determine the change due to the contact lens. This value is the difference between the patient's corneal curvature and the base curve of the contact lens. Add the value of the base curve of the contact lens to the change in refraction produced by the contact lens to get the patient's true corneal power. This method is applicable only to patients with at least 20/80 vision.

O   **If the original refraction and keratometric measurements prior to refractive surgery were available, how would you calculate the true corneal power?**

Determine the refractive effect of the surgery (original spherical equivalent minus the present post-refractive spherical equivalent) and then subtract this from the original keratometry.

❍   **What is a common complication seen when doing cataract extraction in a patient with a posterior polar cataract?**

Intraoperative posterior capsular rupture is a common complication when performing cataract surgery in these patients.

❍   **A patient with strabismic amblyopia and a new posterior subcapsular cataract comes for consultation. His best-corrected visual acuity is 20/60 and a laser interferometer estimates a Snellen potential acuity of 20/25. What advice should be given to this patient regarding the improvement in visual acuity that is likely to occur with surgery?**

The potential acuity estimates of laser interferometer devices are often falsely high in the setting of amblyopia. Some effort should be made to determine the patient's best-corrected visual acuity prior to cataract development as this is the best predictor of visual acuity following surgery.

❍   **Why do pupils of patients with pseudoexfoliation syndrome dilate submaximally?**

This is probably related to iris infiltration and fibrosis from the pseudoexfoliation.

❍   **What type of cataract is usually seen in retinitis pigmentosa?**

Posterior subcapsular cataract.

❍   **Why do superior clear corneal incisions produce more endothelial cell loss (15%) with phacoemulsification than with temporal clear corneal incisions (7%)?**

Superior incisions are closer to the central endothelium than the more posterior temporal incisions.

❍   **How should a posterior chamber IOL be placed inside the capsular bag if zonular dialysis less than 180 degrees is present?**

The haptics should be placed in the axis of the dialysis.

❍   **How should the posterior chamber IOL be oriented if zonular dialysis less than 180 degrees is present and sulcus fixation is chosen?**

The long axis of the IOL should be placed perpendicular to the axis of the dialysis; i.e. the haptics should be kept away from the region of the dialysis to avoid decentration.

❍   **What is the effect of tight corneal sutures on the corneal shape?**

Tight sutures will flatten the cornea over the suture but steepen the cornea central to the suture along that axis.

❍   **What are signs of a posterior capsular rupture during phacoemulsification?**

Vitreous in the anterior chamber, deepening of the anterior chamber and an area of the posterior capsule that appears clearer than adjacent areas.

○   **What is the incidence of erosion of the polypropylene transscleral suture used in transscleral fixation of posterior IOLs through the scleral flap after 1 year?**

100%.

○   **What are patient risk factors for an intraoperative suprachoroidal expulsive hemorrhage?**

Elevated intraocular pressure, glaucoma, axial length ≥26 mm, intraoperative pulse ≥85 beats per minute, generalized atherosclerosis.

○   **A patient with a history of schizophrenia and psychotic episodes requires cataract surgery. Should you perform this procedure using topical anesthesia or with retrobulbar anesthesia?**

A potentially uncooperative patient is a contraindication to topical anesthesia because unwanted eye movement during inappropriate times may produce serious intraoperative complications. In this case, retrobulbar or peribulbar anesthesia should be used.

○   **Why should large optic IOLs and large capsulorhexis openings are used in diabetic patients undergoing cataract surgery?**

Cataract extraction is highly associated with asymmetric progression of nonproliferative diabetic retinopathy with women, especially obese patients, with a significantly increased risk of progression of retinopathy and worse visual outcomes. These patients may require panretinal photocoagulation in the future, hence the need for large capsulorhexis openings and large-optic IOLs.

○   **What is the most effective chemical preparation of the eye in decreasing the bacterial flora of the conjunctiva prior to ophthalmic surgery without causing toxicity to the ocular surface?**

5% (half strength) povidone-iodine (Betadine) solution.

○   **What is a morgagnian cataract?**

In a morgagnian cataract, the cortex is liquified and opaque. The nucleus is very mobile and hard to emulsify.

○   **What type of posterior chamber intraocular lenses should not be placed in the ciliary sulcus or in patients without an intact, continuous curvilinear capsulorhexis opening?**

Single piece (plate) foldable IOLs can produce pseudophakodonesis if placed in the ciliary sulcus, resulting in pigment release and recurrent iritis. They can migrate out of the capsular bag if an intact, continuous, curvilinear capsulorhexis opening is not present.

○   **What is the average axial length of the adult eye?**

24 mm.

○   **Two days after uneventful corneal incision phacoemulsification and capsular-bag implantation of a foldable acrylic posterior chamber lens, a patient experiences a 3.5 D myopic shift in refraction associated with shallowing of the anterior chamber. Slit lamp examination reveals a capsulorrhexis that is smaller than the optic and central posteriors capsule that is several millimeters behind the optic. What is the diagnosis and treatment?**

The diagnosis is capsular bag distention from sequestered viscoelastic material. The treatment is release of the sequestered viscoelastic by Nd:YAG anterior or posterior capsulotomy.

○   **What concentration of copper in an intraocular foreign body is toxic to the eye?**

Intraocular foreign bodies containing 70 to 90% copper will produce chalcosis while concentrations greater than 90% will incite an acute inflammatory response.

○   **What 4 types of aspiration pumps are employed in the current generation of phacoemulsification machines?**

1. Peristaltic.
2. Diaphragm.
3. Venturi.
4. Rotary vane.

○   **What is a Sommerring's ring?**

It is a proliferation of lens epithelial cells within a closed space at the equatorial regions formed when the edges of the anterior capsule adhere to the posterior capsule following extracapsular cataract extraction or traumatic rupture of the lens capsule.

○   **What surgical mistake most often precipitates iris prolapse during scleral tunnel phacoemulsification?**

Entering the anterior chamber too posteriorly.

○   **What is responsible for the growth of the lens throughout life?**

Proliferation and migration of epithelial cells and their extension from the equatorial lens bow.

○   **What happens to intraocular pressure 1 month after uncomplicated extracapsular cataract extraction using either a manual expression or phacoemulsification technique of nucleus removal?**

In nonglaucomatous eyes, intraocular pressure drops by an average of 2 mm Hg.

❍   **What is the most likely explanation for high intraocular pressure 1 day after uneventful cataract surgery?**

Retained viscoelastic material.

❍   **Which part of the lens capsule is thinnest?**

Central posterior lens capsule.

❍   **Which part of the lens capsule does a capsule forceps during intracapsular cataract extraction grasp?**

Mid-peripheral anterior capsule, either inferiorly when using a tumbling technique or superiorly when using a sliding technique.

❍   **When is an erysophake usually used for intracapsular cataract extraction?**

Intumescent lenses. Enzymatic zonulolysis with alpha chymotrypsin is almost mandatory.

❍   **What is the characteristic histopathologic finding in phacoantigenic uveitis?**

Zonal granulomatous inflammation.

❍   **What are snowflake cataracts associated with?**

Diabetes mellitus.

❍   **What term is used to describe a mature cataract with liquid cortex, an intact capsule, and a freely mobile brunescens nucleus?**

Morgagnian cataract.

❍   **In an infant with rubella syndrome, what characteristic histopathological finding can be found in the lens?**

Retention of lens fiber nuclei within the lens center is characteristic although not pathognomonic of rubella cataracts.

❍   **During cataract surgery, the posterior capsule ruptures and the lens nucleus falls back into the vitreous. How would you manage this case?**

Remove any remaining cortical and nuclear material from the posterior chamber, and perform a vitrectomy. An IOL of choice can be implanted depending on the remaining capsular integrity. The patient is then referred electively to a vitreoretinal surgeon for removal of the nucleus within 7 to 14 days.

❍   **A patient who requires a corneal transplant has a 1+ nuclear sclerotic cataract. Give three reasons why the cataract should be removed concomitantly in this case.**

1. Cataracts may progress more rapidly after corneal transplantation.

2. Topical steroids used after keratoplasty can hasten cataract development.
3. Cataract surgery after corneal transplantation can traumatize the grafted endothelium.

❍ **You decide that your cataract patient with highly hyperopic eyes piggyback IOLs. Which lens should be inserted more posteriorly?**

The higher power lens should be inserted most posteriorly within the capsular bag and the lower power lens either in the bag or in the sulcus to facilitate lens exchange of the lower-power IOL for postoperative refractive adjustment if necessary.

❍ **What is a potential complication of piggyback IOLs that has required IOL explantation in some cases?**

Interlenticular opacification.

❍ **Which type of IOLs do not require irrigation with balanced salt solution after removal from the package?**

Silicone lenses become difficult to handle when wet and do not require irrigation.

❍ **What is the primary advantage of phaco chop techniques over the four-quadrant divide and conquer technique?**

Reduced phacoemulsification time and energy in phaco chop techniques.

❍ **The Leiske and Azar 91-Z intraocular lenses were discontinued because of a high incidence of pseudophakic bullous keratopathy. How would you classify these lenses?**

Closed loop anterior chamber lenses.

❍ **Give 10 relative contraindications to IOL implantation in children.**

1. Microcornea.
2. Microphthalmos.
3. Corneal endothelial dystrophy.
4. Nanophthalmos.
5. Rubella cataract.
6. Uncontrolled glaucoma.
7. Persistent fetal vasculature.
8. Uveitis.
9. Proliferative diabetic retinopathy.
10. Sclerocornea.

❍ **What is flipped in the "chip and flip" nucleofractis technique?**

The epinuclear shell.

❍ **How long should cycloplegics using cyclopentolate or atropine be used in children following cataract surgery?**

1 month.

O   **Why are dispersive viscoelastics, eg. Viscoat and Vitrax, the agents of choice in the setting of a posterior capsular rupture?**

Dispersive agents have little tendency for self-adherence with low molecular weights and low surface tension. They will tamponade the vitreous to the posterior capsule and will tend not to be aspirated from the eye during cortical clean up.

O   **While performing eye surgery under general anesthesia, your anesthesiologist informs you that the patient is showing signs of malignant hyperthermia. What is treatment for this problem?**

Cessation of anesthesia and surgery, administration of dantrolene and general supportive measures.

O   **What neuromuscular blocking agent used during general anesthesia could have triggered the malignant hyperthermia?**

Succinylcholine.

O   **At what potassium level should elective surgical procedures is aborted?**

Over 6 mEq/l or below 3 mEq/l.

O   **Which local anesthetics are amide compounds?**

Lidocaine and bupivacaine.

O   **What is the incidence of retinal detachment following uncomplicated ICCE?**

2-3%.

O   **What is the incidence of retinal detachment following uncomplicated ECCE?**

0.5-2%.

O   **What are predisposing factors to retinal detachment following uncomplicated cataract surgery?**

Axial myopia (>25 mm), lattice degeneration, previous retinal tear or detachment in the operated eye, history of retinal detachment in the opposite eye, and family history of retinal detachment.

O   **What is the incidence of retinal detachment when cataract surgery is accompanied by vitreous loss?**

≥5%.

O   **What optical compromise is associated with multifocal intraocular lenses?**

Depth of focus is improved while contrast is reduced.

❍   **How often does retinal detachment occur in eyes with retained lens fragments in the vitreous cavity following phacoemulsification?**

15%.

❍   **What are the relative contraindications to topical or topical intracameral anesthesia?**

1. A strong blink reflex (uncontrollable lid squeezing).
2. Young age.
3. Mental retardation.
4. Communication difficulty (different language, deaf or hearing impaired).
5. Difficult cases (hard lenses, weak zonules, and small pupils).
6. Very apprehensive patients.

❍   **What size of lens fragments in the vitreous cavity following cataract surgery always requires removal by pars plana vitrectomy?**

≥2 mm.

❍   **Using fluorescein angiography, how often does cystoid macular edema occur in eyes following ICCE?**

Fluorescein angiography demonstrates that CME occurs in 40-60% of eyes after ICCE.

❍   **How often does angiographic CME occur following ECCE surgery?**

1%-11%.

❍   **What is the incidence of CME associated with visual loss (clinical CME) following cataract surgery?**

2%-10% following ICCE and 1%-2% is following ECCE.

❍   **What glaucoma medications are associated with CME in aphakic patients?**

Epinephrine and dipivefrin are associated with cystoid macular edema in patients with aphakic glaucoma or those without intact posterior capsules. Recently, latanoprost has been associated with reversible CME in eyes that have undergone recent intraocular surgery.

❍   **What does the practice of couching refer to?**

It is an ancient form of cataract surgery performed by inserting a needle through the temporal sclera at the pars plana region and dislocating the cataractous lens into the vitreous cavity.

❍   **What are the most common intraocular sources of glare after intraocular lens implantation?**

1. Posterior capsule translucencies.
2. Lens decentration.
3. A large or irregular pupil combined with a small optic.
4. An iridectomy or iridotomy within the lid fissure.
5. A lens positioning hole in the pupillary aperture.

❍   **What is lenticonus?**

It is a localized, cone-shaped deformation of the anterior or posterior lens surface.

❍   **What type of lenticonus is more common, anterior or posterior?**

Posterior lenticonus is more common and is usually unilateral and axial in location.

❍   **What type of lenticonus is associated with Alport syndrome?**

Anterior lenticonus, which is often bilateral.

❍   **What type of lentiglobus is more common and what is it often associated with?**

Posterior lentiglobus is more common than anterior lentiglobus and is usually associated with posterior pole opacities.

❍   **What do lenticonus and lentiglobus appear as on retroillumination?**

They appear as an oil droplet in the red reflex using retroillumination.

❍   **What condition following cataract surgery is characterized by peripheral corneal edema, punctate brown pigment beneath the areas of edematous cornea, and a centrally clear cornea with or without guttata?**

Brown-McLean Syndrome.

❍   **How often do lens opacities develop in patients with aniridia?**

50%-80% of patients with aniridia develops lens opacities within the first two decades of life.

❍   **What is the WAGR complex, and is this a familial or a sporadic condition?**

Wilms tumor, aniridia, genitourinary malformations and mental retardation, which can occur in sporadic cases of aniridia.

❍   **What are cerulean cataracts?**

They are small, bluish opacities located in lens cortex and are nonprogressive. They usually do not cause visual symptoms.

○   **What is a snowflake cataract?**

Snowflake or diabetic cataracts consist of bilateral, multiple gray-white anterior and posterior subcapsular opacities with a snowflake appearance, typically in young patients with uncontrolled diabetes. Maturation and intumescence follow shortly thereafter.

○   **Why is early-morning pachymetry a better indicator of endothelial function than specular microscopy?**

The endothelium is under the greatest stress after the eyelids have been closed during sleep.

○   **What pachymetric corneal thickness is consistent with corneal edema and endothelial dysfunction and increases the likelihood of postoperative corneal edema following cataract surgery?**

≥600 microns.

○   **Three months after extracapsular cataract extraction and intraocular lens implantation a patient has a refractive error of -1.50 +3.00 x 125. The patient has 5 interrupted 10-0 nylon sutures in the anterior sclera at 10, 11, 12, 1, and 2 o'clock. Which suture should the surgeon cut first to reduce astigmatism?**

The axis of the correcting plus cylinder points to the tight suture. Therefore, the suture at 11 o'clock, corresponding to an axis of 120°, should be cut first.

○   **A patient's refractive error 2 months after extracapsular cataract extraction measures +2.00 -4.50 x 090. Seven equally spaced 10-0 nylon sutures span the limbus from 10 o'clock to 2 o'clock. Which suture should the surgeon cut first to reduce astigmatism?**

The patient in this example has 4.5 D of against-the-rule astigmatism. The horizontal corneal meridian is considerably steeper than the vertical meridian. No sutures should be cut, as doing so would only worsen the astigmatism further.

○   **A patient with a corneal laceration has a cataract from the injury. Should the cataract be extracted through the laceration?**

No. This procedure would further injure an already traumatized corneal epithelium.

○   **How should cataract surgery by modified in a case of chronic iridocyclitis to prevent posterior synechiae formation?**

Posterior synechiae are adhesions between the posterior iris and the lens capsule. A lens with a large optic should be placed in the ciliary sulcus to minimize the likelihood of posterior synechiae development. Implantation of a heparin-surface-modified lens may also be helpful.

○   **What is the preferred method of cataract surgery in young children?**

Small-incision cataract aspiration combined with posterior capsulectomy and anterior vitrectomy because the posterior capsule opacifies very quickly in children. Nd:YAG posterior capsulotomy is difficult to perform in children even if the lens capsule has not become fibrotic.

○   **Why is ICCE not recommended for removing cataracts in children?**

Hyaloid-lenticular adhesions present in children will lead to uncontrolled vitreous loss following ICCE.

○   **Does topical anesthesia for cataract surgery eliminate the risk of postoperative ptosis?**

No, because the ptosis results from trauma from a lid speculum or postoperative periorbital inflammation that weakens the levator muscle attachment.

○   **What is postoperative diplopia following cataract surgery under topical anesthesia due to?**

It is the result of anisometropia or decompensation of a preexisting phoria.

○   **When should eyes with postoperative endophthalmitis undergo pars plana vitrectomy in addition to vitreous tap or biopsy and antibiotic injection?**

The Endophthalmitis Vitrectomy Study found that eyes with light perception visual acuity at the time of presentation benefitted from immediate pars plana vitrectomy. Eyes with better vision did not.

○   **What can cause spontaneous lens subluxation?**

1. Syndromes: Marfan's, Weill-Marchesani, Ehlers-Danlos, Stickler's.
2. Metabolic disorders: homocystinuria, hyperlysinemia, and sulfite oxidase deficiency.
3. Familial ectopia lentis.
4. Ocular disorders: aniridia, buphthalmos, keratoconus, and megalocornea.

○   **What is the differential diagnosis of a shallow anterior chamber in the immediate postoperative period?**

1. Wound leak.
2. Pupillary block.
3. Aqueous misdirection.
4. Choroidal effusion.
5. Suprachoroidal hemorrhage.
6. Capsular block.

○   **When should the ophthalmologist perform combined cataract and glaucoma surgery rather than staged procedures or cataract surgery alone?**

1. Severe glaucomatous optic neuropathy and the inability to withstand a postoperative pressure spike.
2. Poor control of intraocular pressure by medications alone.
3. Poor compliance with or tolerance of medical therapy.
4. Inability to tolerate multiple surgical procedures.

NEURO-OPHTHALMOLOGY

○ **What is the normal CSF pressure?**

≤ 200 mm.

○ **What is Gradenigo's sign?**

Suppurative otitis media with VI nerve paralysis, ipsilateral facial pain in the distribution of the V nerve and ipsilateral facial paralysis.

○ **How can the photostress recovery test be used to distinguish between macular and optic nerve disease in an eye with decreased vision?**

Patients with vision better than 20/80 and maculopathy will take 90-180 seconds to recover pretest vision after looking at a bright light for 10 seconds, while patients with vision better than 20/80 and optic nerve disease will have a recovery time of less than 60 seconds.

○ **What layers of the lateral geniculate body do crossed fibers pass to?**

They pass to layers 1, 4 and 6.

○ **How many nuclei does the trigeminal nerve possess, and what are their functions?**

There are four trigeminal nuclei:
1. Motor nucleus.
2. Mesencephalic involved in proprioception.
3. Main sensory nucleus in the pons, which is involved with light touch.
4. Spinal nucleus, the nucleus of the descending track, which is responsible for pinprick and temperature sensation.

○ **Nystagmus is defined by which component?**

Fast component.

○ **What is the origin of the different components of nystagmus?**

The slow component is vestibular in origin and is based on the direction of endolymph flow; the fast phase is compensatory and arises from the reticular formation.

○ **What cells produce myelin for retrobulbar optic nerve fibers?**

Oligodendrocytes.

O   **What does Meckel's cave contains?**

It contains the trigeminal nerve ganglion, which consists of cell bodies of the bipolar cells whose axons form the trigeminal nerve.

O   **What is the reason why macular vision is sometimes spared in posterior cerebral artery occlusion?**

Occipital cortex subserving macular function may be supplied by the middle cerebral artery.

O   **What is Foster-Kennedy syndrome, and what is it classically due to?**

Unilateral papilledema and contralateral optic atrophy characterize it. It is classically due to a tumor compressing one optic nerve and causing contralateral papilledema because of obstructive hydrocephalus.

O   **What is the most frequent cause of a pseudo-Foster-Kennedy syndrome?**

Ischemic optic neuropathy.

O   **What will muscle biopsy of a patient with Kearns-Sayre syndrome show?**

"Ragged red fibers."

O   **Why should edrophonium not be given to a patient where Kearns-Sayre syndrome is in the differential diagnosis?**

Cardiac conduction abnormalities, including heart block producing sudden death, may be present in patients with Kearns-Sayre syndrome and may require insertion of a pacemaker. Edrophonium can cause bradycardia in these patients and is therefore contraindicated.

O   **How do you confirm the presence of a Horner's syndrome?**

Cocaine, which prevents the reuptake of norepinephrine in the third order neuron ending at the pupil, will cause the normal pupil to dilate. An abnormality in the sympathetic pathway will prevent norepinephrine release, thus preventing cocaine from causing pupillary dilation.

O   **How can you distinguish between a preganglionic and a postganglionic Horner's syndrome?**

If the lesion is postganglionic, there will be less stored norepinephrine available for release in the nerve terminals adjacent to the iris dilator muscle fibers. Hydroxyamphetamine, which stimulates the release of norepinephrine in these nerve terminals, will therefore produce less pupillary dilation in the eye with postganglionic Horner's syndrome compared to an eye with preganglionic Horner's syndrome or a normal eye.

❍   **What type of VEP is used to test visual acuity in preverbal children?**

Pattern VEP.

❍   **What innervates Müller's muscle in the eyelid, and in what diseases is it affected?**

Müller's muscle, which raises the eyelid, is a smooth muscle innervated by the sympathetic nervous system and is affected by thyroid disease and Horner's syndrome.

❍   **When do myelinated nerve fibers at the optic nerve occur?**

When oligodendroglial cells, which make myelin and are normally not found in the lamina cribrosa, are present within the lamina cribrosa and retina.

❍   **A patient presents with a visual acuity of 20/80 OD. What tests could you do to check for factitious visual loss in this patient?**

Red-green glasses, fogging refraction, and stereo acuity are used to check for mild visual deficits up to 20/100. The rocking mirror test, optokinetic nystagmus and the base-up prism test are more useful for visual acuity worse than 20/100.

❍   **A patient develops a III nerve palsy with contralateral hemiparesis. What is your diagnosis?**

Weber syndrome, caused by occlusion of the interpeduncular branches of the basilar artery that disrupts the cerebral peduncle and the III nerve nuclei on one side of the midbrain.

❍   **What is the differential diagnosis of myelinated nerve fibers?**

1. Papilledema.
2. Cotton wool spots.
3. Congenital anomalies, e.g. retinal astrocytomas, hamartomas, Morning glory syndrome.

❍   **What are tilted discs?**

They are a bilateral condition caused by oblique insertion of the optic nerve into the globe. The disc appears oval or D-shaped with the axis frequently oblique. There may be an inferior crescent, situs inversus of the retinal blood vessels, hypopigmentation of the inferonasal fundus, myopia and oblique astigmatism.

❍   **Describe the visual field changes that can be produced by tilted discs.**

Visual field defects may be present in the upper temporal quadrants and, if bilateral, may be mistaken for those caused by chiasmal lesions on cursory examination. However, visual field defects caused by tilted discs do not respect the vertical midline.

❍   **What are optic disc drusen?**

Optic disc drusen are hyaline-like material buried within the substance of the optic nerve head. They are often bilateral and familial. The vision is typically normal. The optic cup is usually absent and the disk margin has a lumpy appearance. When the drusen emerge from the surface of the disc, they have a pearl-like, waxy appearance.

O   **In what groups of patients are optic disc drusen more commonly found in?**

1. Caucasians.
2. Patients with angioid streaks.
3. Patients with retinitis pigmentosa.

O   **What special investigations can you request to diagnose optic disc drusen?**

Optic disc drusen exhibit autofluorescence prior to injection of fluorescein dye. After injection of dye, they become hyperfluorescent and are well outlined. Optic disc drusen are also well seen using the CT scan and B-scan ultrasound.

O   **How can optic disc drusen cause impairment of vision?**

While uncommon, some patients can develop peripapillary choroidal neovascularization.

O   **How can optic disc pits cause visual impairment?**

A serous macular detachment can occur that may be easily mistaken for a central serous retinopathy, resulting in permanent damage to the macula if left untreated.

O   **What is the risk of developing serous macular detachments from congenital optic disc pits?**

50%.

O   **How would you treat this complication of optic disc pits?**

Laser photocoagulation of the temporal disc can be tried. In unresponsive cases, vitrectomy with gas tamponade may be required.

O   **What are the signs and symptoms of giant cell arteritis?**

Headache, fatigue, arthralgia, myalgia, and jaw claudication, associated with tenderness and diminished or absent pulse of the temporal artery.

O   **A patient presents with inability to look up, large pupils with light-near dissociation, Collier sign, and convergence paralysis. What is your diagnosis?**

This patient has Parinaud's syndrome (supranuclear upward gaze, convergence and accommodative palsy) and is caused by a lesion on the quadrigeminal plate of the dorsal midbrain. In children, this can be caused by aqueduct stenosis, pinealoma and meningitis. In young adults, demyelination, trauma and arteriovenous malformations can produce this while midbrain strokes, mass lesions and posterior fossa aneurysms are the more common causes among the elderly.

○   **What are the findings of pseudotumor cerebri?**

1. Increased intracranial pressure on lumbar puncture.
2. Normal neuro-imaging studies.
3. Normal CSF.

○   **What is the normal value for cerebrospinal fluid protein?**

It should not exceed 40 mg/ml.

○   **What cranial nerve palsy may occur in patients with increased intracranial pressure such as pseudotumor cerebri?**

VI nerve palsy.

○   **What are the causes of pseudotumor cerebri?**

1. Obesity.
2. Pregnancy.
3. Oral contraceptives.
4. Nalidixic acid.
5. Tetracycline.
6. Vitamin A.
7. Rapid withdrawal of systemic steroids.

○   **How would you workup a patient whom you suspect has pseudotumor cerebri?**

Inquire about medications used in the medical history. Do a systemic examination, including blood pressure and temperature. Perform a complete ocular examination, including pupillary assessment and optic nerve evaluation. Any patient with papilledema requires a CT scan or MRI scan as soon as possible. If that is normal, the patient should have a lumbar puncture performed. Visual field testing should also be done to document any changes to the visual field.

○   **When and how would you treat a patient with pseudotumor cerebri?**

Treatment is indicated for severe headaches or evidence of progressive visual acuity or visual field loss. Treatment consists of weight loss if overweight, oral acetazolamide, stopping any causative medication, and optic nerve sheath decompression or a lumboperitoneal shunt in unresponsive patients.

○   **What is Foster-Kennedy Syndrome?**

It consists of an optic atrophy in one eye and optic disc edema in the contralateral eye. This is caused by an intracranial tumor such as a frontal lobe tumor raising intracranial pressure and causing edema in one optic nerve while compressing the optic nerve of the other eye.

○   **What are the visual field findings of Foster Kennedy syndrome?**

There is an enlarged blind spot in the eye with optic disc edema and a central or cecocentral scotoma in the contralateral eye with the optic atrophy.

O   **What other conditions can produce findings similar to the Foster Kennedy syndrome?**

Pseudo-Foster Kennedy Syndrome can be produced by ischemic optic neuropathy or advanced glaucomatous optic neuropathy or a previous episode of optic neuritis resulting in optic atrophy in one eye and with a new episode of optic nerve swelling in the opposite eye.

O   **What are the types of optic neuritis?**

1. Retrobulbar neuritis, which is the most common type in adults and is most frequently, associated with MS.
2. Papillitis, which is the most common type in children.
3. Neuroretinitis, characterized by papillitis in association with a macular star figure composed of hard exudates and is most frequently associated with viral infections and cat-scratch fever, as well as syphilis and Lyme disease. In most cases it is self-limiting and resolves within 6-12 months.

O   **Can multiple sclerosis cause a neuroretinitis?**

No.

O   **What is the most common presenting symptom of multiple sclerosis (MS)?**

Optic neuritis (25%).

O   **What percentage of MS patients develops optic neuritis during their lifetime?**

In a retrospective study, nearly 100% of patients dying of MS had optic nerve demyelination, but only 55% developed clinical optic neuritis.

O   **How is the diagnosis of MS confirmed?**

MRI scan of the brain looking for demyelinating lesions and lumbar puncture (look for oligonal IgG bands in the CSF).

O   **What is Uhthoff's phenomenon?**

Decreased visual acuity produced by an increase in body temperature.

O   **What are the causes of optic neuritis?**

1. Demyelinating disease (most common).
2. Infectious causes, e.g. cat scratch fever, Lyme disease, syphilis, cryptococcal meningitis in AIDS patients, sinus infections.
3. Parainfectious, e.g. following viral illness or vaccination.

❍ **Does bilateral simultaneous optic neuritis occur with MS?**

Rarely. One must consider instead other causes such as Leber's hereditary optic neuropathy, methanol toxicity, Devic's neuromyelitis optica, etc.

❍ **What is Devic's neuromyelitis optica?**

Acute or subacute optic neuritis associated with transverse myelitis either simultaneously or sequentially.

❍ **What are the possible ocular manifestations of multiple sclerosis?**

Optic neuritis, internuclear ophthalmoplegia, pars planitis and periphlebitis, extraocular muscle palsies (in decreasing order VI, III, IV).

❍ **What are the MRI criteria for making the diagnosis of demyelinating lesions in the brain?**

1. Two or more white matter plaques which are periventricular in location.
2. Ovoid in shape, arranged at right angles to the corpus callosum as if radiating from it.
3. ≥ 3 mm in size.
4. Appear brighter on T2-weighted scans. Acute lesions may be highlighted using gadolinium on T1-weighted scans.

❍ **What is the sensitivity of MRI in detecting MS lesions?**

90-97%.

❍ **What other conditions can produce MRI findings similar to MS?**

Behçet's disease, HIV, sarcoidosis, ischemia, systemic lupus erythematosus.

❍ **What were the conclusions of the Optic Neuritis Treatment Trial?**

1. Patients with optic neuritis should undergo a cranial MRI to rule out demylinating white matter lesions consistent with MS.

2. Additional laboratory testing is not necessary for typical optic neuritis but should be considered for atypical cases

3. Treatment with IV methylprednisolone for 3 days followed by oral steroids hastens recovery of optic neuritis but does not change the final visual outcome.

4. Oral steroids alone in conventional doses are not recommended because of the increased rate of new attacks of optic neuritis.

❍ **How long will IV steroid therapy of optic neuritis reduce the risk of developing MS?**

Two years.

❍   **What segment of the optic nerve is most frequently injured following closed head trauma?**

Intracanalicular portion.

❍   **In general, what abnormality found in the ocular examination is most specific for optic nerve disease?**

Relative afferent pupillary defect.

❍   **A 23-year-old patient with a ventriculoperitoneal shunt develops an upgaze paresis, light near dissociation of the pupils, and convergence retraction nystagmus in attempted upgaze. Where is the lesion? What is the significance of the finding?**

The lesion is at the level of the dorsal midbrain. In a patient with a shunt, the constellation of findings consistent with the Parinaud's dorsal midbrain syndrome suggest shunt malfunction.

❍   **Is optic nerve sheath decompression indicated for non-arteritic anterior ischemic optic neuropathy?**

The Ischemic Optic Neuropathy Decompression Trial (IONDT) was a multicenter, randomized, controlled clinical trial that determined that optic nerve sheath decompression was not effective and possibly harmful to patients with non-arteritic anterior ischemic optic neuropathy.

❍   **A patient with neurofibromatosis type I develops gradually progressive proptosis, loss of vision, and optic atrophy of the right eye. Magnetic resonance imaging reveals a fusiform enlargement of the right optic nerve. What is the most likely diagnosis?**

Right optic glioma.

❍   **What are the causes of internuclear ophthalmoplegia (INO)?**

1. Multiple sclerosis (bilateral INO)- young adults.
2. Brainstem stroke (unilateral INO)- elderly.
3. Brainstem tumor.
4. Head trauma.
5. Wernicke's encephalopathy.

❍   **What is the structural appearance of the disc at risk for the development of non-arteritic anterior ischemic optic neuropathy?**

The disc at risk is a small disc with a small crowded appearance and a small cup to disc ratio.

❍   **Where is the lesion that produces INO?**

INO is produced by a disruption of the medial longitudinal fasciculus ipsilateral to the impaired adduction.

❍   **What is Adie's tonic pupil?**

This is a dilated pupil usually occurring in females and is associated with diminished deep tendon reflexes. Adie's pupil can be unilateral or bilateral. The pupil may show denervation supersensitivity and constrict with 0.125% pilocarpine. The pupil may show segmental constriction on slit lamp exam. In chronic cases, the pupil can become miotic and nonreactive.

❍   **An afferent pupillary defect (APD) usually results from damage to the ipsilateral optic nerve or retina. Can an APD result from lesions in other locations?**

An APD may occur in lesions of the optic chiasm/tract prior to the departure of the pupil fibers to the midbrain.

❍   **A 40-year-old patient develops diplopia. There is an adduction deficit in the right eye with abducting nystagmus in the left eye on attempted gaze to the left. The remainder of the eye exam is normal Where is the lesion? What is the most likely etiology?**

This patient has an internuclear ophthalmoplegia (INO) on the right. The most likely etiologies are demyelinating disease in a young person and stroke in an elderly person, but other entities involving the medial longitudinal fasciculus including neoplasm, infection or inflammation may cause an INO.

❍   **What is an Argyll-Robertson pupil?**

A small and irregular pupil that constricts with accommodation but not to light stimulation. This can be a sign of neurosyphilis.

❍   **A 68-year-old female presents with sudden loss of vision in one eye. She also reports an ipsilateral headache, scalp tenderness and pain in her jaw with chewing. What tests should be run to make the diagnosis?**

Biopsy of the temporal artery. This patient most likely has temporal arteritis or giant cell arteritis. A Westergren sedimentation rate of over 50 mm/hr suggests this diagnosis.

❍   **Should high dose oral prednisone be delayed until the biopsy of the temporal artery is made?**

No. The biopsy may still be positive even after one week of systemic steroid use. The patient is at risk for loss of vision in the opposite eye unless systemic steroids are started.

❍   **What are causes of isolated IV nerve palsies?**

1. Congenital.
2. Closed head trauma, which frequently causes bilateral palsies.

3. Vascular diseases, eg. Hypertension, diabetes mellitus.
4. Idiopathic.

○   **What are the main clinical features of a left IV nerve palsy?**

1. Defective depression of the left eye in adduction.
2. Left hypertropia in primary gaze.
3. Positive Bielschowsky test with deviation increasing on head tilt to the left shoulder.
4. Left excyclotropia.
5. Compensatory head posture consisting of right head tilt, right face turn and chin depressed.

○   **What is the significance of vertical fusional amplitudes of greater than 5 prism diopters in a patient with IV nerve palsy?**

It suggests a congenital IV nerve palsy.

○   **What is the parent artery of the ophthalmic artery?**

Internal carotid artery.

○   **A 60-year-old patient presents with acute onset of right ptosis, exotropia, intorsion on downgaze, limited elevation and depression and a dilated right pupil. What is your diagnosis?**

Right III nerve palsy.

○   **What are the important causes of an isolated III nerve palsy?**

1. Vascular disease.
2. Trauma.
3. Aneurysm at the junction of the posterior communicating artery and the internal carotid artery.
4. Idiopathic.

○   **A 58-year-old hypertensive woman complained of double vision. Neuro-ophthalmic examination was normal except for no adduction past midline of the right eye and abducting nystagmus of the left eye. Examination two months later revealed ptosis OU (right eye worse than left), no adduction and nystagmus on abduction of the right eye, and limited adduction, abduction and elevation of the left eye. What is the likely etiology of her motility problems?**

Although the initial presentation suggested an internuclear ophthalmoplegia (medial longitudinal fasciculus lesion), this adduction paresis resolved. The patient later has ptosis and external ophthalmoplegia. All of the above should raise the possibility of ocular myasthenia gravis (OM). The initial motility problem was a myasthenic pseudo-internuclear ophthalmoplegia OM should be considered in any case of ocular motor weakness without pupil involvement because MG may mimic any pattern of neurogenic paresis. Any extraocular muscle may be selectively impaired, especially the medial rectus, and weakness characteristically increases with sustained effort. Myasthenia can mimic pupil sparing third nerve palsies, superior division third nerve palsies, abducens nerve palsies, trochlear nerve palsies internuclear ophthalmoplegia, the one-and-a half syndrome, horizontal or vertical gaze palsy, double elevator palsy, and complete external ophthalmoplegia. The Tensilon test in this patient was positive.

○   **A patient presents with a ptosis and ipsilateral miosis of the pupil and has pain in the ipsilateral arm. Where is the lesion?**

The clinical diagnosis is Horner's syndrome. This can be confirmed with topical pharmacologic testing with cocaine drops. If the involved pupil does not dilate then the patient has an ipsilateral Horner's syndrome. The presence of arm pain suggests that the lesion involve the sympathetic chain at the level of the brachial plexus. An apical lung tumor (Pancoast tumor) should be suspected in this setting.

○   **What are the features of a left VI palsy?**

1. Left esotropia in primary gaze.
2. Defective abduction.
3. Horizontal diplopia, which is worse on, left lateral gaze.
4. Compensatory face turns to the left.

○   **What are important causes of isolated VI nerve palsies?**

1. Vascular disease.
2. Tumors.
3. Demyelination.
4. Raised intracranial pressure.
5. Basal skull fracture.

○   **A 33-year-old patient presents with central loss of vision in the right eye, a right afferent pupillary defect and a supertemporal defect in the left eye. The remainder of the examination is normal. Where is the lesion?**

A lesion at the junction of the right optic nerve and chiasm could involve the inferonasal fibers from the left eye (Wilbrand's knee) as they travel for a short course anteriorly into the right optic nerve. Although the anatomic existence of the knee itself has recently been called into question, the localizing significance of the junctional scotoma remains valid.

○   **What are the typical features of cluster headache?**

Periodic attacks of severe, unilateral head pain referred to the orbital or periorbital regions, associated with at least one autonomic symptom (miosis, ptosis, conjunctival hyperemia, rhinorrhea)

○   **A patient with normal vision presents with bilateral small, irregular pupils that do not react to light but constrict normally to convergence effort. What is the diagnosis?**

This patient demonstrates light near dissociation of the pupils. Tertiary syphilis causing Argyll-Robertson pupils should be suspected and syphilis serology should be ordered.

○   **What are the ocular features of myotonic dystrophy?**

1. Christmas tree cataracts.
2. Light-near dissociation of pupillary response.
3. Pigmentary retinopathy.
4. Ocular hypotony.
5. Lid lag.
6. Low voltage ERG.

○   **A 55-year-old patient with diplopia presents with an inability to elevate, depress, or adduct the left eye. The ipsilateral lid is ptotic and the pupil is not reactive to light. There are no other neurologic signs or symptoms. Where is the lesion and what is the evaluation?**

The diagnosis is an isolated pupil-involved third nerve palsy. This patient should undergo an evaluation to exclude an aneurysm of the posterior communicating artery including cerebral arteriography.

○   **A 35-year-old fashion model weighing 90 lbs. was brought to the emergency room because of slowly progressive confusion and imbalance of several days' duration. She is disoriented and confused and frequently repeated herself and has an unsteady gait. She has a full range of eye motion and no ocular misalignment. However, she has a primary position upbeat nystagmus, which became downbeating with convergence, and mild horizontal end gaze nystagmus. What is the likely etiology for her confusion and eye findings?**

The patient probably has Wernicke's encephalopathy caused by thiamine deficiency. Although most often seen with nutritional deprivation associated with chronic alcoholism, the disorder may also be seen with eating disorders, bulimia, hyperemesis gravidarum, and maintaining low weight. Characteristic findings include the classic triad of ophthalmoplegia (bilateral lateral rectus weakness), ataxia, and mental changes. The ocular motor signs are quite varied in Wernicke's disease and include bilateral abducens palsies, gaze-evoked or primary position vertical nystagmus, various combinations of horizontal and vertical gaze palsies and internuclear ophthalmoplegia, convergence disorders and ocular bobbing. Thiamine therapy must be urgently instituted.

○   **What can cause light-near dissociation of pupillary responses?**

1. Argyll-Robertson pupils.
2. Parinaud's dorsal midbrain syndrome.
3. Myotonic dystrophy.
4. Adie's tonic pupil syndrome (usually unilateral).
5. Aberrant regeneration of the III nerve.
6. Juvenile-onset diabetes.
7. Encephalitis.
8. Herpes zoster ophthalmicus (rare).

9. Chronic alcoholism.

○   **A patient with diplopia has an inability to elevate, depress, abduct or adduct the left eye. The left pupil is smaller than the right pupil is. The left eyelid is ptotic. Where is the lesion?**

This patient has a third, fourth, and sixth nerves paresis. The pupil is smaller due to presumed involvement of the oculosympathetic pathway within the cavernous sinus. Neuroimaging studies should be directed to this location.

○   **A 60-year-old man has a history 18 months ago of radiation to the brain for a malignant neoplasm. He now complains of progressive, bilateral painless visual loss for several weeks. There is bilateral impaired visual acuity, bilateral impaired color vision, bilateral constricted visual fields, and normal optic discs. MR imaging shows no evidence of optic pathway compression by the brain tumor. What should be considered?**

The patient may well have radiation optic neuropathy that presents with acute, gradual or progressive painless visual loss that may be unilateral or bilateral. Acuity may be 20/25 to NLP, variable color deficits are present, and there is often visual field abnormalities. Initially the optic nerves may be normal or show pallid edema; later the nerves become atrophic. There may be associated signs of radiation retinopathy, including microaneurysms, hemorrhages, exudates, telangiectasias, venous stasis, cotton wool patches, arteriolar narrowing, neovascularization and neovascular glaucoma, and focal retinal pigment epithelial loss. The onset of the optic neuropathy is months to years after the radiation therapy (usually within three years). Optic pathway compression by the original neoplasm must always be a consideration and evaluated by appropriate neuroimaging. Sometimes hyperbaric oxygen treatments started early in the course may be beneficial and slow down progression.

○   **What are the causes of Horner's syndrome?**

1. Intrathoracic: Pancoast tumor, aneurysms of the aorta and carotid artery, enlarged mediastinal lymph nodes.
2. Neurological disease: Wallenberg's syndrome, syringomyelia, cluster headaches, cervical cord trauma and tumors.
3. Neck lesions: surgery, tumors, and glands.
4. Congenital (associated with heterochromia).
5. Idiopathic.

○   **A 75-year-old woman presents with acute loss of vision, an afferent pupillary defect and a normal appearing optic nerve in the right eye. What is the next most appropriate step?**

An acute retrobulbar optic neuropathy in this elderly woman may represent posterior ischemic optic neuropathy. An evaluation for giant cell arteritis (including erythrocyte sedimentation rate and temporal artery biopsy) is indicated. Other causes for a retrobulbar optic neuropathy including compressive, infiltrative and inflammatory etiologies have to be considered as well but the evaluation should be directed towards excluding giant cell arteritis.

○ **A 25-year-old woman is noted to have anisocoria. Her left pupil remains at 8 mm in both bright and dim light, while her right pupil size is 5 mm in dim light and 2 mm in bright light. With near fixation, her right pupil constricts to 2 mm, while her left pupil very slowly constricts to 6 mm. What is your diagnosis?**

Adie's tonic pupil.

○ **What test can you perform to confirm the diagnosis of Adie's tonic pupil?**

The pupil will show denervation supersensitivity and constrict to 0.05% pilocarpine.

○ **A patient with a third nerve palsy develops signs of aberrant regeneration. Can this be an ischemic palsy?**

Aberrant regeneration of the third nerve is virtually never associated with an ischemic palsy and alternative etiologies should be considered.

○ **A 60-year-old woman presents with painless progressive loss of vision, an afferent pupillary defect, optic atrophy, and opticociliary shunt vessels in the right eye. What is the most likely diagnosis?**

The classic triad of progressive visual loss, optic atrophy, and opticociliary shunt vessels is very suggestive of optic nerve sheath meningioma. The shunt vessels represent retinochoroidal collaterals.

○ **What are the clinical features of Kearns-Sayre syndrome?**

1. Chronic progressive external ophthalmoplegia (CPEO) initially involving upgaze then lateral gaze.
2. Bilateral progressive ptosis.
3. Heart block.
4. Pigmentary retinopathy.
5. Onset before age 20 years.

○ **Do patients with Kearns-Sayre syndrome complain of diplopia?**

No. The CPEO is symmetrical.

○ **A 40-year-old woman has a history of bilateral lid retraction, mild bilateral proptosis, and vertical diplopia secondary to thyroid ophthalmopathy (Graves' disease). She now complains of unilateral progressive visual loss for the last 2 weeks. Acuity is 20/40 and 20/30, respectively, color vision is depressed on the left, a left relative afferent pupillary defect is evident, and the discs are normal bilaterally. The anterior segment appears normal. What is causing the visual impairment?**

The patient has optic neuropathy secondary to her thyroid ophthalmopathy. Optic neuropathy with thyroid ophthalmopathy is usually caused by apical compression of the optic nerve by enlarged extraocular muscles and can cause permanent visual loss. The discs may be swollen, normal, or atrophic. Treatment possibilities include high doses of oral or intravenous corticosteroids, orbital irradiation, orbital decompression, or a combination of these procedures.

○ **A patient has a complete ptosis of the right upper eyelid. Can this be a Horner's syndrome?**

The sympathetic innervation to the eyelid supplies the Müller's muscle. Oculosympathetic paresis results in only 1-2 mm of ptosis. A complete ptosis on a neurogenic basis suggests a third nerve palsy and is not consistent with a Horner's syndrome.

○ **A 45-year-old patient presents with painless variable diplopia and ptosis. There is moderate weakness of eyelid closure bilaterally. The pupils and the remainder of the exam are normal. What is the next most appropriate evaluation?**

Myasthenia gravis may mimic any pupil-spared, non-proptotic, painless ophthalmoplegia. It may occur with or without ptosis. An edrophonium (Tensilon) test may reverse the ptosis and ophthalmoplegia but a positive Tensilon test is not pathognomonic for the disorder nor does a negative test exclude myasthenia.

○ **A 16-year-old patient presents with variable diplopia. Examination reveals episodes of a large variable esotropia associated with miosis of the pupil and a bilateral abduction deficit. During the intervals between these episodes the eyes appear straight and abduction is normal. What is the most likely diagnosis?**

Convergence spasm. A true sixth nerve palsy would not demonstrate the large variability and normal alignment intermittently. Miosis of the pupils is the clinical clue that the convergence effort is being stimulated to create the deviation.

○ **What does De Morsier's syndrome consist of?**

1. Optic nerve/disc hypoplasia.
2. Absence of the septum pellucidum.
3. Hypothalamic-pituitary abnormalities (hypoglycemic seizures and growth retardation).

○ **A 45-year-old diabetic complains of blurred vision bilaterally. Neuro-ophthalmologic exam reveals visual acuity of 20/50 OD and 20/40 OS. The optic discs are moderately swollen and hyperemic bilaterally and mild bilateral macular edema is present. What is causing the disc swelling?**

Although papilledema from increased intracranial pressure is a concern, the patient likely has diabetic papillopathy, which may be unilateral or bilateral. Patients may have type I or type II diabetes. Disc swelling is mild to moderate, consistently hyperemic, and, on an average, resolves within four months. Macular edema is a frequent associated finding.

The differential includes papilledema from increased intracranial pressure, neovascularization of the disc, anterior ischemic optic neuropathy, and optic neuritis.

○ **What ocular findings are suggestive of craniocervical junction abnormalities?**

1. Downbeat nystagmus.
2. Periodic alternating nystagmus.

○ **A 30-year-old man with a history of chronic lymphocytic leukemia (CLL) complains of painless, bilateral visual impairment. Acuity and color visions are diminished bilaterally, the pupillary reaction is sluggish bilaterally, but the discs are normal. What should be considered?**

Progressive visual loss from optic nerve infiltration may be a clinical manifestation of leukemia, including CLL. The discs may be normal or swollen and progressive optic atrophy with loss of acuity and visual fields often occurs. MR imaging with gadolinium may reveal optic nerve involvement and meningeal involvement and spinal tap to document meningeal infiltration by the leukemia are warranted. Optic nerve irradiation may result in improvement.

○ **Where does the abducens nerve run within the cavernous sinus in relation to the internal carotid artery?**

It lies lateral to the artery in the sinus.

○ **A 55-year-old diabetic patient develops acute onset of proptosis, chemosis, and ophthalmoplegia. A black eschar is seen on the palate. What is the most likely diagnosis?**

An acute ophthalmoplegia with orbital signs in a diabetic patient is Mucormycosis until proven otherwise. Early recognition is crucial as the disease may be life threatening.

○ **What is spasmus nutans?**

This is a triad consisting of
1. Asymmetrical, small amplitude pendular nystagmus
2. Head bobbing
3. Torticollis
It starts 4 months to one year of age and is self-limiting, although CT or MRI scans should be done to exclude intracranial pathology.

○ **What are causes of spasmus nutans?**

1. Idiopathic.
2. Empty sella syndrome.
3. Glioma of the anterior visual pathways.
4. Porencephalic cyst.

○   **A 75-year-old white female presents with acute loss of vision, an afferent pupillary defect and a swollen and pale optic nerve. She complains of headache, scalp tenderness and weight loss. What is the evaluation and treatment?**

This patient has anterior ischemic optic neuropathy. The constitutional symptoms and signs suggest the diagnosis of giant cell arteritis. An erythrocyte sedimentation rate should be performed, steroid therapy should be started, and the patient should be scheduled for a temporal artery biopsy.

○   **What are the causes of periodic alternating nystagmus?**

1. Cerebellar disease.
2. Multiple sclerosis.
3. Ataxia-telangiectasia.
4. Arnold-Chiari malformation.
5. Trauma.
6. Phenytoin.

○   **A 60-year-old white male alcoholic develops painless, progressive bilateral simultaneous loss of vision. His visual acuity is 20/200 in both eyes, there is a cecocentral scotoma in each eye and the optic nerves show mild temporal pallor. What is the most likely diagnosis?**

The differential diagnosis for a painless progressive bilateral optic neuropathy includes infectious, inflammatory, infiltrative, demyelinative, compressive, and hereditary (Leber's hereditary optic neuropathy). The clinical history however is most compatible with toxic/nutritional amblyopia. Toxins such as drugs or heavy metals should be excluded and the patient should be evaluated for vitamin B12 and folate deficiency. A compressive lesion should be excluded with neuroimaging.

○   **Where do the III, IV and ophthalmic division of the V cranial nerve enter the orbit?**

Through the superior orbital fissure.

○   **A patient who recently had a stroke presents with vertical oscillations of the eyes with simultaneous palatal muscle contractions. What does the patient have and where is the lesion causing it?**

The patient has ocular myoclonus, which is usually seen after a brainstem or cerebellar infraction.

○   **What are the causes of downbeat nystagmus?**

1. Craniocervical junction lesions, eg. Arnold-Chiari malformation, syringobulbia, cerebellar disease, Paget's disease.
2. Drugs, eg. Phenytoin, lithium, barbiturates, carbamazepine.
3. Wernicke encephalopathy.
4. Demyelination.

5. Hydrocephalus.

❍   **A 22-year-old female presents with acute onset of severe headache and a bitemporal hemianopsia. What is the most likely diagnosis?**

Pituitary apoplexy.

❍   **What is upbeat nystagmus usually associated with?**

1. Posterior fossa lesions (pons, medulla, cerebellum).
2. Drugs.
3. Wernicke encephalopathy.

❍   **What happens to the pupil of the abducting eye on lateral gaze?**

There is a physiological dilatation of the pupil.

❍   **If the pupillary response to direct light is brisk and intact, does that mean that the accommodative reflex will also be intact?**

Yes.

❍   **What is thought to be the anatomic cause of light-near dissociation of the pupillary response?**

The ill-defined midbrain center for the near reflex is probably located in a more ventral location than the light reflex (pretectal nucleus), which may be why compressive lesions, eg. Pinealomas preferentially involve the dorsal pupillomotor fibers and initially spare the ventral near reflex fibers.

❍   **What ocular motor abnormalities can be produced by cerebellar disease?**

1. Nystagmus (gaze evoked, rebound, upbeat, downbeat, positional, pendular).
2. Impaired optokinetic nystagmus.
3. Square wave jerks.
4. Saccadic pursuit.
5. Skew deviation.
6. Opsoclonus.
7. Ocular dysmetria.

❍   **A patient is observed to have bizarre conjugate saccadic eye movements in all directions even while asleep. What does this patient have?**

Opsoclonus

❍   **What is the difference between ocular flutter and opsoclonus?**

In ocular flutter, the saccadic oscillations are purely horizontal, while in opsoclonus; the oscillations go in any direction.

○   **What are the causes of opsoclonus and ocular flutter?**

1. Metastatic neuroblastoma in children
2. Viral encephalitis
3. Demyelination
4. Paraneoplastic syndrome (lung cancer)
5. Drug induced (lithium, phenytoin, imipramine, and amitriptyline)

○   **What is ocular dysmetria?**

It is an overshooting or undershooting of the eyes followed by a small amplitude saccadic oscillation before the eyes come to rest at the new fixation point which is provoked when the patient is asked to fixate on a new target.

○   **A 23-year-old patient presents with a constricted visual field to 5 degrees in each eye. The remainder of the ocular exam is unremarkable. A tangent screen in a patient with functional visual field loss will demonstrate what findings?**

A tangent screen at 1 meter and 2 meter (with doubling of the test object size) often demonstrates non-expanded or tunnel visual field (i.e. a 5 degree field at 1 meter and a 5 degree field at 2 meters). This is a non-organic finding.

○   **When asked to look up, a patient exhibits retraction of the globe into the orbit and jerk nystagmus in which the fast phase exhibits a convergence movement. What lesions can produce this finding?**

This is a convergence-retraction nystagmus, which is produced by lesions of the pretectal area, eg. Pinealomas and vascular accidents.

○   **What happens when warm water is poured into the left ear?**

The patient will develop left jerk nystagmus (i.e. fast phase to the left). A useful mnemonic is COWS (cold-opposite, warm-same) indicating the direction of the nystagmus.

○   **What are the causes of anterior ischemic optic neuropathy?**

1. Giant cell arteritis.
2. Hypertension.
3. Collagen vascular disorders, eg. Wegener's granulomatosis, SLE, polyarteritis nodosa.

○   **What are the ocular manifestations of giant cell arteritis?**

Most common: Anterior ischemic optic neuropathy.
Common: Pseudo-Foster Kennedy syndrome (common).
Uncommon: CRAO, extraocular nerve palsies, cotton wool spots, and amaurosis fugax.

Rare: Posterior ischemic optic neuropathy, cortical blindness, and anterior
                   segment ischemia.

○   **A 59-year-old man has had four recent episodes of transient visual loss followed by headache. The episodes are stereotyped and consist of loss of vision in both eyes, always in the left hemifield, followed by right occipital headache. Neuro-ophthalmologic exam reveals a left scotomatous central homonymous field defect. Is this migraine?**

The presence of a small area of bilateral visual loss or a mild bilateral disturbance of vision that progressively increases over 15 or more minutes is highly characteristic of migraine. However, any patient with abnormalities on visual field examination suggesting a retrochiasmal lesion or any patient with atypical migraine-like phenomena, especially patients with visual symptoms that are brief, episodic, unformed, and not associated with the angular, scintillating figures that occur with migraine, requires neuroimaging to investigate the possibility of occipital arteriovenous malformation (AVM), venous sinus thrombosis, or tumor. The patient had a right occipital AVM.

○   **Can a retrochiasmal lesion cause a monocular field defect?**

Although monocular peripheral temporal visual field defects are most often due to retinal or optic nerve disease, a lesion of the peripheral nasal fibers in the anterior occipital lobe may produce a unilateral (monocular) temporal crescent-shaped visual field defect from 60 to 90 degrees.

○   **A 56-year-old man develops unilateral complete third nerve palsy, except the pupil is completely normal. Is an aneurysm likely?**

Third nerve palsy with a normal pupillary sphincter and completely palsied extraocular muscles is almost never caused by aneurysms. This type of third nerve palsy is most commonly caused by ischemia, especially related to diabetes (see above). The probable explanation for pupillary sparing in diabetic third nerve palsy is the lack of damage to the periphery of the nerve where the majority of pupillomotor fibers are thought to pass. Neuroimaging should be performed in patients with no vasculopathic risk factors or in patients who do not improve by 12 weeks of follow-up. Patients with this type of third nerve palsy should be observed at 24- to 48-hour intervals for one week because some patients with aneurysms may develop delayed pupil involvement. Vasculopathic risk factors, especially diabetes mellitus, hypertension, and increased cholesterol, should be sought and controlled. Patients over the age of 55 years, especially those with other symptoms suggestive of giant cell arteritis (e.g., headache, jaw or tongue claudications, polymyalgia rheumatica symptoms) should have a sedimentation rate. Temporal artery biopsy should be performed if the sedimentation rate is elevated or other systemic symptoms suggestive of giant cell arteritis are present. Myasthenia gravis may rarely mimic this type of third nerve palsy so a Tensilon test should be considered, primarily in patients with fluctuating or fatiguing ptosis or ophthalmoplegia.

○   **What type of pupillary defect will be produced by a pure optic tract lesion?**

Contralateral afferent pupillary defect together with a complete homonymous hemianopia.

○ **After a brainstem stroke, a patient complains of diplopia. On examination he can move neither eye to the left. On attempted right gaze, abduction is full in the right eye but there is no adduction of left eye. What has happened?**

The patient has a one-and-a-half syndrome. In the one-and-a-half syndrome, there is conjugate gaze palsy to one side ("one") and impaired adduction on looking to the other side ("and-a-half"). As a result, the only horizontal movement remaining is abduction of one eye, which may exhibit nystagmus in abduction. The responsible lesion is in the pons and involves the paramedian pontine reticular formation (PPRF) or abducens nucleus and the adjacent medial longitudinal fasciculus (MLF) on the side of the complete gaze palsy. Patients with the one and a half syndrome often have exotropia of the eye opposite the side of the lesion (paralytic pontine exotropia) because, due to the gaze palsy, the eyes tend to drift to the side opposite the lesion, but adduction in this direction is limited by the MLF lesion.

○ **What are the lengths of the different parts of the optic nerve?**

Intraocular = 1 mm
Intraorbital = 25 mm
Intracanalicular = 10 mm
Intracranial = 17 mm
The mnemonic for remembering these numbers is the telephone number 125-1017.

○ **A patient acutely presents with a III nerve palsy and a contralateral hemitremor. What is the diagnosis?**

Benedikt syndrome, which is an involvement of the III nerve fasciculus as it passes through the red nucleus in the midbrain.

○ **A previously healthy child with repetitive, new onset rapid involuntary multivectorial rapid eye movements (saccades) should be evaluated for what conditions?**

Opsoclonus describes multidirectional involuntary saccadic eye movements that may occur after viral encephalitis, with toxins, in cerebellar or brainstem disease, and is associated with a paraneoplastic effect in children with occult neuroblastoma.

○ **What are the most common causes of a centrocecal scotoma?**

1. Toxic optic neuropathy.
2. Optic pit with serous retinal detachment.

○ **What are the most common types of visual field defects produced by ischemic optic neuropathy?**

1. Altitudinal field defect (inferior > superior).
2. Arcuate visual field defect.

❍   **A medical student tells you that the patient you are about to see had horizontal jerk nystagmus beating to the left. You see the patient several minutes later and you find that the patient has horizontal jerk nystagmus beating to the right. What is a more likely explanation?**

The patient probably has periodic alternating nystagmus (PAN). With PAN, the eyes exhibit primary position horizontal nystagmus, which, after 60 to 120 seconds, stops for a few seconds and then starts beating in the opposite direction. PAN may be congenital, but it is often acquired and due to disease processes at the craniocervical junction, especially processes that damage the nodulus and uvula of the cerebellum. PAN is thus thought to be produced by dysfunction of the GABA-ergic velocity-storage mechanism and may be controlled in most, but not all patients, by the GABA-B agonist baclofen.

❍   **What type of visual field defect does optic neuritis typically produce?**

Central scotoma, although any type of monocular visual field defect can be produced.

❍   **What type of visual field defect does nutritional optic neuropathy produce?**

Bilateral central scotoma.

❍   **A 23-year-old male presents with bilateral simultaneous painless loss of vision. The visual acuity is 20/400 in each eye, there is a dense central scotoma in each eye, and mild disc hyperemia in both eyes. The patient's brother and maternal uncle had similar visual loss. What is the most likely diagnosis?**

Leber's hereditary optic neuropathy is characterized by bilateral rapidly progressive central visual loss. It is a mitochondrial disorder and therefore all female carriers pass the mutation to all of their offspring but affected males can not transmit the disorder. There is no effective therapy available.

❍   **What is the most common cause of binasal hemianopsia?**

Glaucoma.

❍   **A 75-year-old patient presents develops the acute onset of a markedly constricted visual field to 10 degrees in each eye. The remainder of the ocular exam is normal. A tangent screen at 1 and 2 meters demonstrates an organic and appropriate expansion of the visual field. What is the next most appropriate evaluation?**

This patient could have cortical visual impairment and a neuroimaging study should be performed. A cerebrovascular accident would be the most likely etiology.

❍   **What happens to the optokinetic nystagmus (OKN) response if there is a lesion affecting the optomotor pathways in the posterior hemisphere?**

The OKN response will be diminished when targets are rotated towards the side of the lesion or away from the hemianopia.

❍   **What does the combination of OKN asymmetry and a homonymous hemianopia suggest?**

There is a parietal lesion, often caused by a neoplasm.

❍   **What is characteristic of an ophthalmoplegic migraine?**

Recurrent, transient III nerve palsy which begins after the headache. It usually starts before the age of 10 years.

❍   **What type of headache can produce a transient or permanent postganglionic Horner's syndrome?**

Cluster headache.

❍   **A middle-age woman develops the acute onset of mild eyelid swelling, conjunctival chemosis, proptosis, and dilated conjunctival vessels. She also complains of pulsatile tinnitus. Vision is normal. What etiology is likely?**

The clinical findings are suggestive of a spontaneous dural carotid-cavernous sinus fistula. Cerebral angiography is indicated.

❍   **What are the clinical features of temporal lobe lesions?**

1. Upper quadrantanopia (pie in the sky).
2. Contralateral hemiparesis and hemisensory disturbance.
3. Paroxysmal olfactory and gustatory hallucinations (uncinate fits).
4. Formed visual hallucinations.
5. Seizures.
6. Receptive dysphasia.

❍   **A 59-year-old man complains of episodes lasting minutes of monocular transient visual loss (TVL) only on exposure to bright sunlight. Ophthalmologic exam is normal. What is the likely etiology of the episodes of visual loss?**

In some patients, monocular TVL may occur when the patient is exposed to bright light. These patients usually have severe, ipsilateral carotid occlusive disease. Bilateral, simultaneous TVL induced by exposure to bright light may rarely occur with bilateral severe carotid stenosis or occlusion. The light-induced TVL probably reflects the inability of a borderline ocular circulation to sustain the increased retinal metabolic activity associated with light exposure.

❍   **What are the clinical features of parietal lobe lesions?**

1. Inferior quadrantanopsia (pie in the floor).
2. Agnosia.
3. Visual perception difficulties (right parietal lesions).
4. Right-left confusion.
5. Acalculia (left parietal lesions).
6. OKN abnormalities.

○ **A 23-year-old female presents with an irregular 6 mm right pupil that does not respond to light stimulus but reacts briskly to convergence effort. There is a sector paresis of the iris sphincter and pilocarpine 1/8% constricts the right pupil but not the left pupil. What is the most likely diagnosis?**

Adie's tonic pupil. There is a 4% chance per year of bilateral involvement. The condition is benign and usually requires no therapy.

○ **What are the features of occipital lobe lesions?**

1. Macular-sparing congruous homonymous hemianopsia (posterior cerebral artery occlusion).
2. Congruous homonymous macular defects (injury to tip of occipital cortex).
3. Formed visual hallucinations.
4. Anton syndrome (denial of cortical blindness).
5. OKN abnormality (rare).

○ **What are the features of optic tract lesions?**

1. Incongruous homonymous hemianopsia.
2. Wernicke hemianopic pupil.
3. Optic atrophy.
4. Contralateral pyramidal signs.

○ **What associated condition should you suspect might be present in a patient who develops an acute III nerve palsy after trivial head trauma without loss of consciousness?**

The development of a III nerve palsy following trivial head trauma should alert you to the possibility of an associated basal intracranial tumor that has stretched and tethered the nerve trunk.

○ **What is the cause of the optic disc edema in papilledema?**

Cessation of axonal transport with swelling and enlargement of axons.

○ **In what age group does optic glioma usually occur in?**

Ninety percent occur in the first two decades of life and typically affects young girls.

○ **What systemic disease can be associated with optic glioma in 25-50% of patients?**

Neurofibromatosis (NF-1).

○ **What does CT scan of the orbit show in a patient with optic nerve glioma?**

Fusiform enlargement of the optic nerve and "kinking."

○ **What is the most common ophthalmic sign produced by extracranial carotid dissection?**

Horner's syndrome.

❍   **What is the treatment for patients with optic nerve gliomas?**

Excision is done if the tumor is growing, especially if the vision is poor and the proptosis is cosmetically unacceptable. Radiotherapy is performed if there is intracranial extension of tumors that are beyond surgical excision.

❍   **What is the prognosis of patients with malignant gliomas?**

The average survival period after diagnosis is 6 to 9 months. Malignant gliomas occur more frequently in adults than in children.

❍   **A 67-year-old man notes poor vision after awakening from lumbar laminectomy. Visual acuity is poor bilaterally, pupillary reaction to light is poor in both eyes, and the discs are swollen bilaterally. What is the likely etiology for the patient's visual loss?**

The patients likely has bilateral anterior ischemic optic neuropathies (AION) as a complication of surgery. This complication is not rare, may occur unilaterally or bilaterally, and may occur after almost any type of major surgery. A combination of hypotension and anemia has been noted in most previously well documented cases of AION after nonophthalmic procedures. Disc edema may be absent, mild or pronounced and the onset of visual loss may be immediate or delayed in appearance by several days after surgery.

❍   **A 28-year-old obese woman describes headaches for three months and episodes lasting "seconds" of unilateral or bilateral loss of vision. The episodes of visual loss occur 20 to 30 times per day and occasionally are precipitated by sudden changes in posture. Funduscopic examination reveals papilledema. What is the cause of the episodes of transient visual loss (TVL)?**

Episodes of TVL lasting less than 60 seconds may occur in patients with papilledema secondary to increased intracranial hypertension. These transient obscurations of vision may occur in one or both eyes (individually or simultaneously) and typically last only a few seconds. The episodes may be precipitated by changes in position and are thought to be related to the effects of increased intracranial pressure on the flow of blood to the eye, perhaps where the central retinal artery penetrates the optic nerve sheath to enter the substance of the nerve.

❍   **A 40-year-old woman notes episodes of transient monocular visual loss that only occur in certain gaze postures. Between episodes the vision is normal. Where is the lesion causing gaze-evoked TVL located and what etiologies should be considered?**

Patients who experience TVL evoked by eccentric position of gaze (gaze-evoked TVL) usually have an intraorbital mass that intermittently compresses the circulation to the optic nerve or retina. The most common lesions are cavernous hemangiomas or optic nerve sheath meningiomas, but other lesions have included osteomas, neurofibromas, gliomas, medial rectus granular myoblastoma, varices, orbital trauma, and metastases.

❍   **What is the classic triad of signs of optic nerve sheath meningiomas?**

1. Visual loss.
2. Optic atrophy.
3. Opticociliary shunt vessels.

❍   **A 24-year-old woman develops acute visual loss in the right eye. Examination reveals decreased acuity and decreased color vision in the affected eye with a relative afferent pupillary defect. Funduscopic exam revealed disc swelling in the right eye with a macular star and 2+ vitreous cells. The left eye was normal. What entities should be considered, and what is the patient's chance of developing multiple sclerosis in the future?**

The patient has neuroretinitis or optic disc edema with a macular star (ODEMS). The clinical features include sudden visual loss, swelling of the optic disc, peripapillary and macular exudates, which may occur in a star pattern, and cells in the vitreous. Although usually idiopathic, infectious etiologies for this syndrome, especially syphilis, Lyme disease, cat scratch disease, and toxoplasmosis, should be considered. The macular exudate likely results from primary optic nerve disease and not from inflammation in the retina. Patients who demonstrate acute papillitis with a normal macula should be reevaluated within two weeks for the development of a macular star. Unlike optic neuritis, the presence of a macular star militates strongly against the subsequent development of multiple sclerosis.

❍   **What conditions can optociliary shunt vessels occur in?**

1. Optic nerve sheath meningiomas.
2. Optic nerve gliomas (rarely).
3. Vascular occlusive disease of the retina.
4. Long-standing primary open angle glaucoma.

❍   **What does CT scan of the orbit show in a patient with optic nerve sheath meningioma?**

Tubular thickening and calcification of the optic nerve (railroad track sign).

❍   **What percentage of all meningiomas do primary optic nerve sheath meningiomas represent?**

Two percent.

❍   **Do optic nerve sheath meningiomas and optic nerve gliomas occur more frequently in males or females?**

Females.

❍ **A 25-year-old nurse is evaluated for acute anisocoria and headache. The left pupil is 4 mm and reacts well to light but the left pupil is 9 mm and fixed to light. Extraocular motility is normal. What is the likely cause of the anisocoria?**

Nurses, physicians, and other health care workers are particularly prone to inadvertent or intentional exposure to pharmacologic mydriatics. The pupil size with pharmacologic blockade is often quite large. In poorly reactive pupils of uncertain origin, topical pilocarpine 1% can be used as a test for pharmacologic blockade. A pupil dilated from a third nerve palsy will constrict to pilocarpine 1% but a pupil with a parasympathetic pharmacologic blockade will not constrict.

❍ **Where does optic nerve hypoplasia more commonly occur in?**

1. Children of diabetic mothers.
2. Fetal exposure to quinine, antiepileptic medications or LSD.
3. DeMosier's syndrome (absence of septum pellucidum, hypothalamic-pituitary abnormalities).

❍ **What neuro-ophthalmic manifestations may a patient with ataxia telangiectasia or Louis-Bar syndrome present with?**

Reduced voluntary eye movements and an intact oculocephalic maneuver.

❍ **What immune deficiencies may be present in ataxia telangiectasia?**

Affected children have thymic hypoplasia, decreased serum IgA, increased susceptibility to infections, and an increased incidence of leukemia and lymphoma.

❍ **A 40-year-old patient develops the acute onset of intermittent shimmering or fluttering of the right eye lasting seconds to minutes at a time. Examination during the episode demonstrates fine intorsion movements of the right eye. The remainder of the exam is normal. What is the most likely diagnosis?**

Superior oblique myokymia.

❍ **The pupils in a patient with anisocoria react normally to light. What are the possible causes of the anisocoria?**

Anisocoria with normally active pupils may be due to essential anisocoria or Horner syndrome. The two can be differentiated by instilling 10% cocaine drops into both eyes. The Horner pupil will not dilate while the essential anisocoria pupils will dilate well.

❍ **What is progressive supranuclear palsy?**

It is a degenerative disorder characterized by supranuclear ophthalmoplegia affecting vertical gaze, dysarthria, axial rigidity, dementia, pseudobulbar palsy, and Parkinsonism that responds poorly to levodopa.

❍ **What is Wallenberg syndrome?**

1. Nystagmus.
2. Horner's syndrome.
3. Contralateral hemiparesis.
4. Ipsilateral ataxia.
5. Contralateral loss of pain and temperature sense.

❍   **A patient with an isolated III nerve palsy complains of periorbital pain. Is the III nerve palsy caused by diabetes or by an aneurysm?**

The presence of pain is not helpful in differentiating between a diabetic and an aneurysmal III nerve palsy because both are frequently accompanied by pain.

❍   **What is the most common cause of pseudo-Argyll Robertson pupils?**

AR pupil is an irregular miotic pupil with light-near dissociation and is caused by syphilis. Pseudo AR pupil can result from aberrant neuronal regeneration and is most commonly caused by diabetes.

❍   **A patient with left sixth nerve palsy also has a left Horner syndrome. Where is the lesion?**

The lesion is in the left cavernous sinus where the sympathetic fibers to the eye join the sixth nerve for a short distance.

❍   **A patient with bilateral occipital infarcts denies that he is blind yet is unable to read the largest letter on the Snellen chart. What is this condition called?**

Anton's syndrome, which is cortical blindness from bilateral occipital infarcts, associated with denial of blindness.

❍   **Are the pupils affected in Anton's syndrome?**

No, they are normal in this condition.

❍   **While practicing aikido in a dojo, a patient receives a blow to the left side of the neck and presents with mild left ptosis; a constricted left pupil and ipsilateral jaw pain. What should you suspect could be present in this case?**

Traumatic cervical carotid artery dissection producing an ipsilateral Horner's syndrome.

❍   **What are the causes of an enlarged blind spot?**

Chronic papilledema, optic disc drusen, glaucoma, peripapillary myelinated nerve fibers, juxtapapillary choroiditis, myopic peripapillary chorioretinal degeneration, tilted disc.

❍   **A patient is knocked unconscious when hit in the forehead by a baseball bat. After the injury, he complains of binocular vertical diplopia. On examination, there is a right hypertropia on left gaze and a left hypertropia in right gaze. Head tilt to the right reveals a right hypertropia and head tilt to the left reveals a left hypertropia. What has happened?**

The patient has developed bilateral fourth nerve palsies. The long course of the fourth nerve around the midbrain, near the edge of the tentorium, makes this nerve particularly vulnerable, and a severe blow to the forehead may cause a contrecoup contusion of one or both fourth nerves against the rigid tentorium. Severe frontal trauma may also cause bilateral fourth nerve palsies by contusion of the anterior medullary velum where both nerves cross.

O   **How long does it take for the second eye to be involved in Leber's hereditary optic neuropathy?**

Usually within several weeks to months.

O   **A patient with Graves' ophthalmopathy (thyroid eye disease) is noted to be exotropic. Is this from the Graves' disease?**

Unlikely. Graves' disease mainly affects the inferior rectus, medial rectus, and superior rectus muscles, in that order, and causes a restrictive myopathy. Lateral rectus muscle involvement is very rare and, thus, an exotropia should raise the possibility of associated myasthenia gravis with medial rectus paresis. There is an increased risk of myasthenia gravis in patients with Graves' disease.

O   **A 35-year-old woman relates episodes lasting minutes of transient distortion of one pupil. During the spells there is peaked elongation of the pupillary aperture. Neuro-ophthalmologic examination between episodes is normal. What is going on?**

The patient has tadpole pupils. Patients with tadpole pupils report episodes of pupillary distortion that are ordinarily brief, lasting less than five minutes in most, which may occur repeatedly in a single day. Horner's syndrome is a precursor in about half, a third of patients are migraineurs, and a small number have Adie's tonic pupils. The peaked elongation of the pupillary aperture is characteristic. This pupillary phenomenon is not associated with any serious illness.

OPTICS AND REFRACTION

○   **What optical property of the cornea prevents visualization of the angle structures and is overcome by using a goniolens?**

Total internal reflection.

○   **A patient wearing a –5.0 D contact lens desires spectacles. If the resulting vertex distance will be 15 mm, what will be the resulting power of the new spectacle lens?**

Focal length of contact lens = 100/(-5) = -20 cm
Focal length of new spectacles = -20 cm + 1.5 cm = -18.5 cm
Power of new lens = 100/(-18.5)= -5.4 D

○   **An aphakic patient wearing +10 D lenses desires contact lenses. If the vertex distance is 10 mm, what will be the power of the contact lenses?**

Focal length of spectacle lens = 100/(+10) = 10 cm
Focal length of contact lens = 10 cm – 1 cm = 9 cm
Power of contact lens = 100/9 = +11.11 D

○   **At what distance will an object 0.25 meters in front of a +6.0 D lens come to focus?**

U = 1/u = 1/(-0.25 M) = -4.0 D
P = +6.0 D
V = U + P = (-4) + (+6) = +2 D
v = 1/V = 1/2 = 0.5 M or 50 cm

○   **A point source of light 1/3 of a meter to the left of a +2 D lens will have its image focus at what distance and where?**

U = 1/u = 1/(-0.33 M) = -3 D
P = +2 D
V = U + P = -3 + 2 = -1 D
v = 1/V = 1/(-1) = -1.00 meters
The image is 1 meter to the left of the lens.

○   **Where would the image of an object 0.5 meters from a –10.00 D lens come to focus?**

U = 1/u = 1/(-0.5) = -2 D
P = -10 D
V = U + P = (-2) + (-10) = -12 D

163

v = 1/V = 1/(-12) = 0.0833 meters or -8.3 cm

O   **What type of image is formed in the previous problem?**

It is a virtual image (because it has a minus sign).

O   **What is the linear magnification of the image in the previous question, and is it upright or inverted?**

M = v/u = U/V = (-2)/(-12) = +1/6
The image is upright (+ sign) and 1/6 the size of the object.

O   **A patient looks at a magazine through a 10 D magnifier held 4 cm from the page. Where is the image located?**

U = 1/u = 100/(-4) = -25 D
P = +10 D
V = U + P = (-25) + (+10) = -15
v = 1/V = 1/(-15) = 0.067 meters = -6.7 cm
The image is on the same side of the lens as the printed page.

O   **What is the index of refraction of the cornea?**

1.376

O   **What is the strength of a prism, which displaces a light beam 150 mm when the image is measured at 50 cm from the prism?**

Prism diopter = amount of displacement in cm / distance in meters
= 15 cm/0.5 = 30 prism diopters

O   **What are the relationships of the incident and emergent light rays for the maximum angle of deviation and the minimum angle of deviation for a prism?**

The angle of incidence must be equal to the angle of emergence in the minimum angle of deviation, while they must be as different as possible with the maximum angle of deviation.

O   **A child wearing her full cycloplegic refraction has 15 prism diopters of esophoria at 0.5 meter. With a –2.00 D lens over her glasses, the esophoria increases to 25 prism diopters. Calculate the AC/A ratio using the lens gradient method.**

(prism deviation *without* the lens – prism deviation *with* the lens)/ lens power
= (25 – 15) / 2 = 10/2 = 5 : 1

O   **What type of phoria will be induced if a base-in prism is held in front of an orthophoric patient's eye?**

Esophoria (A base out prism will be required to neutralize the phoria-inducing base-in prism, the same way that a base-out prism is required to neutralize an esophoria/tropia.

Tip: The direction of the strabismus can be determined from the direction of the CORRECTING prism).

○   **What type of phoria will be induced by a base-up prism held in front of an orthophoric patient's eye?**

Hyperphoria in that eye or hypophoria in the contralateral eye.

○   **What type of phoria will be induced if both eyes look through base-down prisms of equal strength?**

None. A phoria is induced only if there is a difference in the amount of deviation of the light beam between the two eyes and/or if there is a difference in the direction of the deviation of the light beam between the two eyes.

○   **What type of phoria is induced by base-out prisms held in front of both eyes in an orthophoric patient?**

Exophoria.

○   **What type of phoria is induced by a base-in prism held in front of the right eye and a base-out prism held in front of the left eye if the two prisms are of equal strength?**

None.

○   **If a 1 prism diopter base-out prism is held in front of the right eye and a 2 prism diopter base-out prism is held in front of the left eye, how much phoria will be induced?**

3 prism diopter exophoria. If the prisms are pointing in opposite directions, then the amount of phoria produced is equal to the sum of the powers of the two prisms.

○   **If a 3 prism diopter base-out prism is held in front of the right eye and a 10 diopter prism base-in prism is held in front of the left eye, how much phoria is induced?**

7 prism diopter esophoria. If both prisms are pointing to the same direction, then the amount of phoria produced is equal to the difference between the two prisms.

○   **If a 10 prism diopter base-up prism is held in front of the right eye and a 7 prism diopter base-up prism is held in front of the left eye, how much phoria is induced?**

3 prism diopter right hyperphoria.

○   **If a 3 prism diopter base-down prism is held in front of the right eye and a 3 diopter prism base up prism is held in front of the left eye, how much phoria is produced?**

6 prism diopter right hypophoria or 6 prism diopter left hyperphoria. By convention, the eye with the hyperdeviation is described.

○   **What is the power of a spherical lens which displaces a light ray 20 cm when measured at 0.5 meter when the ray passes through a point 15 mm below the lens' optical center?**

Power of the prism = displacement in cm/distance in meters
Prism diopter = 20 cm/0.5 meters = 40 prism diopters

Prentice rule:
Prism diopter = hD, where h is the displacement from the optical center in cm and D is the power of the lens in diopters

40 prism diopters = (1.5 cm) x (power of the lens)
Power of the lens = (40 prism diopters)/1.5 cm = 26.7 D

○   **How much prism is induced if a patient looks through a +10.00 D lens 20 mm below its optical center?**

Prentice rule: prism diopter = hD

Prism diopter = (2 cm)(10.00 D)
= 20 prism diopter base up

○   **How much prism is induced if a patient looks through a –4.00 D lens 7 mm below its optical center?**

Prism diopter = (0.7 cm)(-4.00 D) = 2.8 prism diopter base down.

○   **How much phoria is induced if a –6.00 D lens is held in front of the left eye such that the optical center of the lens is 5 mm lateral to the visual axis?**

Prism diopter = (0.5 cm)(-6 D) = 3 prism diopter base in
This lens therefore produces an esophoria.

○   **A patient has a refraction of –5.00 D OD and –10.00 D OS with a PD of 65 mm and adds of +2.50 D. What is the horizontal phoria induced if the glass spectacle PD is 70 mm and equally centered?**

OD = (0.25 cm)(-5.00 D) = 1.25 prism diopter base in
OS = (0.25 cm)(-10.00 D) = 2.5 prism diopter base in

Total phoria = 1.25 + 2.5 = 3.75 prism diopters of esophoria

○   **What is the vertical phoria through the bifocals in the previous problem if the optical center of the bifocals is 10 mm below the optical center of the distance prescription?**

Because the add is equal in both eyes, it can be ignored here. The left eye has –5.00 D more power than the right eye, so:

Prism diopters = (1 cm of displacement) x (–5.00 D) = 5 prism diopters base down OS

This patient has a 5 prism diopter left hypophoria or a 5 prism diopter right hyperphoria.

Note that the hyperphoria occurs in the eye with the less minus (or more plus) correction.

❍ **How would you reduce the induced vertical prism in anisometropes such as in the previous problem?**

Use slab-off over the bifocal segment of the more minus or less plus lens.

❍ **What is slab-off?**

It is a process that removes a piece of glass shaped like a base-down prism from the lower part of the lens, thus creating a base-up prism effect without altering the dioptric power. Because the more minus lens of the pair of glasses induces the greater base-down effect, the slab-off must be ground on that lens. Typically, one can achieve a maximum slab-off prism of about 3 prism diopters base-up.

❍ **A patient whose anisometropia is fully corrected in his distance upper segment develops a substantial right hyperphoria when reading through his bifocal segment. Which lens will probably require slab-off?**

The left lens.

Note: The prism in CR-39 plastic slab-off bifocals is base-down, so in the anisometropic prescription the slab-off is used on the less minus or more plus bifocal. They are available in prism powers up to 6 prism diopters base-down. Therefore, if one were to use CR-39 plastic bifocals in this case, you would use it in the right lens.

❍ **In general, when should an induced vertical phoria in the normal reading position (8-10 mm below the distance optical centers) be corrected with slab-off?**

Induced vertical phorias greater than 1.5-2 prism diopters should be corrected. If it is less, it is unlikely to cause symptoms.

❍ **How would a base-up bifocal add affect image jump and object displacement in a hyperope?**

It will decrease image jump and increase object displacement.

❍ **How would a base-up bifocal add affect image jump and object displacement in a myope?**

It will decrease image jump and decrease object displacement.

❍   **How would a base-down bifocal add affect image jump and object displacement in a hyperope?**

It will increase image jump and minimize object displacement.

❍   **What is the most common and annoying problem of bifocals?**

Image jump.

❍   **Give two examples of base-down bifocal add designs.**

Ultex and Kryptok.

❍   **How can you best minimize image jump in bifocal design?**

Use a bifocal that has the segment's optical center near the segment top.

❍   **What is a simple magnifier?**

It is a plus lens held between the eye and the object, which is 25 cm away from each other.

❍   **If we use a +20.00 D lens as a simple magnifier, what is its magnification?**

Simple magnification = D/4
= 20/4 = 5X

❍   **What is the power of a 3X magnifying lens?**

D = simple magnification x 4
D = (3)(4) = 12.00 D

❍   **What is the angular magnification of a Galilean telescope with a +10.00 D objective lens and a –40.00 D eyepiece, and is the image erect or inverted?**

Angular magnification = eyepiece/objective
= -40/10 = 4X (erect since Galilean telescopes produce only erect images)

❍   **How much accommodation would be required to view an object at 1 meter if viewed through the telescope above?**

Total accommodation through telescope = (normal accommodation required for that distance)(angular magnification of the telescope)^2
= (1.00 D at 1 meter)(4)^2
= (1)(16) = 16.00 D

❍   **How much accommodation will be required to view the moon from your rooftop using the Galilean telescope above?**

None.

❍ **What power of telescope will be required for a patient with 20/400 vision to be able to read the 20/40 line of a Snellen chart at a distance of 20 feet?**

10X (The 20/400 line is 10X larger than 20/40 line)

❍ **How do you define legal blindness?**

Visual acuity equal to or less than 20/200 or 6/60 in the better eye.

❍ **What are the relationships between the posterior and anterior vertex powers of plus and minus lenses?**

|Posterior vertex power| > |total vertex power| > |anterior vertex power| for both minus and plus lenses

❍ **Why are spectacles placed with the posterior surface toward the lensometer?**

The posterior surface is used as a reference point, and this is called the posterior vertex power. It has also become synonymous with standard vertex refracting power.

❍ **In which direction are the principal planes for plus and minus meniscus lenses displaced?**

Anteriorly for plus, posteriorly for minus.

❍ **If a myopic patient wearing spectacles switches to contact lenses, does the perceived image get larger or smaller?**

Larger.

❍ **Does the patient in the previous problem use more or less accommodation while wearing contact lenses?**

More.

❍ **If a hyperopic patient switches to contact lenses, does the image size get larger or smaller while wearing contact lenses?**

Smaller.

❍ **Does the hyperopic patient above use more or less accommodation while wearing contact lenses?**

Less.

❍ **Which type of contact lens-wearing patient is more likely to experience presbyopic symptoms, a myope or a hypermetrope?**

Myope.

○   **What is the spherical equivalent of a Jackson cross cylinder?**

Zero.

○   **Is the prescription –0.75 + 1.50 x 90 a Jackson cross cylinder?**

Yes.

○   **Is the prescription +1.00 –2.00 x 36 a Jackson cross cylinder?**

Yes.

○   **Is the prescription –2.50 + 3.50 x 180 a Jackson cross cylinder?**

No (spherical equivalent = -0.75 D).

○   **Is the cross cylinder +1.00 x 180 combined with –2.50 x 90 equivalent to the prescription in the previous problem?**

Yes (note: use power crosses to solve these types of problems involving cross cylinders and stenopeic slits).

○   **What is the spherical equivalent of the following cross cylinder: +1.00 x 45 combined with –3.00 x 135?**

Spherical equivalent of cross cylinders = (min + max)/2
= (+1.00 – 3.00)/2 = -1.00 D

○   **How would you write the prescription for the cross cylinder in the previous problem in plus cylinder form?**

-3.00 +4.00 x 45

○   **A patient is refracted using a stenopeic slit with the following results:**
Slit placed vertically (90°) = +1.00 D
Slit placed horizontally (180°) = -2.00 D

Assuming that the working distance has already been taken into account, what is the equivalent prescription?

+1.00 –3.00 x 90 or –2.00 + 3.00 x 180
(Note: You can solve these types of problems either with power crosses or by imagining that you are refracting these patients with the slit beams of the retinoscope oriented in the above positions and obtaining these results.)

○   **A patient has the following refraction using stenopeic slits:**
Slit placed vertically (90°) = -2.00 D
Slit placed horizontally (180°) = -1.50 D
Assuming the working distance has already been taken into account, what is the equivalent prescription?

-2.00 + 0.50 x 90 or –1.50 –0.50 x 180

○   **Retinoscopy of a patient's eye yields the following results (working distance included):**
+1.00 @ 90
+2.00 @ 180
What is the proper prescription?

+2.00 –1.00 x 180 or +1.00 + 1.00 x 90

○   **A patient has a spectacle correction of –5.00 +2.00 x 90. What is the actual refractive error of the eye's optical system?**

+5.00 –2.00 x 90 or +3.00 + 2.00 x 180

(Note: This is a favorite trick question in board exams.)

○   **What does the spherical equivalent of a sphero-cylinder lens accomplish with regards to the image formed in the retina?**

It places the circle of least confusion on the retina.

○   **What is the spherical equivalent of the following prescription: -5.00 +5.00 x 180?**

Spherical equivalent = sphere + (cylinder/2)
= -5.00 + (+5.00/2) = -5.00 + (+2.50)
= -2.50 D

○   **What is the spherical equivalent of the following prescription: +0.75 + 2.00 x 90?**

+1.75 D

○   **If you decide not to give a patient his full cylinder correction, what must you maintain when you rewrite the prescription using a smaller cylinder correction?**

You must maintain the spherical equivalent of the original prescription in the new prescription so that the circle of least confusion will remain on the retina.

○   **A patient's spectacle correction is +2.00 + 3.00 x 180. If you decide to reduce the cylinder correction by 1 diopter, what should the resulting prescription be?**

(Sphere + (cylinder reduction/2)) combined with (cylinder – cylinder reduction) x axis
or
(S + (L/2)) combined with (C-L) x axis

= (+2.00 + (+1.00/2)) combined with (+3.00 –(+1.00)) x 180
= +2.50 +2.00 x 180

❍   **What is the spherical equivalent of both prescriptions in the previous problem?**

+3.50 D

❍   **A patient's spectacle correction is –1.00 –1.50 x 90 OD and plano - 5.00 x 90 OS. If you reduce the cylinder correction by half in the left eye, what should the resulting prescription be?**

= (0 + (-2.50/2)) combined with (-5.00 –(-2.50)) x 90
= -1.25 –2.50 x 90

❍   **When fitting an astigmatic patient with a soft contact lens, how would you adjust the spectacle correction to get the contact lens power required?**

You must first convert the prescription to its spherical equivalent before calculating the spectacle's focal length and the equivalent contact lens focal length and power.

❍   **A patient's spectacle correction is –5.00 +2.00 x 90 with a vertex distance of 10 mm. What is the soft contact lens prescription?**

Spherical equivalent = -4.00 D
Spectacle focal length = 100/(-4.00) = -25 cm
Contact lens focal length = -25 cm + (-1 cm for vertex distance) = -26 cm
Contact lens power = 100/(-26) = -3.85 D

❍   **How do you fit an astigmatic patient with a gas permeable contact lens?**

When fitting with hard or gas permeable contact lenses, first convert to a minus cylinder prescription, use the sphere in your calculations and ignore the cylinder correction when calculating the equivalent contact lens power. Finally, adjust the prescription depending on how much steeper than the "flattest K" do you want to fit the lens using the SAM rule (Steeper Add Minus).

❍   **What is the gas permeable contact lens power for a spectacle correction of +12.00 +1.00 x 90 and a vertex distance of 10 mm?**

Step 1: Convert to minus cylinder
        = +13.00 -1.00 x 180

Step 2: Find the focal length of the sphere
        = 100/(+13.00) = 7.69 cm

Step 3: Find the focal length of the contact lens
        = 7.69 -1.0 cm (for vertex distance) = 6.69 cm

Step 4: Find the power of the contact lens
        = 100/6.69) = +14.95 D

❍   **The spectacle correction of a patient is –7.50 +2.50 x 45 with a vertex distance of 10 mm and a K reading of 44.50 @ 45 and 42.00 @135. What should the lens**

power be if one wishes to fit a gas permeable contact lens 1.00 D steeper than the "flattest K?"

Step 1: Convert to minus cylinder
           = -5.00 -2.50 x 135

Step 2: Find the focal length of the sphere
           =1/(-5.00) = -20 cm or -0.2 meters

Step 3: Find the focal length of the contact lens
           = -20 cm +(-1.0 cm for the vertex distance) = -21 cm or -0.21 meters

Step 4: Find the power of the contact lens
           =100/(-21) = -4.76 D

Step 5: For +1.00 D steeper than the flattest K, add -1.00 D to compensate (SAM rule or Steeper Ad Minus)
           =-4.76 D + (-1.00 D) = -5.76 D

❍ **What is the power of a plano +1.00 x 180 lens if measured at 30 degrees from the horizontal axis of the spectacle?**

+0.25 D (Note: the power of a cylinder measured at an oblique axis is 1/4 of the full power at 30 degrees from the cylinder's axis, 1/2 at 45 degrees, and 3/4 at 60 degrees)

❍ **What is the power of a +2.00 +2.00 x 90 lens if measured 60 degrees from the vertical axis?**

+2.00 D sphere + (2.00 D cylinder)(0.75) = +2.00 + 1.50 = +3.50

❍ **What is the power of the lens above at the 180 degree meridian or, in other words, perpendicular to the axis of its cylinder?**

+4.00 D

❍ **What is the chromatic interval between visible blue and red light in the eye?**

1.25 D

❍ **What is the effective prescription of –10.00 D lens with a pantoscopic tilt of 10 degrees?**

-10.10 D –0.31 D x 180

❍ **A pantoscopic tilt of 20 degrees in a plus lens will induce a plus or minus cylinder at axis 180°?**

Plus cylinder (if the lens is minus, minus cylinder at axis 180 will be induced).

❍ **What type of distortion does a high myope experience with his glasses?**

Barrel distortion.

○ **What type of distortion does an aphake experience wearing aphakic spectacles?**

Pincushion.

○ **Why is curvature of field the only desirable lens aberration in the eye?**

The curved image formed by a spherical lens will approximately match the curvature of the retina.

○ **Describe the image formed by a convex mirror.**

Virtual, erect, minified.

○ **What is the minimum height of a plano mirror necessary for a person to completely visualize himself?**

One half of his height.

○ **What is a Purkinje Sanson image?**

It is the reflected image formed on the anterior and posterior surfaces of the cornea and lens.

○ **Which Purkinje image is inverted, real and minified?**

Purkinje image 4 or the one formed on the posterior surface of the lens is inverted, real and minified. Purkinje images 1 to 3 are all erect, virtual and minified.

○ **Which Purkinje image is the only one used clinically and serves as the basis for the Hirschberg, Krimskey, keratometer and placido disc?**

Purkinje image 1 or the image formed on the anterior surface of the cornea.

○ **What is the refracting power of the air-cornea interface if the average radius of curvature of the cornea is 8 mm and the index of refraction of the cornea is 1.376?**

$P_s = (n' - n)/r$ where n' = corneal index of refraction, n = index of refraction of air and r = corneal radius of curvature in meters

$= (1.376 - 1.00)/0.008 = 47$ D

○ **Why is the total power of the cornea less than the power of the anterior corneal surface?**

The total power of the cornea is the sum of the powers of both the anterior and posterior surfaces, and the posterior surface has a negative value. The index of refraction of the cornea is 1.376 and the tear and aqueous both have an index of refraction of 1.336. If the anterior central radius of curvature is 7.7 mm and the posterior is 6.9 mm, the total power of the cornea is the sum of the power of the air-tear, the tear cornea and the cornea-aqueous interface. This works out to 43.6 D + 5.3 D –5.8 D = 43.1 D

❍   **What is the reflecting power of the cornea?**

P_{mirror} = -2/r where r = the radius of curvature

= -2/0.008 = -250 D

❍   **Which part of the eye has the most powerful refractive surface?**

Air to cornea (or corneal tear film)

❍   **What is the index of refraction of aqueous humor?**

1.336

❍   **If the blood sugar of a diabetic patient rises, what happens to his refractive error?**

He becomes increasingly myopic.

❍   **What can happen to the refractive error of a patient who develops a central serous retinopathy?**

He can become more hyperopic.

❍   **A patient receives a scleral buckle during retinal detachment surgery. What will be the effect on his refractive error?**

He can become more myopic.

❍   **What is the distance between the retina and the nodal point in the schematic eye?**

17 mm.

❍   **An object 50 cm from the nodal point of the eye is 5 cm tall. What is the retinal image height?**

x/17 mm = 50 mm/500 mm

x = 17(0.1) = 1.7 mm

❍   **What is the size of the scotoma formed by the optic disc on the Goldmann perimeter if the horizontal width of the optic disc is 1.5 mm and the testing distance is 33 cm?**

1.5 mm/17 mm = y/330 mm

y = 29.12 mm

○   **What is the size of a retinal lesion if it produces a scotoma 20 cm across on a tangent screen 2 meters in front of a patient?**

1.7 mm.

○   **What is the average depth of the anterior chamber?**

3.6 mm.

○   **What is the axial length of the schematic eye?**

22.5 mm.

○   **What is the near point of accommodation (NPA)?**

It is the nearest point that a patient can see clearly and is the reciprocal of his total accommodative power or accommodative reserve.

○   **The nearest point a young emmetrope can see without glasses is 7 cm. What is his accommodative reserve?**

Accommodative reserve = 1/NPA = 1/0.07
= 14.3 D

○   **A 65-year-old emmetrope wearing +2.50 D readers has a near point of accommodation of 25 cm. What is his near point of accommodation without glasses?**

NPA with +2.50 Rx = 25 cm or +4.00 D
NPA without +2.50 Rx = +4.00 –2.50 = +1.50 D of accommodative reserve or 66.7 cm

○   **The patient above wishes to have glasses for reading material at 50 cm. What should the appropriate power of the reading spectacles be?**

Reading distance of 50 cm requires +2.00 D.
Accommodation required for comfortable reading = accommodative reserve/2
= +0.75 D

Reading Rx = +2.00 – 0.75 = +1.25

○   **A –5.00 myope has atropine 1% drops instilled in his eye. What would the only distance that he could still see clearly without glasses?**

20 cm.

○   **If a +4.00 D hyperope has atropine drops instilled into his eye, what would be the only distance that he could still see clearly without glasses?**

None.

❍ **A –2.00 D myope is completely cylopleged. What will be the power of the contact lens required seeing an object at 20 cm in front of his eye clearly?**

+3.00 D

❍ **What is Knapp's Rule?**

No matter what the amount of axial ametropia (myopia or hyperopia), a proper corrective lens located at the anterior focal point of the eye will produce retinal images of the same size.

❍ **What is the percentage of aniseikonia in a patient with an IOL in one eye?**

2.5%.

❍ **What is the approximate percentage of aniseikonia in a monocular aphake wearing a contact lens?**

8%.

❍ **What is the percentage of aniseikonia in a monocular aphake wearing spectacles?**

25%.

❍ **How can you reduce aniseikonia produced by a plus lens?**

Decrease vertex distance, reduce the front base curve of the lens, and decrease thickness of the lens (minimal effect on aniseikonia).

❍ **How can you reduce aniseikonia produced by a minus lens?**

Decrease vertex distance, increase the front base curve, and increase lens thickness (minimal effect on aniseikonia).

❍ **How would you minimize meridional aniseikonia in an astigmatic patient when writing your prescription?**

Prescribe minus cylinders.

❍ **A monocular aphake wearing a +14.00 D contact lens who sees 20/20 wishes to have a secondary intraocular lens implant. What should the power of the IOL be if you implant it 5 mm behind the anterior corneal surface?**

Focal length of the contact lens = 1/14.00 = 7.1 cm
Focal length of the IOL required = 7.1 cm – 0.5 cm = 6.6 cm
Power of IOL in aqueous = index of refraction of aqueous/focal length of IOL
=133.6/6.6 = +20.2 D

❍   **What is the most important finding that you should look for in the first follow-up visit of a patient whom you just fitted with contact lenses?**

Central punctate staining.

❍   **If the both the anterior and posterior focal lines in an astigmatic eye lie in front of the retina, then what type of astigmatism does the eye have?**

Compound myopic astigmatism.

❍   **If the anterior focal line lies in front of the retina while the posterior focal line lies behind the retina, then what type of astigmatism does the eye have?**

Mixed astigmatism.

❍   **If the anterior focal lines lie on the retina while the posterior focal line lies behind the retina, what type of astigmatism is present?**

Simple hyperopic astigmatism.

❍   **What is the magnification of the direct ophthalmoscope?**

The eye acts as a simple magnifier, which means that
Angular magnification = 60 D/4
= 15X

❍   **Using a direct ophthalmoscope, you note that it takes a shift of 3D to focus on the top of a swollen optic disc. What is the height of the optic nerve head?**

Each diopter corresponds to approximately 1/3 mm in axial length, so 3 D would be about 1 mm in height.

❍   **What is the actual and the perceived axial magnifications of the aerial image produced by an indirect ophthalmoscope when using a +20.00 D viewing lens?**

An indirect ophthalmoscope functions like an astronomical telescope. Lateral magnification gives an indication of image size, while axial magnification gives a sense of the height or depth of the image. The pupillary distance is reduced four fold by the binocular eye piece. Stereopsis is also reduced, and the axial magnification is perceived to be four fold less.

Step 1: Calculate lateral magnification
        = 60 D (eye)/20 D (viewing lens) = 3X

Step 2: Calculate axial magnification
        = (linear magnification)^2 = (3X)^2 = 9X

Step 3: Calculate perceived axial magnification
        = 9X/4 = 2.25X

❍ **What is the actual and the perceived axial magnifications of the aerial image produced by an indirect ophthalmoscope when using a +30.00 D viewing lens?**

Step 1: Calculate lateral magnification
= 60 D (eye)/30 D (viewing lens) = 2X

Step 2: Calculate axial magnification
= (linear magnification)^2 = (2X)^2 = 4X

Step 3: Calculate perceived axial magnification
= 4X/4 = 1X

❍ **Using a 90 D lens in front of a slit lamp, what is the axial magnification produced when viewing the fundus?**

Lateral magnification = 60/90 = 0.67X
Axial magnification = (2/3)^2 = 0.44X

❍ **Using a 78 D lens in front of a slit lamp, what is the axial magnification produced when viewing the fundus?**

Lateral magnification = 60/78 = 0.77X
Axial magnification = (0.77)^2 = 0.59X

❍ **Which handheld lens will give you the impression of greater height of the optic nerve head when viewing a patient with papilledema through a slit lamp, a 90 D lens or a 78 D lens?**

78 D lens.

❍ **Which lens will give you the impression of greater height of a choroidal melanoma when doing indirect ophthalmoscopy, a 15 D lens or a 30 D lens?**

15 D lens.

❍ **What happens to the size of the aerial image and the retinal image as you move closer to the viewing lens when doing indirect ophthalmoscopy?**

The aerial size remains the same, which is why many retinal specialists recommend standing as far away from the viewing lens for ease in visualization. However, the retinal image size increases as you get closer, although visualization becomes more difficult because your light source is not coaxial but oblique.

❍ **How large an area of the cornea do most keratometers measure?**

Central 3 mm area.

❍ **An emmetropic swimmer, who is not wearing swimming goggles, opens his eyes underwater. What is his refractive state underwater?**

He becomes hyperopic.

○   **What is the power of an IOL (n = 1.491, radius of curvature = 7.5 mm) inside an eye if you fill the anterior chamber with air?**

P = (n' – n)/r where r is radius of curvature in meters

IOL in aqueous (n= 1.336)
P = (1.491-1.336)/0.0075 = +20.67 D

IOL in air (n = 1)
P = (1.491 –1)/0.0075 = +65.47 D

○   **Where is the patient's far point located with respect to the observer performing retinoscopy at neutralization?**

Observer's pupil.

○   **What steps can you take to increase the movement of a contact lens on a patient's cornea?**

1. Increase the base curve radius
2. Make the lens smaller
3. Add more peripheral curve
4. Decrease the weight of the lens
5. Increase the peripheral curve radius

○   **During cataract surgery, you lose vitreous and are forced to put in an anterior chamber IOL. The posterior chamber lens that you were originally planning to insert had an A constant of 118 and a power of 20 D for emmetropia. If the AC IOL has an A constant of 115, what should the IOL power be for postoperative emmetropia?**

+17.0 diopters.

○   **A cataract patient's eye has an axial length of 23.5 mm and keratometry measurements of 43.00 D @ 180 and 44.00 D @ 90. If you use the original SRK formula, what IOL power will produce emmetropia if you use an IOL with an A constant of 118.5?**

Power for emmetropia = A constant –2.5(axial length in mm) –0.9(average K readings)

= 118.5 –2.5(23.5) –0.9((43+44)/2)

= +20.57 diopters

○   **What is the difference between a prolate-shaped cornea and an oblate-shaped cornea?**

A prolate-shaped cornea is flatter in the periphery than in the central cornea, while an oblate-shaped cornea is steeper peripherally.

○   **What is the advantage of the cornea having a prolate shape?**

It corrects for spherical aberrations as light is refracted through the peripheral cornea.

○   **What does refractive surgery do to the shape of the cornea?**

It turns the cornea's shape to an oblate configuration, thereby increasing optical aberrations and causing glare and decreased contrast sensitivity, which worsen when the pupil dilates under low light conditions.

○   **A new patient seen at the Low Vision clinic has a distance visual acuity of 20/200. What reading add can be first tried initially?**

Kestenbaum's rule of taking the reciprocal of the Snellen distance visual acuity can be used to get a good initial approximation of the reading add. In this case, one can start this patient on a trial +10.00 D reading add.

○   **What are the advantages to aiming for a myopic postoperative refraction when planning for cataract surgery in a hyperopic patient with age-related macular degeneration who has 20/200 vision, moderate nuclear sclerosis and mild posterior subcapsular cataracts?**

A myopic postoperative refraction offers near-point focus without glasses for less demanding close activities such as grooming, facilitates higher plus adds and does not interfere with peripheral visual acuity or with routine mobility.

○   **If the spectacle lenses of a hypermetrope is moved forward while viewing a distant object, can accommodation compensate for the increased blur produced?**

No. Moving a plus spectacle lens forward moves its secondary focal point forward, increasing its effective plus power when viewing a distant object. This will blur distant objects but bring intermediate-distance objects into better focus. Accommodation can only further increase plus power; thus increased accommodation cannot compensate for this.

○   **A patient with a refraction of +5.00 D OU and a P.D. of 50 mm is given glasses with a P.D. of 60 mm by mistake. How much dioptric convergence power will the patient be required to exert in order to read at 33 cm?**

20 prism diopters.

○   **How can image jump best be minimized when designing bifocals?**

Choose a bifocal type with the segment's optical center near the segment top.

○   **A −2.00 D myope is totally cyclopleged. What power contact lens must you place on his cornea in order for him to see an object clearly at 25 cm?**

+2.00 D

○   **A myope has a spectacle correction of –4.00 + 1.50 x 90. What is the optical characteristic of this patient's eye?**

+4.00 –1.50 x 90

○   **A telescope has a +2.00 D objective and a –10.0 D eyepiece. What type of telescope is this, and what is the magnification and direction of the image?**

This is a Galilean telescope.

Magnification = -eyepiece/objective = -(-10)/2 = 5X

Since this number is positive, the image is erect.

○   **An aphakic patient corrected with +12.5 D spectacles at a vertex distance of 1.7 cm is corrected to emmetropia with a +16.00 D IOL. How much magnification was the patient experiencing with his aphakic glasses prior to surgery?**

Correction of an aphakic eye with spectacles results in a Galilean telescope. In this patient,

Objective = +12.5 D
Eyepiece = -16.0 D
Magnification = -(-16)/12.5 = +1.28

Images therefore appeared 28% larger to this patient when using these aphakic glasses prior to secondary IOL implantation.

○   **An emmetropic low vision patient with a visual acuity of 20/200 comes to your clinic and wants to be able to read the 20/40 line. You have a Galilean telescope with an eyepiece that is –20 D but it is missing an objective lens. What power objective lens does this patient need in order to use this telescope?**

The magnification required for the 20/40 line to appear the size of a 20/200 line is 5X. The objective lens required in this Galilean telescope to produce such a magnification is therefore:

Objective = -eyepiece/magnification = -(-20)/5 = +4.0 D

ORBIT AND OCULOPLASTICS

○ **A child is accidentally shot in the eye with a BB gun. What type of imaging procedure should be performed to localize the foreign body?**

CT scan is the procedure of choice to locate an intraocular or intraorbital metallic foreign body. A MRI scan is contraindicated if a metallic foreign body is suspected because the strong magnetic field could cause movement of the foreign body and additional injury.

○ **How is levator function evaluated?**

The patient is asked to look up and down and the excursion of the upper eyelid is measured.

○ **What is normal levator function?**

Approximately 13 mm or more of eyelid excursion.

○ **What is good levator function?**

Approximately 8 to 13 mm of movement.

○ **What is fair levator function?**

Approximately 4 to 8 mm of function.

○ **What is poor levator function?**

Less than 4 mm of eyelid movement.

○ **Why is it important to know the levator function of an eyelid?**

Levator function determines the type and amount of surgery that need to be performed.

○ **Eyelid sling procedures are generally used for what amount of levator function?**

Less than 4 mm.

○ **In the transconjunctival approach to lower eyelid blepharoplasty, is the orbital septum incised?**

In the transconjunctival approach, the palpebral conjunctiva and lower eyelid retractors are incised. The orbital septum is anterior to the extraconal fat in the eyelid and is not incised.

❍   **What structures are encountered if one makes an incision 1 cm above the upper tarsus?**

Skin, orbicularis muscle, orbital septum, orbital fat, levator aponeurosis, Müller's muscle, conjunctiva.

❍   **Why is it important to incise the orbital septum when performing surgery on the levator aponeurosis for ptosis repair?**

The levator aponeurosis is posterior to the pre-aponeurotic fat. In order to adequately expose the aponeurosis, the septum must be incised and the pre-aponeurotic fat gently dissected from the anterior surface of the aponeurosis.

❍   **A 3-year-old patient present with unilateral congenital ptosis. The eyelid margin bisects the visual axis and the levator function appears to be 3 mm. What surgical procedure is indicated to correct this ptosis?**

A fascia lata sling with either autogenous or banked fascia.

❍   **What is the principle visual concern in this age group?**

Occlusion amblyopia due to disruption of the visual axis.

❍   **Would there be as much concern if the ptosis were bilateral?**

Patients can develop amblyopia with unilateral or bilateral severe ptosis. In bilateral cases, however, there may be a head tilt to allow the patient to look under the eyelids.

❍   **What would be the procedure of choice if the levator function were 7 mm instead of 3 mm?**

A levator resection.

❍   **How is the amount of resection determined?**

It is based both on the amount of ptosis and the levator function. Tables exist for determining the exact amount of resection. In general, 6 to 7 mm of aponeurosis and muscle should be excised to correct each 1 mm of ptosis.

❍   **What is the embryologic origin of the orbital bones?**

Cranial neural crest cells.

❍   **A 75-year-old patient presents with slowly progressive unilateral ptosis of unknown duration. Examination of the involved eye reveals a margin reflex distance-one of 0 mm, levator function of 17 mm, and a margin crease distance of 14. What is the origin of this ptosis?**

Dehiscence of the levator aponeurosis. This is a classic presentation for age-related aponeurotic ptosis.

○   **When should skin sutures be removed from areas of good blood supply (i.e. face and neck)?**

Within 4 to 5 days.

○   **What is the absorption rate of chromic gut sutures?**

20 days.

○   **A 30-year-old patient complains of a bump in his left upper lid. An umbilicated, dome shaped nodule with multiple whitish inclusions is found on the lid, and a follicular conjunctivitis is present. What is the treatment and what will histopathology of the lesion show?**

The patient has molluscum contagiosum. The treatment of choice is excision biopsy or curettage of the lesion. Antiviral agents are not effective in the treatment of these lesions. The histopathology will show large eosinophilic intracytoplasmic inclusion bodies.

○   **What are the most common complications of ptosis surgery?**

Overcorrection, undercorrection, corneal exposure due to lagophthalmos, abnormal eyelid crease, abnormal eyelid conformation and curve, eyelash loss.

○   **What is the most common cause of bilateral proptosis in adults?**

Thyroid orbitopathy.

○   **What is the importance of the neosynephrine test in evaluating age-related ptosis?**

The neosynephrine test using either 2.5% or 10% neosynephrine is a test of Müller's muscle (superior tarsal muscle) function. A positive response (eyelid elevation) is essential if a conjunctiva-Müller's muscle excision is to be utilized to repair the ptotic eyelid.

○   **What are the most common procedures to correct age-related ptosis with good levator function?**

Aponeurosis repair and/or resection, Conjunctiva-M¸llerís muscle excision, and tarsectomy (Fasanella-type procedure).

○   **What is the upper lid retraction produced by Grave's disease due to?**

Overreaction of Müller's muscle.

○   **If a pin is inserted into the upper eyelid 4 mm above the lashes, what eyelid structures are encountered from anterior to posterior?**

Skin, orbicularis muscle, levator aponeurosis, tarsus, and conjunctiva.

❍ **In unilateral congenital ptosis requiring a fascia lata sling, should any procedure be performed on the opposite normal eye?**

Either nothing, in which case the asymmetrical postoperative appearance and function should be explained to the patient and his/her family or a sling procedure can be placed in the normal side to achieve symmetry between the two sides.

❍ **Where is the valve of Hasner located?**

Underneath the inferior turbinate of the nose.

❍ **Do pleomorphic adenomas of the lacrimal gland have a true capsule?**

They are not truly encapsulated, but compression of surrounding orbital tissues occurs which can simulate a capsule.

❍ **A 45-year-old female recently had cervical fusion. It was noted after surgery that one of the patients' eyelids was ptotic. Why? What other findings would be expected? What surgical procedures can be used to correct this problem?**

Horner's syndrome due to damage to the sympathetic nerves in the neck is common after neck surgery. It is associated with miosis and dyshydrosis as well as ptosis. Cocaine and hydroxyamphetamine testing is indicated to show the exact location of the lesion. Repair involves either levator aponeurosis surgery or a conjunctiva-Müller's muscle excision.

❍ **What innervates Müller's muscle?**

Müller's muscle, which elevates the upper lid about 2 mm, is innervated by the sympathetic system.

❍ **An ill-appearing patient presents with a fever of 104° F, bilateral chemosis, III nerve palsy and a history of sinusitis. What is the most likely diagnosis?**

Cavernous sinus thrombosis.

❍ **If a pin is inserted into the upper eyelid 10 mm above the lashes in the area of the eyelid crease, what structures are encountered from anterior to posterior?**

Skin, orbicularis muscle, levator aponeurosis, Müller's muscle, and conjunctiva.

❍ **What are Touton giant cells?**

Touton giant cells have a central zone of eosinophilic cytoplasm surrounded by an inner ring of multiple nuclei and an outer clear zone containing lipid. They are usually found in lipid granulomas or xanthomas of diseases such as juvenile xanthogranuloma and fibrous histiocytoma.

❍ **What infectious organism is the most common cause of chronic canaliculitis?**

Actinomyces.

❍ **What is the treatment for jaw-winking ptosis with fair levator function?**

Excision of the levator aponeurosis and fascia lata sling ptosis correction.

❍ **What infectious organisms are the most common causes of acute dacryocystitis?**

S. pneumoniae, staphylococcus and *H. influenza*

❍ **What are the main clinical features of an orbital blowout fracture?**

1. Periocular signs, eg. Ecchymosis, edema and subcutaneous emphysema.
2. Infraorbital nerve anesthesia.
3. Enophthalmos.
4. Diplopia.

❍ **Are most medial wall orbital blowout fractures associated with a floor fracture?**

Yes. Isolated medial wall fractures are relatively rare. Entrapment of the medial rectus can give rise to defective adduction and abduction.

❍ **What are the indications for surgical intervention in a patient with a blowout fracture?**

Surgical repair is performed 10-14 days after the injury if the patient has persistent diplopia when looking straight ahead or when attempting to read, if he has unacceptable enophthalmos or if a large fracture involving half or more of the orbital floor is present.

❍ **In which Le Fort fractures is CSF rhinorrhea commonly seen?**

Le Fort II and III.

❍ **What is the significance of visualizing a large vascular channel at the superior tarsal border during ptosis surgery from via a skin approach?**

The vessel is the peripheral arterial arcade traveling beneath the levator aponeurosis and on the surface of Müller's muscle. When this vessel is visualized, the levator aponeurosis is dehisced.

❍ **What sling materials should be considered in an adult with chronic progressive external ophthalmoplegia?**

A silicone rod will allow the eyelid to close more easily. Patients with CPEO and similar diseases such as myasthenia gravis may have decreased orbicularis muscle function.

❍ **What other procedures can be used to elevate the eyelids in patients with poor levator function and decreased orbicularis function?**

A Fasanella-type tarsectomy or a small levator resection is useful for minimally elevating the eyelids in these patients. Some surgeons advocate blepharoplasty alone so as not to compromise eyelid closure.

O   **What nerves pass through the superior part of the superior orbital fissure?**

1. Lacrimal nerve.
2. Frontal nerve.
3. Trochlear nerve (CN IV).

O   **How many millimeters above the superior tarsal border can Whitnall's (superior transverse) ligament be visualized?**

Approximately 15 to 20 mm.

O   **What nerves pass through the inferior part of the superior orbital fissure?**

1. Oculomotor nerve (CN III).
2. Abducens nerve (CN VI).
3. Nasociliary nerve (CN V).

O   **What is acanthosis?**

It is an increase in the prickle cell layer due to increase in mitotic activity of the basal cells.

O   **In the immediate postoperative period what are the appropriate management options for overcorrected ptosis?**

Suture release, downward eyelid massage, and eyelid stretching over a Desmarres retractor.

O   **In the late postoperative period what surgical procedure is usually performed to correct overcorrected ptosis?**

Levator recession and scar release. These procedures can be performed either from a posterior or anterior approach.

O   **How many extraconal fat compartments are present in the upper eyelid and how many in the lower eyelid?**

There are two extraconal fat compartments in the upper eyelid and three in the lower. The lacrimal gland substitutes for the lateral fat compartment in the upper eyelid.

O   **What is the most common type of rhabdomyosarcoma in children?**

Embryonal rhabdomyosarcoma.

O   **Which type of rhabdomyosarcoma has the worst prognosis?**

Alveolar type.

❍ **Where are the most common locations for rhabdomyosarcoma in the orbit?**

Retrobulbar followed by superior and inferior.

❍ **What part of the orbit does alveolar rhabdomyosarcoma usually present?**

Inferiorly.

❍ **What does a CT scan of rhabdomyosarcoma reveal?**

CT shows a poorly defined mass of homogeneous density, adjacent bony destruction and invasion of paranasal sinuses.

❍ **What is the management for rhabdomyosarcoma?**

Biopsy to confirm the diagnosis, followed by radiotherapy and chemotherapy.

❍ **Which is the weakest wall in the orbit?**

The medial wall is the weakest orbital wall. It includes the lamina papyracea of the ethmoid bone, the thinnest bone in the orbit, which predisposes it to fractures and secondary orbital infections due to ethmoidal sinusitis.

❍ **A 75 year-old man presents with a one-year history of unilateral Bell's palsy. He is complaining about ocular irritation. Which options are available to manage his symptoms?**

Artifical tear ointment, gold weight placement in the upper eyelid, tarsorrhaphy, dental spring placement in both the upper and lower eyelid, lower eyelid resuspension, and placement of a fascia lata in the eyelid to hold them shut.

❍ **What is the origin of the upper eyelid crease and fold?**

Fibers of the levator aponeurosis inserting into the subcutaneous tissues just inferior to the orbital septum. The skin above the crease is less firmly attached to the underlying tissues than the skin below the crease allowing it to fold over the crease when the eyelid is open.

❍ **What is the surgical significance of the eyelid crease?**

The normal adult crease is 10-12 mm above the eyelid margin and is where the upper eyelid incision should be made during ptosis and blepharoplasty procedures to hide the incision postoperatively. A high eyelid crease usually indicates a levator aponeurosis dehiscence.

❍ **What is the cause of involutional ectropion?**

Eyelid laxity.

❍   **What are the underlying pathologies for involutional lower eyelid entropion?**

Horizontal eyelid laxity, dehiscence of the capsulopalpebral fascia, and pre-septal orbicularis muscle hypertrophy.

❍   **Is bilateral inflammatory pseudotumor more common in children or in adults?**

Unilateral involvement is the rule in adults, while in children bilateral involvement occurs in 30%. In adults, a careful evaluation should be performed to rule out a systemic vasculitis and lymphoma.

❍   **Where is the most common location for an orbital meningocele?**

Above the medial canthus.

❍   **What is the most common form of congenital ptosis?**

Myogenic congenital ptosis is the most common form and results in a fibrotic levator muscle with or without fat infiltration that is unable to function.

❍   **A child with a sinus infection presents with left proptosis, swollen eyelid and an inferolaterally displaced globe. What is the most likely diagnosis?**

Orbital cellulitis and abscess associated with ethmoid sinusitis.

❍   **What is the most common bacterial agent likely to lead to orbital cellulitis and CNS infection in infants and young children?**

H. influenzae.

❍   **What is the most common bacterial agent implicated in orbital cellulitis in adults?**

Staphylococcus.

❍   **What are the potential complications of orbital cellulitis?**

1. Intracranial complications: cavernous sinus thrombosis, brain abscess, and meningitis.
2. Subperiosteal abscess.
3. Ocular: exposure keratitis, optic nerve inflammation, increased IOP, retinal vascular occlusion.

❍   **At what age group does capillary hemangioma usually present?**

During the first year of age. More than 50% are present by the first two months of life.

❍   **What systemic disease may be associated with congenital encephaloceles?**

Neurofibromatosis type 1.

○   **What structures pass through the inferior orbital fissure?**

1. Pterygopalatine ganglion.
2. Maxillary nerve.
3. Pterygoid nerve.
4. Inferior ophthalmic vein.

○   **What structures pass through the optic foramen?**

1. Optic nerve.
2. Ophthalmic artery.
3. Sympathetic fibers from the carotid plexus.

○   **What syndrome consists of thrombocytopenia, strawberry skin nevi and subglottic hemangioma?**

Kasabach-Merritt syndrome.

○   **What is distichiasis?**

It is an extra row of lashes present in the orifices of the Meibomian glands.

○   **Where do dermoid cysts usually present in the orbit in children?**

Anterior upper temporal orbit.

○   **What is the most common benign orbital tumor in adults?**

Cavernous hemangioma.

○   **What are the ocular features of Crouzon's syndrome?**

1. Proptosis with shallow orbits.
2. Blue sclera.
3. Strabismus.
4. Congenital cataract.
5. Optic atrophy.
6. Hypertelorism.

○   **Where is the most common location for sebaceous cell carcinoma?**

Sebaceous gland carcinoma occurs more commonly in the meibomian glands of the upper eyelid. These can be extremely aggressive both locally and systemically.

○   **What bone forms the lacrimal fossa?**

Frontal.

○   **Where does Whitnall's ligament insert in the orbit?**

It inserts 10 mm above Whitnall's tubercle.

○ **What bones form the medial orbital wall?**

Ethmoid, lacrimal, sphenoid and maxillary.

○ **Which is the strongest wall of the orbit?**

Lateral wall, made up by the zygoma and the greater wing of the sphenoid.

○ **What is the embryonic origin of the lacrimal gland?**

Surface ectoderm.

○ **Where is Rosenmüller's valve located?**

Common canaliculus.

○ **A 23-year-old burn victim presents with an ectropion of the lower eyelid. What is the most likely etiology for this?**

This patient most likely has a cicatricial ectropion due to scarring of the anterior lamella of the eyelid.

○ **What is the most reasonable treatment for this problem and why?**

Burn patients usually have a vertical deficiency of eyelid skin due to their injury and the subsequent scarring of the eyelid. Skin grafts are required to replace deficient skin.

○ **What are some of the important concepts to remember when skin grafting?**

The amount of graft tissue should be at least twice what is required as graft shrinkage is common. The scar tissue and other eyelid tissues must be extensively released to adequately graft the eyelid. The lid should be placed on maximum stretch during the healing process to ensure adequate graft coverage.

○ **Describe the course of the infraorbital nerve within the orbit.**

The infraorbital nerve, which is a branch of the trigeminal nerve (CN V), travels via the infraorbital canal anteriorly from the infraorbital groove and exits the orbit about 4 mm below the inferior orbital rim.

○ **What is a tripod fracture?**

It is a fracture of the zygoma away from the face.

○ **How do patients with a tripod fracture present?**

They have a variably depressed lateral wall and cheek, depending on the degree of zygomatic rotation away from the face.

❍ **What symptom characteristically occurs in patients with tripod fractures?**

Pain with mouth opening or chewing because of impingement of the zygomatic bone on the coronoid process of the mandible.

❍ **What bone forms the optic foramen and optic canal?**

Lesser wing of the sphenoid.

❍ **What are the causes of entropion after ptosis repair?**

Over aggressive excision of tarsus, improper suture placement, improper sling placement.

❍ **A 36-year-old patient presents with eyelid retraction following orbital rim fracture repair after a motor vehicle accident. What is the appropriate intervention?**

Release of the eyelid retractors and scar tissue and placement of an interpositional graft.

❍ **What is the most frequent cause of unilateral proptosis in adults?**

Thyroid orbitopathy.

❍ **A 50-year-old patient presents with bilateral lacrimal gland enlargement. The chest X-ray is normal, and the abdominal CT shows a retroperitoneal mass. What is the most likely diagnosis?**

Malignant lymphoma.

❍ **What is the most common cause of unilateral proptosis in children?**

Orbital cellulitis.

❍ **What is the appearance of vitreous in T1- and T2-weighted MRI images?**

Vitreous appears dark in T1-images and bright in T2-images.

❍ **What is the appearance of orbital fat in T1- and T2-weighted MRI images?**

It appears bright in T1-images and dark in T2-images.

❍ **What is the best view to obtain when requesting for a plain radiograph of a patient with orbital trauma?**

Waters view is the single best method for demonstrating the maxillary sinuses, as well as fractures of the maxilla, inferior rim, floor and zygomatic arches.

❍ **Why is MRI a poor choice for imaging blowout fractures?**

MRI clearly demonstrates soft tissue details of a blowout fracture better than CT, but the absence of a cortical bone signal makes it a poor choice for visualization of fractures.

❍ **Does an orbital floor fracture usually occur medial or lateral to the infraorbital nerve?**

Medial to the infraorbital nerve.

❍ **What is the best way to distinguish a restrictive motility disorder from a paretic disorder following a blowout fracture?**

Forced-duction testing.

❍ **What is the most common intracranial tumor to spread to the orbit?**

Sphenoid wing meningioma.

❍ **What is the most common type of Le Fort fracture?**

Le Fort II.

❍ **What kinds of ocular complications can result from a Le Fort II fracture?**

Orbital emphysema, enophthalmos, optic nerve trauma and motility disturbances.

❍ **What are some of the materials that have been used for interpositional spacers?**

Hard palate, ears cartilage, nasal septal cartilage and attached mucosa, tissue-banked sclera.

❍ **Which of these materials shrinks the most? The least?**

Sclera shrinks the most and cartilage the least.

❍ **If there is a linear scar of the eyelid associated with eyelid retraction what repair option might be considered?**

Scar excision with Z-plasty to correct the linear nature of the scar?

❍ **From which areas should eyelid skin grafts be obtained?**

The upper eyelid skin is the thinnest in the body. The best match is from the opposite upper eyelid. Second choice would be the post-auricular area. Third choice would be the supraclavicular area or from the inner part of the arm.

❍ **A patient involved in a motor vehicle accident presents with a ruptured globe and a significant blowout fracture. How would you manage his eye injuries?**

Repair the globe immediately and delay the repair of the orbital floor fracture by 2 to 4 weeks.

❍ **What does a low HS-TSH level indicate?**

It indicates either thyrotoxicosis or a thyroid operating independent of pituitary control.

○   **What is the significance of a high or rising HS-TSH blood level after thyroid suppression therapy?**

This may be associated with an exacerbation of thyroid orbital disease.

○   **How do you make the presumptive diagnosis of euthyroid Graves' disease?**

This may be made on the basis of typical clinical findings and analysis of abnormal orbital anatomy by CT or MR imaging in the presence of normal TRH tests and normal blood levels of HS-TSH.

○   **What extraocular muscles are commonly involved in Graves' disease?**

The inferior recti are most commonly involved, followed by medial recti then the superior recti and lateral recti muscles.

○   **What is the correct procedure for correcting a cicatricial entropion?**

A horizontal blepharotomy with rotation sutures to rotate the eyelid segment away from the globe.

○   **What are the purposes of posterior lamellar grafts?**

To replace lost posterior lamellar tissue and by doing so correct eyelid retraction or cicatricial entropion doe to inadequate tissue.

○   **What is the most common disease causing eyelid retraction?**

Thyroid-related orbitopathy.

○   **Describe the appearance of the extraocular muscles affected by Graves' disease with imaging studies.**

In the early acute phase, muscle enlargement may be diffuse, and inflammation may extend anteriorly to involve the tendinous insertions. As the disease progresses, muscle enlargement is more confined to the muscle belly, and the tendon assumes a thinner contour.

○   **While interpositional eyelid spacers work well to correct lower eyelid retraction associated with thyroid-related orbitopathy, what procedure should be considered for correcting upper eyelid retraction?**

Recession of the levator aponeurosis. A myotomy of the levator can also be considered. Recession of Müller's muscle should also be carried out. If recession of the levator is not adequate to lower the eyelid, a scleral graft can be placed as an upper eyelid spacer.

○   **What non-surgical interventions are available for managing post-traumatic or iatrogenic eyelid retraction?**

Intralesional steroid injections and massage.

○   When performing a dacryocystorhinostomy, what bony structures are removed during the osteotomy?

During the osteotomy, the lacrimal sac fossa and the superior nasal wall of the nasolacrimal duct are removed, which includes the entire lacrimal bone and part of the maxillary bone.

○   What is epiblepharon?

It is a horizontal fold of skin and pretarsal muscle that overrides the lid margin, causing a misdirection of the eyelashes toward the globe.

○   What non-surgical interventions are available for managing a chalazion?

Intralesional steroid injections, a tetracycline, hot compresses.

○   How many millimeters does Müller's muscle normally elevate the upper eyelid?

2 mm.

○   What is the treatment for fibrous histiocytoma?

Fibrous histiocytoma is a tumor that affects middle aged patients and causes slowly progressive proptosis and diplopia. Aggressive surgical excision is necessary because this tumor has a tendency to recur locally.

○   What is the classic triad of Hand-Schüller-Christian disease?

1. Exophthalmos.
2. Lytic lesions of the skull.
3. Diabetes insipidus.

○   Of the different manifestations of histiocytosis X (Langerhans cell histiocytosis), which one has the worst prognosis and which has the worst?

Letterer-Siwe disease results in systemic spread of abnormally proliferating histiocytes with rapid death; while eosinophilic granuloma, where disease is confined to isolated bony lesions, has the best prognosis.

○   A 54-year-old golfer presents with a 6mm necrotizing lesion of the eyelid. What is the most likely diagnosis?

Basal cell carcinoma although other forms of skin cancer cannot be excluded.

○   What surgical intervention should be considered?

A biopsy to confirm the diagnostic impression.

❍ **What does the grey line in the eyelid represent and what is its significance?**

This represents the most posterior pretarsal orbicularis muscle fibers (muscle of Riolan). A vertical incision made here will split the eyelid into anterior (skin and orbicularis) and posterior (conjunctiva and tarsus) layers.

❍ **What are the signs of orbital apex syndrome?**

1. Decreased visual acuity.
2. External and internal ophthalmoplegia.
3. Decreased sensation.

❍ **What is the horizontal length of the eyelid?**

About 29 or 30 mm.

❍ **What is the vertical height of the upper eyelid tarsus and the lower eyelid tarsus?**

10 mm and slightly less than 4 mm, respectively.

❍ **What would be diagnostic for orbital mucormycosis in biopsy specimens?**

The presence of large, nonseptate branching hyphae in biopsy specimens of the orbit is pathognomonic for orbital mucormycosis. There is ischemic necrosis due to arteriolar invasion.

❍ **How does orbital mucormycosis spread to the intracranial cavity?**

Via the ophthalmic artery.

❍ **Why is the treatment of pleomorphic adenomas or benign mixed tumor of the lacrimal gland complete excision without incisional biopsy?**

Incisional biopsy may seed tumor cells into the orbit. Also, incompletely excised tumors may undergo malignant transformation.

❍ **What is the cause of congenital dacryoceles, and what is the treatment?**

Congenital dacryoceles are due to an obstruction of the nasolacrimal duct with amniotic fluid or mucus filling the dilated lacrimal sac. Probing performed during the first year of life results in a cure rate of greater than 90%.

❍ **What are the most common clinical features of carotid-cavernous fistula?**

Proptosis, chemosis, bruit, ocular motor nerve palsies, increased IOP and retinopathy.

❍ **What re the most common causes of painful external ophthalmoplegia?**

Thyroid disease, TB, sarcoidosis, Wegener's granulomatosis, metastatic breast, prostate or GI cancer, Tolosa-Hunt syndrome, diabetes mellitus, cavernous sinus thrombosis and mucormycosis.

O   **What is the most common orbital tumor in childhood?**

Capillary hemangioma, which is absent at birth, appears by one year of age, increases in size and disappears by age 5 years. It can produce occlusion or meridional amblyopia.

O   **What is the most common orbital tumor in adults?**

Cavernous hemangioma.

O   **What is the treatment of choice for cavernous hemangiomas?**

Surgical excision.

O   **What does orbital CT scanning of an optic nerve glioma show?**

Fusiform enlargement of the optic nerve.

O   **What is the incidence of neurofibromatosis in a child with an optic nerve glioma?**

25 to 50%.

O   **How long do adult patients with optic nerve gliomas live after being diagnosed with the tumor?**

Most of these patients die within 6-12 months. This tumor is benign in children, although it can involve the more posterior structures such as the optic chiasm and sella turcica.

O   **What can be expressed from canaliculi infected with *Actinomyces*?**

Yellow sulfur granules.

O   **What is the difference in the insertion of the levator aponeurosis between Caucasian and Oriental eyelids?**

In Caucasians, the orbital septum joins the levator aponeurosis about 3 mm superior to the tarsus of the upper lid. In Oriental eyes, these two structures join along the anterior surface of the tarsus.

O   **What is the normal position of the eyebrow in a male and in a female?**

In men, the eyebrow is usually at or just below the superior orbital rim, while in women it is above the superior orbital rim.

O   **What is a reliable sign of penetration of the orbital septum during eyelid surgery or evaluation of eyelid trauma?**

Presence of fat in the surgical field.

❍ **What bones form the orbital floor?**

Maxillary, zygomatic and palatine bones.

❍ **What muscle separates the medial from the central fat compartment in the lower eyelid?**

The inferior oblique muscle.

❍ **What is the significance of eyebrow ptosis in blepharoplasty surgery?**

Eyebrow ptosis may exaggerate the amount of dermatochalasis that is present and contribute to superior visual field loss. Correcting eyebrow ptosis prior to skin excision will reduce the amount of skin excision required.

❍ **What is the most common cause of congenital obstruction of the nasolacrimal duct?**

Membranous blockage at the valve of Hasner.

❍ **What is hypertelorism?**

Increased distance between the medial orbital walls.

❍ **What is telecanthus?**

Increased distance between the medial canthi of the eyelids as a result of abnormally long medial canthi tendons.

❍ **A 4-year-old presents to your office with a mass at the superolateral aspect of the right orbit. The CT scan shows a well-defined, cystic structure with normal bony landmarks. What is your diagnosis?**

Dermoid cyst.

❍ **What is Horner's syndrome?**

It is produced by interruption in sympathetic innervation to the eye and is characterized by miosis, mild ptosis, anhidrosis, and enophthalmos.

❍ **Why does lower eyelid retraction occurs following inferior rectus recession?**

Lockwood's ligament, the inferior suspensory ligament for the globe, is attached to the inferior rectus muscle sheath, the capsulopalpebral fascia, and the inferior oblique muscle. When the inferior rectus muscle is recessed, the other muscles attached to it via Lockwood's ligament also are moved posteriorly leading to eyelid retraction.

❍ **What is the Fasanella-Servat procedure?**

It is a transconjunctival resection of the upper border of the tarsus together with the lower border of Müller's muscle used to correct mild ptosis due to Horner's syndrome and very mild congenital ptosis.

O   Why does superior rectus muscle resection result in ptosis?

The superior rectus muscle, levator aponeurosis and muscle, and the superior oblique tendon are all attached to Whitnall's ligament, the superior suspensory ligament for the globe and eyelid structures. Resecting the superior rectus muscle causes the ligament to move anteriorly resulting in a forward movement of the levator aponeurosis with a resultant ptosis.

O   How do you perform the Jones 1 test, and how do you interpret its results?

The Jones 1 test differentiates a partial obstruction of the lacrimal passages from hypersecretion of tears. Fluorescein is instilled into the conjunctival sac. After 5 minutes, a cotton-tip bud moistened in 4% cocaine is inserted under the inferior turbinate at the opening of the nasolacrimal duct. Fluorescein recovered from the nose indicates that the drainage system is patent, and the test is considered positive. No further tests are then necessary. If no dye is recovered, there is either a partial obstruction somewhere along the lacrimal drainage passages or failure of the lacrimal pump mechanism. The Jones 2 test is then performed.

O   How do you do the Jones 2 test, and how do you interpret the results?

This test identifies the probable site of partial obstruction after a negative Jones 1 test. Topical anesthetic is instilled into the conjunctival sac and any residual fluorescein is washed out. The drainage system is then irrigated with saline. If fluorescein-stained saline is recovered from the nose, there is a partial obstruction to the nasolacrimal duct; and the test is considered positive. If no fluorescein is recovered, the obstruction lies in the upper drainage system (punctum, canaliculi or common canaliculus) or there is a defective lacrimal pump mechanism.

O   What are the lengths of the various parts of the lacrimal drainage system in adults?

1. Ampulla (2 mm).
2. Canaliculus (8 mm).
3. Nasolacrimal sac (10 mm).
4. Nasolacrimal duct (12 mm).

O   What is the treatment for acute dacryocystitis?

Broad-spectrum systemic antibiotics and warm compresses. Irrigation and probing is contraindicated. A dacryocystorhinostomy may be necessary once the infection has been controlled.

O   When is insertion of a Jones tube indicated during a DCR?

A Jones tube is inserted when there is absence of canalicular function.

❍   **When should probing be performed in a child with congenital nasolacrimal duct obstruction?**

Probing is not done until the child is 12-18 months old because spontaneous recanalization occurs in about 95% of cases.

❍   **What is the cure rate of congenital nasolacrimal duct obstruction with probing?**

90% are cured after the first probing, and an additional 6% by the second probing.

❍   **If probing fails to cure the nasolacrimal duct obstruction, when should a DCR be performed?**

Patients who fail two technically satisfactory probings and insertion of silastic tubes or balloon dilation of the nasolacrimal duct can be treated by DCR between the ages of 3 and 4 years.

❍   **What condition is epicanthus inversus associated with?**

Blepharophimosis syndrome.

❍   **A 500 lb man complains of chronic left eye redness and irritation. On examination, you note that the upper eyelid is loose and easily everted. Papillary conjunctivitis is present in the affected tarsus. What is your probable diagnosis and treatment for this condition?**

Floppy eyelid syndrome causing eversion and trauma to the lids during sleep and a chronic papillary conjunctivitis of the exposed tarsal conjunctiva. This can be treated with horizontal lid shortening if the condition is severe.

❍   **A 17-year-old female presents with recurrent episodes of painless, nonpitting edema of her upper eyelids since puberty, which resolves spontaneously after a few days. What are the diagnosis, and what complications can occur from this?**

The patient has blepharochalasis, a rare condition that can cause stretching of the skin so that it has the appearance of wrinkled cigarette paper, weakening of the orbital septum with fat herniation, and aponeurotic ptosis.

❍   **When do you suspect that lid retraction is present?**

Lid retraction is suspected when the upper lid margin is level with or above the superior limbus of the eye.

❍   **What are the attachments of the medial canthal tendon?**

The superficial head of the pre-tarsal and pre-septal portions of the orbicularis muscle tendon insert onto the anterior lacrimal crest while the deep heads of the tendons insert into the posterior lacrimal crest. The orbital portion of the orbicularis muscle inserts into the anterior lacrimal crest. The lacrimal sac is invested between the deep and superficial head of the tendon.

О   **Why is it important to understand the anatomy of the medial canthal tendon?**

With blinking, the tendon squeezes the lacrimal sac pushing tears into the nose. Eyelid laxity can reduce the pumping action of the eyelids resulting in tearing. In addition, making an incision into the tendon can damage the lacrimal sack and cause tearing.

О   **What is dermatochalasis?**

It is characterized by redundancy of the upper eyelid skin among elderly patients.

О   **A 3-year-old child is brought to you for droopy eyelids. You find that the patient has a moderate ptosis, telecanthus, short horizontal palpebral apertures, lateral ectropion of the lower eyelids, poorly developed nasal bridge, hypolastic superior orbital rims, and epicanthus inversus. You notice that the father has a similar appearance. What is your diagnosis, and what complication can result from this disorder?**

The patient and the father have the blepharophimosis syndrome, a rare congenital disorder that is an autosomal dominant trait. Amblyopia can develop in 50% of patients.

О   **How would you treat a patient with blepharophimosis syndrome?**

Correction of the epicanthus and telecanthus followed a few months later by bilateral frontalis suspension for the ptosis.

О   **What are the attachments of the lateral canthal tendon?**

The lateral canthal tendon is in fact a raphe or interdigitation of muscle fibers. It is attached to the lateral orbital tubercle on the inner surface of the lateral orbital wall, slightly posterior to the lateral orbital rim.

О   **Why is it important to understand the anatomy of the lateral canthal raphe?**

During a tarsal strip procedure to reduce eyelid laxity, failure to adequately reposition the lateral tarsal strip to the inside of the orbital rim and at an appropriate level in comparison to the opposite side can cause a gap between the globe and the eyelid as well as an abnormal tilt to the horizontal fissure.

О   **A child present to you with left upper lid ptosis. The upper eyelid retracts when the child opens her mouth. What is your diagnosis and treatment?**

Marcus Gunn jaw-winking syndrome, which is treated with bilateral levator excision and frontalis brow suspension.

О   **What is the margin-reflex distance (MRD), and what is the normal value?**

It is the distance between the upper lid margin and the light reflex of the pupil with the patient looking directly at a penlight held by the examiner. The normal MRD is about 4 mm.

○   **How often is the eye involved in myasthenia gravis, and what are the eye manifestations?**

The eye is involved in 90% of cases and is the presenting feature in 60%. Ocular manifestations include ptosis, diplopia, and nystagmoid movements on extremes of gaze.

○   **What tests can you do to evaluate a patient for myasthenia gravis?**

1.   Tensilon (edrophonium) test.
2.   Electromyography.
3.   Presence of antibodies to acetylcholine receptors.
4.   CT or MRI of the anterior mediastinum to rule out a thymoma.

○   **How do you perform the Tensilon test?**

This test should never be performed without an assistant and a resuscitation tray in case of sudden cardiorespiratory arrest.

1.   Obtain baseline measurements of the ptosis or a Hess test in patients with diplopia.
2.   Inject a test dose of 0.2 ml (2 mg) edrophonium HCl.
3.   After 60 seconds, inject the remaining 0.8 ml (8 mg), provided there is no hypersensitivity.
4.   Take measurements and compare the results within 5 minutes.

○   **Does a negative Tensilon test result eliminate the possibility of myasthenia gravis?**

No.

○   **How often are antibodies to acetylcholine receptors present in patients with myasthenia gravis?**

90% of cases.

○   **How much of an eyelid can be removed via a wedge resection allowing the resulting defect to be closed primarily?**

About one-fourth to one-third of the eyelid, depending upon the amount of eyelid laxity that is present. In some older individuals as much as 40 percent of an eyelid can be removed and the defect closed primarily.

○   **If slightly extra eyelid tissue is needed to close a defect what is the simplest option?**

A canthotomy and cantholysis of the eyelid tendon with allow closure of a defect involving as much as 50 percent or more of an eyelid.

○   **When is a Tenzel flap used to close eyelid defects?**

A Tenzel semicircular flap is used to close defects involving more than a third but less than half of the eyelid.

○   **What is the Hughes procedure?**

This is a procedure used to correct lower eyelid defects greater than 50% that involves taking a tarsoconjunctival flap from the upper eyelid, leaving behind 3 to 4 mm of the upper tarsus intact, and advancing the flap to correct a lower eyelid defect.

○   **What potential complications can result from steroid injections to shrink a capillary hemangioma?**

Skin depigmentation, fat atrophy, eyelid necrosis, and, rarely, central retinal artery occlusion.

○   **What is loss of cohesion between epidermal cells with breakdown of intercellular junctions, creating spaces within the epidermis, called?**

Acantholysis.

○   **How do you define hyperkeratosis?**

Hyperkeratosis is a thickening of the stratum corneum or keratin layer, usually by too rapid growth and maturation of the epidermis.

○   **What is acanthosis?**

Thickening of the squamous cell layer.

○   **What is retention of nuclei in the stratum corneum called?**

Parakeratosis.

○   **What is dyskeratosis?**

Occurrence of keratin in the basal cell layer or deeper layers of the prickle cell layer.

○   **After being struck in the eye with a racquetball, a patient goes to the emergency room and complains of increasing pain, swelling and worsening of vision. On examination, the visual acuity is 20/200 in the injured eye and proptosis is present. The patient is unable to close his lid and the orbit is tense to palpation. An afferent pupillary defect is present. The fundus examination shows pulsation of the central retinal artery. What is your diagnosis and how would you manage this case?**

The patient has an orbital hemorrhage with compression of the optic nerve. A lateral canthotomy with inferior cantholysis should be performed immediately, followed by high dose corticosteroids and orbital imaging.

○ **What are the indications for removal of intraorbital foreign bodies?**

Indications for surgical removal include organic foreign bodies or foreign bodies located in the anterior orbit. Observation may be done if the foreign body is inert and located in the posterior orbit.

○ **How often do capillary hemangiomas spontaneously involute?**

70 to 80% of cases of capillary hemangiomas will spontaneously involute.

○ **A twelve-year-old girl presents with sudden onset of painful proptosis, decreased motility, periocular swelling, subconjunctival hemorrhage and chemosis after sneezing. She gives a history of intermittent mild proptosis with upper respiratory tract infections. What is the probable diagnosis?**

Orbital lymphangioma.

○ **What is the treatment for the nevus flammeus of Sturge-Weber syndrome?**

Yellow dye laser (wavelength 577 or 585 nanometers).

○ **What are the ocular side effects of botulinum toxin therapy for essential blepharospasm?**

Ptosis, strabismus, lagophthalmos, and ectropion or entropion depending on tone of the eyelids prior to injection.

○ **What radiologic and clinical findings would suggest a malignancy of the lacrimal gland?**

Bone destruction, pain, calcification of the mass and irregular borders of the mass are all suggestive of a malignant process.

○ **A 50-year-old patient presents with unilateral proptosis. The CT scan reveals an encapsulated intraconal mass. What is the probable diagnosis?**

Cavernous hemangioma.

○ **What is the presence of opticociliary shunt vessels in a 65-year-old woman with progressive loss of vision in her right eye, proptosis, and an afferent pupillary defect highly suggestive of?**

The presence of opticociliary shunt vessels is highly suggestive but not pathognomonic of orbital meningioma.

○ **A 22-year-old patient presents with an intermittent, nonpulsatile proptosis of his right eye that increases with the valsalva maneuver. What is your diagnosis?**

Orbital varices.

○   **A three-month-old infant is presented to your office with proptosis. The parents state that it increases whenever the child cries. The eye is noted to be displaced forward and laterally. The proptosis is pulsatile, but no thrill or bruit is detected. What is the probable diagnosis?**

Anterior encephalocele.

○   **A 40-year-old patient presents with a painless, rapidly growing lesion with a central crater on his lower eyelid for the past three weeks. What is the diagnosis and what can this be confused with if an incomplete excisional biopsy is performed?**

This history is classic for a keratoacanthoma, a nonmalignant lesion which can be confused with squamous cell carcinoma if incomplete biopsy is done.

○   **What is a Cutler-Beard procedure?**

It is an eyelid-sharing procedure that uses the skin and muscle from the lower eyelid for reconstruction of upper eyelid defects.

○   **What is a complication of a bridge of eyelid tissue as is done in both the Cutler-Beard procedure and the horizontal blepharotomy for repair of cicatricial entropion?**

Tissue necrosis and loss of the bridge.

○   **An 18-year-old girl presents with a whitish yellow subconjunctival mass on the temporal aspect of her right eye extending to the lateral canthus, which she has had since childhood. She is planning to become a model and wishes to have the lesion removed. What is the probable diagnosis, and how would you treat this?**

This is a dermolipoma, which is composed of fat and fibrous tissue and occurs, usually in the first decade of life. Excision is done only for cosmetic reasons or if it causes functional problems. Only the anterior and visible portion of the tumor should be removed since complete excision is risky due to tumor extension into the orbit. Care should be taken to avoid damaging extraocular muscles and the lacrimal gland.

○   **What is the differential diagnosis of proptosis present at birth?**

1. Congenital encephalocele, which may be associated with neurofibromatosis type 1.
2. Syndromes associated with shallow orbits, eg. Crouzon's, Apert's.

○   **What are the most common eyelid side effects seen with injection of botulinum for hemifacial spasm or blepharospasm?**

Ptosis, ectropion, and lagophthalmos.

○   **When excising a basal cell carcinoma, how much normal tissue around the lesion should be removed?**

At least a 3 mm area of normal appearing tissue should be removed as well as the obvious tumor.

○ **How much normal tissue should be removed with a squamous cell carcinoma? A meibomian gland carcinoma?**

4 mm and 6 mm as these are significantly more aggressive tumors than a basal cell carcinoma.

○ **What are the most successful methods for ensuring complete tumor removal in skin cancer?**

Mohs surgery or frozen section control of tissue margins.

○ **How often does neuroblastoma metastasize to the orbit?**

40% of cases, which typically presents with abrupt onset of proptosis accompanied by lid ecchymosis.

○ **What is the preferred treatment for large capillary hemangiomas involving the eyelid and associated with astigmatism or occlusion of the visual axis?**

Intralesional steroids although the use of systemic steroid has also been advocated.

○ **What are the ocular features of Crouzon's syndrome?**

1. Very shallow orbits with proptosis.
2. Optic atrophy.
3. Blue sclera.
4. Strabismus.
5. Congenital cataract.

○ **What effect can carbon dioxide lasers have on the eye?**

Exposure to a 10,600 nm wavelength can cause corneal opacification because the energy is largely absorbed on the surface of the eye.

○ **What are two methods for correcting epicanthal folds?**

Either an Y to V plasty or Mustard's double opposing Z-plasty.

○ **What tissue can substitute for a lateral canthal raphe when that tissue is lost during trauma or surgery and the eyelid needs to be resuspended?**

Either adjacent periosteum or, if there is sufficient eyelid laxity, tarsus.

PEDIATRIC OPHTHALMOLOGY AND STRABISMUS

○ **What is the difference between a phoria and a tropia?**

A phoria is a latent misalignment of the eyes while a tropia is a manifest deviation. Under certain conditions such as fatigue, a phoria may breakdown into a tropia.

○ **Is strabismus during the first few months of life common?**

Strabismus during infancy occurs in approximately one-third of infants during the first six months of life.

○ **What causes the appearance of pseudoesotropia?**

A wide nasal bridge and/or prominent epicanthal folds.

○ **How can pseudoesotropia be differentiated from true esotropia?**

Using the corneal light reflex or alternate cover test when possible.

○ **What is the generally accepted definition of congenital, or infantile, esotropia?**

An esotropia that develops before six months of life and is documented prior to one year of age.

○ **What is the characteristic angle of deviation in infantile esotropia?**

It is large, usually at least 30 prism diopters and averaging 40 prism diopters.

○ **What can often be documented in parents of children with infantile esotropia?**

Reduced binocular vision. This has been suggested to be a subthreshold effect of the "gene(s)" that cause the disorder.

○ **How can equality of vision be ascertained in children with infantile esotropia?**

By evaluating fixation preference and observing for the presence or absence of cross-fixation.

○ **What was Worth's theory regarding the etiology of infantile esotropia?**

Worth's "sensory" theory stated that the esotropia was due to a deficit in the "fusion" center in the brain and that because there was no way to provide this absent neural function, treatment was hopeless.

❍   **What was Chavasse's theory regarding the etiology of infantile esotropia?**

Chavasse believed the cause was mechanical. In his "motor" theory, binocular function could be restored if the eyes were surgically aligned.

❍   **What is considered a favorable sensory result in children treated for infantile esotropia?**

Monofixation syndrome.

❍   **Define the monofixation syndrome.**

Alignment within 10 prism diopters, a central facultative scotoma, peripheral fusion with fusional vergence amplitudes and possible stereopsis (reduced).

❍   **What is the benefit of the monofixation syndrome?**

It provides motor fusion to help maintain ocular alignment.

❍   **What is cross-fixation?**

When a child with a large angle esotropia uses the crossed or esotropic eye to look to the contralateral side.

❍   **With what may cross-fixation be confused?**

Because the child cross-fixates, the contralateral eye will appear not to abduct in side gaze. Therefore, cross-fixation may lead to the erroneous diagnosis of unilateral or bilateral sixth nerve palsy.

❍   **How can normal abduction be demonstrated in an infant who cross-fixates?**

A doll's head maneuver or occluding one eye will allow the demonstration of normal abduction.

❍   **What is the typical refractive error of a child with congenital esotropia?**

The same as the general population of the same age.

❍   **What are the goals in the treatment of congenital esotropia?**

Reduce the deviation to allow the development of binocular vision.

❍   **When is surgery performed on children with congenital esotropia?**

In general, surgery is performed after amblyopia, if present, is treated and once the angle of deviation is felt to be stable. If an accommodative component may be present, this should be treated prior to surgery.

❍   **What is the mean axial length of the eye of a full term neonate?**

16.8 mm ± 0.6 mm.

❍ **How long are the four recti muscles?**

40 mm.

❍ **When the eye is abducted, what are the primary and secondary actions of the superior oblique?**

When the globe is abducted, the superior oblique acts primarily as an incycloductor and secondarily as an abductor.

❍ **What are the primary and secondary actions of the inferior rectus when the eye is abducted 23 degrees?**

In 23 degree abduction, the muscle plane coincides with the optical axis and the inferior rectus becomes a pure depressor.

❍ **What are the limitations of the cover test for detecting heterotropias?**

Deviations less than 1 degree may escape detection with this test, and small-angle strabismus with eccentric fixation may not perform a detectable fixation movement when the sound eye is covered.

❍ **In the Hirschberg test, how many degrees of ocular deviation correspond to each millimeter of deviation?**

7 degrees.

❍ **What does a patient with right esotropia and anomalous retinal correspondence see when performing the Hering-Bielschowsky afterimage test?**

The vertical afterimage will appear displaced to the left of the horizontal afterimage.

❍ **When performing a Worth four-dot test, a patient reports seeing four lights. What does this result indicate?**

Peripheral fusion with orthophoria or a small-angle esotropia with anomalous retinal correspondence (ARC).

❍ **A patient reports seeing two vertically aligned red lights when performing the Worth-four dot test. What does this result indicate?**

Suppression OS.

❍ **What is the advantage of using Bagolini glasses to test for retinal correspondence?**

It allows examination of retinal correspondence under nearly normal conditions of seeing without dissociation of eyes, while the position of the eyes can be checked with the cover test. Small suppression scotomas can be detected when the patient notes a gap in the luminous stripe.

○   **When and how is the neutral density filter test performed?**

The neutral density filter test is performed before occlusion treatment to differentiate between functional and organic amblyopia. Neutral density filters (Kodak No. 96; ND 2.00 and 0.50) of sufficient density to reduce visual acuity in normal eyes to 20/40 are placed before the amblyopic eye. This will reduce acuity by one or two lines, leave it unaffected, or even slightly improve vision if the amblyopia is functional. Visual acuity is often markedly reduced when organic amblyopia is present.

○   **How long are the tendons of the medial rectus and the lateral rectus?**

The medial rectus tendon is 4 mm, while the lateral rectus tendon is 8 mm long.

○   **Which extraocular muscle has the shortest muscle length but the longest tendon?**

Superior oblique has a muscle length of 32 mm and a tendon 26 mm long.

○   **A three-month-old infant of normal birth weight is noted to have a funnel-shaped retinal detachment emanating from the optic nerve in her left eye during examination. What is the most likely diagnosis?**

Persistent hyperplastic primary vitreous.

○   **Treacher-Collin's syndrome (mandibulofacial dysostosis) is characterized by hypoplasia of what embryologic structures?**

Those derived from the first and second branchial arches.

○   **What are the differences between Apert's syndrome and Crouzon's syndrome?**

Syndactyly of the hands, a significant incidence of cleft palate and more serious facial deformities are present in Apert's syndrome.

○   **Where is the origin of the inferior oblique?**

Floor of the orbit.

○   **What is the 4 prism base-out prism test used for?**

Detection of small central suppression scotomas (1 to 2 degrees) in patients with small angles of esotropia, microstrabismus or previous surgical correction of a larger deviation.

○   **What is the embryologic origin of the temporal portion of the sclera?**

Mesoderm.

○ **Describe the features of cryptophthalmos.**

This condition represents failure of normal lid formation where the skin forms a continuous layer over the anterior surface of the eye. There is no cornea and the lens sits in an anomalous anterior chamber without iris or ciliary body. The retina and optic nerve are usually normal.

○ **Which extraocular rectus muscle is supplied by only one branch of the anterior ciliary artery?**

The lateral rectus is supplied by one branch of the anterior ciliary artery. The other recti muscles receive two branches of the anterior ciliary artery.

○ **How much does the anterior segment perfusion come from the anterior and posterior ciliary arteries?**

The seven anterior ciliary arteries supply 50% while the two posterior ciliary arteries supply the other 50%.

○ **What is the definition of polymorphism?**

Two or more alleles with a frequency greater than 1% in a given population.

○ **What are the causes of congenital iris heterochromia with the involved iris lighter in color?**

Congenital Horner's syndrome and Waardenburg's syndrome

○ **A 15-year-old female with a white forelock, fusion of the eyebrows, deafness and lateral displacement of her inner canthi and puncta presents to your clinic for a routine eye exam. What may you find on ocular examination?**

This patient has Waardenburg's syndrome, an autosomal dominant disorder. The patient will have iris heterochromia, and unilateral fundus hypopigmentation may also be present.

○ **What are some causes of congenital iris heterochromia with the involved iris darker in color?**

1. Ocular melanocytosis.
2. Oculodermal melanocytosis.
3. Sector iris hamartoma.

○ **A mentally retarded child presents to you with congenital cataracts, small crystalline lenses that appear disk shaped, and glaucoma. What is the probable diagnosis?**

Lowe's (oculocerebrorenal) syndrome, which consists of microspherophakia, congenital cataract, glaucoma, and aminoaciduria.

❍   **Where do the recti muscles insert from the limbus?**

The medial rectus inserts 5.5 mm from the limbus, inferior rectus 6.5 mm, lateral rectus 6.9 mm, and superior rectus 7.7 mm.

❍   **What is Hering's law?**

Hering's law states that equal and simultaneous innervation flows to muscles that act in the same direction of gaze. This is the reason why secondary deviations are greater than primary deviations in paralytic strabismus.

❍   **What is the incidence of congenital rubella syndrome after intrauterine infection?**

Intrauterine infections during the first 3 months of pregnancy result in a 50% incidence of rubella embryopathy, whereas infections after the fourth gestational month rarely result in the full rubella syndrome.

❍   **What are the ocular manifestations of congenital rubella?**

1. Cataract
2. Microphthalmos
3. Keratitis
4. Glaucoma
5. Pigmentary retinopathy

❍   **What is the most common ocular manifestation of congenital rubella?**

Pigmentary retinopathy, which is present in 40% of patients. It has a "salt and pepper" appearance.

❍   **How often do cataracts occur in children with congenital rubella syndrome?**

Cataracts are present in 20% of patients and are bilateral 75% of the time.

❍   **What immunological abnormalities are associated with ataxia-telangiectasia?**

Patients with ataxia-telangiectasia have low to absent levels of IgA and low to normal levels of IgG, resulting in increased susceptibility to sinopulmonary infections and increased risk of malignancy, such as lymphoma.

❍   **What eye manifestations may be seen in ataxia-telangiectasia?**

Supranuclear gaze palsies and conjunctival telangiectasias.

❍   **What part of the eye is the sclera thinnest and why is this important to know?**

The sclera is thinnest just posterior to the rectus muscle insertions (0.3 mm). This is especially important to remember when doing surgery on the extraocular muscles or using a superior rectus bridle suture, since taking too deep a pass with the needle can perforate the globe.

○ **A five-year-old child with a 1 mm anterior polar cataract OD has a best-corrected visual acuity of 20/80 OD and 20/30 OS. Her cycloplegic refraction is +4.25 D OD and +1.50 D OS. She has an exophoria of 5 diopters with distance fixation and none at near. What is the most likely cause for her poor vision?**

Anisometropic amblyopia.

○ **Which is more likely to manifest a concomitant vertical deviation, a dissociated vertical deviation (DVD) or inferior oblique overaction?**

Dissociated vertical deviation.

○ **What are the ocular associations of aniridia?**

1. Glaucoma (50%).
2. Congenital nystagmus.
3. Lenticular: cataract, upward subluxation, absence, and persistent pupillary membrane.
4. External: pannus, microcornea, sclerocornea, epibulbar dermoids, and corneolenticular adhesions.
5. Posterior: foveal hypoplasia, coloboma, disc hypoplasia.

○ **How many sporadic cases of aniridia can be associated with Wilm's tumor during early childhood?**

As many as one-third of sporadic cases of aniridia are associated with Wilm's tumor.

○ **What is Miller's syndrome?**

1. Aniridia.
2. Wilm's tumor.
3. Deletion of short arm of chromosome 11.

○ **What malignancy is the long arm 13 deletion (13q14) syndrome associated with?**

Retinoblastoma.

○ **Does a positive family history of aniridia increase or decrease the risk of developing Wilm's tumor in a child with aniridia?**

A positive family history of aniridia significantly decreases the likelihood of developing Wilm's tumor during childhood.

○ **What are the ocular features of Lowe's oculocerebrorenal syndrome?**

1. Congenital cataracts.
2. Congenital glaucoma.

3. Microphakia.

○   **Which of the abnormalities involving the sex chromosomes produces characteristic ophthalmic findings?**

Turner's syndrome, which can manifest with nystagmus, blue sclera, strabismus, prominent epicanthal folds, ptosis, and color vision deficits.

○   **A four-year old child with optic nerve hypoplasia OS has a best-corrected visual acuity of 20/30 OD and 20/200 OS. Her cycloplegic refraction is +1.50 D OU. What is the best treatment option for this patient?**

Occlusion therapy.

○   **What are the ocular features of Alport's hereditary nephritis syndrome?**

1. Anterior lenticonus.
2. Cataract.
3. Albipunctatus-like retinal lesions.

○   **In what congenital syndrome are Brushfield's spots commonly found in?**

Down's syndrome.

○   **Which extraocular muscle has the shortest tendon, and which extraocular muscle has the longest tendon?**

The medial rectus has the shortest tendon, measuring 3.7 mm, while the superior oblique has the longest at 20 mm.

○   **What is the differential diagnosis of proptosis present at birth?**

1. Congenital encephalocele.
2. Shallow orbit syndromes, eg. Apert's, Crouzon's.

○   **A one-year-old child presents with a capillary hemangioma associated with thrombocytopenia. What syndrome does this child have?**

Kasabach-Merritt syndrome.

○   **What signs are strongly suggestive of occult metastatic intracranial neuroblastoma in a child and require urgent referral to a pediatric neurologist?**

1. Opsoclonus.
2. Ocular flutter.
3. Acute cerebellar ataxia.

○   **What is Sherrington's law?**

It states that increased innervation to an extraocular muscle is accompanied by a decrease in innervation to its antagonist muscle.

O   **What is the innervation of the yoke muscle of the right inferior rectus?**

Left IV nerve.

O   **A pregnant woman is exposed to chickenpox during the third month of her pregnancy. What ocular abnormalities can occur in her fetus as a result?**

One-fourth of cases of maternal infection with varicella result in intrauterine infection with almost all occurring in the first two trimesters. Chorioretinitis is the most common ocular finding. Other manifestations include Horner's syndrome, cataract, optic nerve hypoplasia and microphthalmia. Systemic manifestations include hypoplastic limbs, delayed development, cicatricial skin lesions and small size for gestational age.

O   **A three-year-old boy is referred to you by his pediatrician for poor vision. He has a history of progressive deafness and mental retardation and a male cousin with a similar condition. On examination, the patient has bilateral vitreous hemorrhages and retinal detachments. What is the most likely diagnosis?**

Norrie's disease.

O   **What are the characteristics of nonrefractive esotropia?**

An esodeviation that is greater at near than distance fixation.

O   **What is the pathogenesis of nonrefractive esotropia?**

A high accommodative convergence to accommodation (AC:A) ratio. The effort to accommodate elicits an abnormally high accommodative convergence response.

O   **How may the AC:A ratio be determined?**

It may be calculated using the gradient or heterophoria methods. Clinically, the ratio is determined to be high if the near esodeviation is greater than the distance esodeviation by at least 10 prism diopters.

O   **What are some methods of managing a patient with nonrefractive esotropia?**

If the distance deviation is small or non-existent, possible management methods include the use of bifocal lenses, miotics, surgery or simple observation.

O   **What is accommodative esotropia?**

A convergent deviation associated with activation of the accommodative reflex.

O   **What are the forms of accommodative esotropia?**

Refractive, nonrefractive and partial or decompensated.

❍   **What causes refractive esotropia?**

A level of hyperopia that elicits an amount of accommodation and associated accommodative convergence that can not be overcome by fusional divergence mechanisms.

❍   **What is the preferred treatment of refractive accommodative esotropia?**

Full hyperopic correction as determined by cycloplegic refraction.

❍   **What is the characteristic refractive error of children with refractive accommodative esotropia?**

A level of hyperopia greater than the average population of the same age.

❍   **What is the typical age of presentation of refractive accommodative esotropia?**

Between two to three years of life. Rarely, it may occur prior to one year of age.

❍   **What is partial or decompensated accommodative esotropia?**

An esotropia that is not completely eliminated by the use of anti-accommodative therapy. It also describes an esodeviation that is initially eliminated with anti-accommodative treatment but then redevelops and can not be corrected by increasing the hyperopic prescription.

❍   **What is the cause of partial accommodative esotropia?**

It usually develops when there has been a delay between the onset of an accommodative esotropia and anti-accommodative treatment.

❍   **What is the indication for treatment of partial accommodative esotropia?**

When the non-accommodative portion is greater than 10 pd, surgery is indicated to reduce the deviation to enhance the development of binocular vision.

❍   **When should probing of the nasolacrimal duct be considered in a child suspected of having a congenital nasolacrimal duct obstruction or dacryostenosis?**

12-18 months of age.

❍   **What other ocular deviations can be associated with congenital esotropia?**

Dissociated vertical deviations (DVD) and inferior oblique overactions have been reported in up to 90% of patients with congenital esotropia. Parents must be warned that this can occur despite surgery for congenital esotropia.

❍   **What is the treatment of choice for bilateral inferior oblique overaction?**

Myectomy or recession of the inferior oblique muscles.

❍ **What is currently the treatment of choice for dissociated vertical deviation?**

Recession of the inferior oblique and reattachment adjacent to the lateral pole of the inferior rectus muscle.

❍ **How often is glaucoma associated with Peter's anomaly?**

More than 50% of patients with Peter's anomaly will develop glaucoma.

❍ **An 18-month-old child with a wandering left eye is found to have an enlarged, excavated optic disc with glial proliferation in its center, peripapillary staphyloma and an abnormal retinal vascular pattern emanating from the optic disc on ocular examination. The other eye is normal. What is your diagnosis, and is this hereditary?**

The patient has morning glory syndrome, which is nonhereditary and usually unilateral.

❍ **How often is retinal detachment associated with morning glory syndrome?**

Retinal detachments have been reported in up to one-third of cases.

❍ **What other ocular abnormalities may be found in eyes with morning glory syndrome?**

It can be associated with aniridia, microphthalmos, foveal hypoplasia and cataract.

❍ **What systemic abnormalities have been reported with morning glory syndrome?**

1. Absent corpus callosum.
2. Basal encephalocele.
3. Pituitary dysfunction.
4. Renal abnormalities.

❍ **What is the most common infectious cause of neonatal conjunctivitis?**

Chlamydia trachomatis.

❍ **What systemic disease can the neonatal chlamydial conjunctivitis be associated with?**

Neonatal chlamydial pneumonitis, which develops during the first 6 weeks of life and is characterized by nasal discharge, cough, and tachypnea.

❍ **What stain would you request for on conjunctival scrapings of suspected chlamydial conjunctivitis, and what will this show?**

Giemsa stain to identify intracytoplasmic inclusion bodies.

○   **What is the treatment of choice for neonatal chlamydial infection of the conjunctiva?**

Oral erythromycin syrup (50 mg/kg/day) in four divided doses for 14 days to treat both the conjunctivitis and pneumonitis. In addition, parents of infected children should be treated with oral tetracycline or erythromycin for 2 weeks.

○   **If the neonatal chlamydial conjunctivitis is left untreated, what ocular complications can result?**

Untreated chlamydial conjunctivitis usually resolves spontaneously after 8-12 months but may result in micropannus and scarring of the tarsal conjunctiva, In addition, these children are at an increased risk of developing a pneumonitis or otitis.

○   **Does topical silver nitrate 1% solution provide adequate prophylaxis against chlamydial conjunctivitis in newborns?**

No. Either topical erythromycin or tetracycline given within 1 hour after birth significantly decreases the chance of developing neonatal chlamydial conjunctivitis.

○   **A five-year-old girl with a history of low-grade fever, malaise and lymphadenopathy complains of decreased vision in her left eye. On examination, you find optic disc edema and a macular star present in her left eye. What is your diagnosis, and what is a common cause for this condition?**

The patient has a neuroretinitis, and recent studies suggest that cat-scratch fever is a common cause. It is confirmed using the ELISA test. Trimethoprim-sulfamethoxazole may shorten the course of the disease. Other known causes of neuroretinitis are syphilis and Lyme disease.

○   **Is this child at greater risk for developing multiple sclerosis later in life?**

No.

○   **What types of refractive errors are associated with X-linked congenital stationary night blindness and Leber's congenital amaurosis?**

75% of patients with Leber's congenital amaurosis have 3 diopters or more of hyperopia, while X-linked congenital stationary night blindness is usually associated with myopia.

○   **A 5-month-old infant is referred to you for evaluation because of poor vision. There is no nystagmus present. The pupils react normally to light, and the fundus appears normal. What is the likely diagnosis?**

Cortical blindness.

○   **An infant presents with nystagmus, poor vision, and small, hypoplastic optic discs. The MRI scan reveals agenesis of the corpus callosum. What is your diagnosis and is this hereditary condition?**

Bilateral optic disc hypoplasia combined with agenesis of the corpus callosum or the septum pellucidum is called septo-optic dysplasia or de Morsier's syndrome. This is generally a nonhereditary condition.

○ **A 15-year-old boy presents with sudden blurring of vision in his left eye. The visual acuity is 20/20 OD and 20/400 OS. A relative afferent pupillary defect is present in the left eye. His fundus examination is shows a hyperemic-looking disc and normal macula in his left eye. A visual field shows a central scotoma and the MRI of the head is normal. What is the most likely diagnosis, and what DNA abnormality is present in this disorder?**

This boy probably has Leber's hereditary optic neuropathy. This is associated with mutations in the mitochondrial DNA in at least three loci: nucleotides 11778, 3460, and 14484.

○ **What ocular abnormality will you most likely find in an infant with shaken baby syndrome, and what intracranial abnormality can be associated with it?**

The most common ocular abnormality associated with shaken baby syndrome is posterior pole retinal hemorrhages. This is usually associated with intracranial hemorrhages.

○ **What type of muscle fibers is found in extraocular muscles that are not found elsewhere in the body?**

Fibrillenstruktur (fast twitch) and Felderstruktur (slow twitch).

○ **What type of neuromuscular innervation does each motor neuron supply to the extraocular muscle fibers?**

The Fibrillenstruktur have en plaque neuromuscular innervation, while the Felderstruktur have en grappe (grapelike) neuromuscular supply.

○ **What are the clinical types of Duane's retraction syndrome?**

Type 1: (most common): limited abduction with normal or mildly impaired adduction.
Type 2: (least common): limited adduction with normal or mildly limited abduction.
Type 3: limited adduction and abduction.

○ **What are other ocular features seen in Duane's retraction syndrome?**

1. Ipsilateral retraction of the globe and narrowing of the palpebral fissure on attempted adduction
2. Upshoot or downshoot occasionally seen

○ **What are the indications for surgery in Duane's syndrome?**

A significant deviation in primary position, an anomalous head position, a large upshoot or downshoot or retraction of the globe that is cosmetically intolerable.

○ **What surgical procedure(s) should be avoided in Duane's syndrome?**

1. Resection of the lateral rectus which will increase the globe retraction.
2. Large medial rectus recessions, which may lead to a large exotropia when the patient looks into the field of gaze of the previously recessed medial rectus (caused by the co-innervation of the lateral rectus).

○   **If a recessive defect occurs in one out of every 5000 persons, what is the chance of an individual being a carrier?**

1 in 71 (get the square root of the frequency and multiply by 2).

○   **What are the three most common causes of unilateral cataracts in the pediatric population?**

1. Trauma.
2. Posterior lenticonus.
3. Persistent hyperplastic primary vitreous.

○   **A child with mild-to-moderate congenital ptosis in her right eye presents with blurred vision in her right eye and assumes a chin-up head position when fixating on a target. She is orthoptic on motility examination. What is the most likely cause of her poor vision?**

This child probably has anisometropic amblyopia. Up to 20% of children with congenital ptosis have significant refractive errors, which can produce this.

○   **Name other disorders on the differential diagnosis of congenital esotropia.**

1. Pseudoesotropia.
2. Duane retraction syndrome.
3. Möbius syndrome.
4. Nystagmus blockage syndrome.
5. Congenital sixth nerve palsy.
6. Early-onset accommodative esotropia.
7. Sensory esotropia.
8. Esotropia in the neurologically impaired.

○   **What other developments should be watched for after surgery for congenital esotropia?**

DVD, inferior oblique overaction (IOOA), recurrent amblyopia, recurrent esotropia and consecutive exotropia.

○   **How can IOOA be treated?**

Treatment is surgical and includes inferior oblique myotomy, myectomy, disinsertion, recession, denervation and extirpation and anterior transposition.

○   **What type of patients with juvenile rheumatoid arthritis has the highest risk for developing chronic anterior uveitis?**

Young ANA-positive, rheumatoid-negative females with pauciarticular (one to four joints) involvement have an estimated risk as high as 91% of developing uveitis.

○ **A patient presents with defective elevation of the left eye in adduction, overaction of the contralateral right superior rectus in abduction and downdrift of the left eye on contralateral right gaze. What is your diagnosis?**

Left Brown's syndrome.

○ **How common is recurrent esotropia following surgery for congenital esotropia?**

It may occur in 25% of patients and is usually accommodative (78%).

○ **What type of inheritance pattern may be found in the majority of cases of congenital cataracts in otherwise healthy newborns with a family history of congenital cataracts?**

An autosomal dominant pattern may be found in 50% or more of cases.

○ **What type of motility disturbances do patients with bilateral superior oblique palsies commonly complain about and demonstrate on examination?**

These patients are able to fuse at primary gaze but complain of difficulty of reading because of esotropia and excyclotorsion on down gaze.

○ **What type of diagnostic procedure is absolutely contraindicated in a patient whom you suspect has retinoblastoma?**

Vitreous or aqueous tap for histopathologic diagnosis.

○ **What percentage of all cases of retinoblastoma is caused by a germinal mutation?**

Approximately 40%.

○ **What is the most common secondary cancer associated with heritable retinoblastoma?**

Osteosarcoma.

○ **What is a trilateral retinoblastoma?**

It is a bilateral retinoblastoma with a pineal blastoma, a calcifying cancer of the pineal gland.

○ **How often are Lisch nodules present in patients with von Recklinghausen's disease?**

Lisch nodules will be present by age 6 years in more than 90% of patients.

❍   **A patient who undergoes strabismus surgery for left esotropia develops diplopia and left exotropia, which worsens on right gaze shortly after surgery. The patient is unable to adduct her left eye. What is your diagnosis and how would you manage this patient?**

The patient has a slipped medial rectus and requires a reoperation to identify the medial rectus and advance it.

❍   **Where is the origin of the superior oblique muscle?**

The superior oblique arises medial to the optic rim between the annulus of Zinn and the periorbita.

❍   **A three-year-old girl presents with a red eye of 1 week duration and poor vision in her left eye. On examination, there appears to be a hypopyon present in the anterior chamber. There is no view of the fundus. What diagnostic procedures should be done prior to performing an anterior chamber tap?**

CT scan or ocular ultrasound must be performed to rule out retinoblastoma, which can present with a pseudohypopyon and mimic uveitis in a young child. An anterior chamber tap into an eye with retinoblastoma can result in systemic spread of the disease and death.

❍   **Describe the characteristics of dissociated vertical deviation (DVD).**

DVD consists of a slow upward deviation of one or alternate eyes. Excyclotorsion can often be seen as the eye rotates upward. DVD may be latent or manifest. DVD occurs in up to 90% of children with a history of congenital esotropia. Its development is unrelated to the development of binocular vision.

❍   **A 5-year-old patient presents with a 15 prism diopter esotropia in primary position, which increases to 25 prism diopters on down gaze and decreases to 7 prism diopters on upgaze. There is no inferior oblique overaction present. How would you surgically manage this patient's strabismus?**

This patient has a V pattern esotropia, which can be corrected in this case with bimedial rectus recession for the esotropia and vertical displacement of the horizontal muscles, infraplacing the medial recti and supraplacing the lateral recti.

❍   **Describe the characteristics of inferior oblique overaction (IOOA).**

IOOA causes a hypertropia of the adducting eye when looking into side gaze. It occurs in up to 80% of patients with a history of congenital esotropia. Its development is unrelated to the development of binocular vision.

❍   **Why can DVD and IOOA be confused on clinical examination?**

Both may produce a hypertropia of the adducting eye in side gaze. This occurs in DVD due to the bridge of the nose breaking fixation and allowing the deviation to be manifest.

❍ **How can DVD and IOOA be differentiated?**

Although both may produce a hypertropia in side gaze, only IOOA will produce a corresponding hypotropia of the abducting eye. Excyclorotation of the hypertropic eye is not seen in IOOA.

❍ **What are the most common causes of VI nerve palsies in children, and how should you manage a child with a recent onset of VI nerve palsy?**

Trauma, congenital abducens nerve palsy, intracranial tumors such as pontine gliomas and cerebellar astrocytomas, and post-infectious causes account for almost 70% of VI nerve palsies in childhood. A complete neurologic workup should be performed and a MRI should be requested if additional abnormalities are found suggesting an intracranial tumor.

❍ **Where does the inferior oblique muscle insert?**

It inserts in the posterior inferior temporal quadrant adjacent to the macula. This is important to remember when working on the inferior oblique and helps to orient the enucleated globe.

❍ **Is Leber's congenital amaurosis commonly associated with high myopia or high hyperopia?**

High hyperopia.

❍ **When measuring the amount of strabismus with free prisms, why is it advisable not to stack prisms together in the same direction?**

Prisms do not add linearly when stacked together in the same direction. For example, stacking a 40 diopter prism with a 30 diopter prism will actually produce a prism displacement of 141 prism diopters. This does not occur, however, if a vertical and a horizontal prism are stacked together.

❍ **When performing the Brückner test to detect ocular misalignment, which eye is the deviating eye?**

In the presence of strabismus, the eye with the brighter light reflex is the deviating eye.

❍ **In general, do infants with congenital or infantile esotropia have a normal or a high AC/A ratio?**

The amount of esotropia is usually the same with both distance and near fixation in congenital or infantile esotropia. In other words, they usually have a normal AC/A ratio.

❍ **How often is Duane's syndrome bilateral?**

15%.

❍ **How often is perceptive deafness present in patients with Duane's syndrome?**

10%.

O   **What is the developmental neurologic abnormality in Duane's syndrome?**

Absence of the abducens nuclei and partial innervation of the lateral rectus by branches from the oculomotor nerves.

O   **What is Panum's area?**

Panum's area describes objects in the visual fields of both eyes that are seen as one object but fall on disparate retinal areas. Objects within Panum's area are seen as one and in stereo while objects outside Panum's area are seen as double.

O   **What is Aicardi syndrome?**

It is seen only in females and consists of chorioretinal lacunae, agenesis of the corpus callosum and infantile spasms.

O   **What are the main forms of neurofibromatosis?**

Type 1 (NF1) or von Recklinghausen disease consists of café-au-lait spots, neurofibromas, plexiform neuromas, iris hamartomas (Lisch nodules), optic gliomas and osseous lesions. It is caused by a gene mutation on chromosome 17 and accounts for 85% of all neurofibromatosis.

Type 2 (NF2) is produced by a mutation in chromosome 22 and produces bilateral acoustic neuromas. Ocular manifestations include cataracts prior to age 30 in two-thirds of patients, extraocular motor defects in 10% of cases and combined hamartomas of the RPE and retina and epiretinal membranes.

O   **What are the characteristics of the esotropia that occurs in patients with Mobius syndrome?**

It occurs early in life and is secondary to bilateral sixth nerve palsies. Forced duction testing is generally positive at the time of surgery.

O   **What is tuberous sclerosis?**

Tuberous sclerosis (Bourneville disease) is an autosomal dominant phacomatosis whose classic triad consists of mental handicap, epilepsy, and adenoma sebaceum. These patients develop astrocytic brain hamartomas in the periventricular area and give rise to epilepsy, mental handicap, and hydrocephalus. They may also develop visceral hamartomas such as rhabdomyomas of the heart and angiomyolipomas of the kidneys.

O   **What is the most common ocular manifestation of tuberous sclerosis?**

About 50% of patients with tuberous sclerosis have retinal or optic nerve astrocytomas, which are bilateral in 15% of cases.

O   **What are Ash leaf spots?**

They are hypopigmented patches of skin in the shape of an Ash leaf involving the trunk, limbs and scalp and are seen in tuberous sclerosis.

O   **What cranial nerve is involved in ophthalmoplegic migraine?**

Ophthalmoplegic migraine typically starts before the age 10 years and is characterized by recurrent, transient III nerve palsy, which begins after the headache.

O   **How would you treat ophthalmoplegic migraine?**

Trial of propranolol or amitriptyline determined as appropriate for the child's age and size by the pediatrician.

O   **How can Brown's syndrome be differentiated from an inferior oblique palsy or unilateral superior oblique overaction?**

1. Brown's syndrome will be forced duction positive in attempted elevation and adduction.
2. Brown's syndrome displays a V pattern in upgaze while superior oblique overaction will demonstrate an A pattern in downgaze.

O   **What are the indications for surgical treatment in Brown's syndrome?**

A hypotropia in primary position, a large downshoot in adduction or a compensatory face turn.

O   **How may Brown's syndrome be surgically treated?**

With a superior oblique tenotomy or tenectomy (with or without simultaneous inferior oblique weakening to avoid postoperative superior oblique palsy), superior oblique recession or placement of a superior oblique spacer.

O   **How may double elevator palsy be differentiated from Brown's syndrome?**

Double elevator palsy will have absent elevation in all fields of gaze whereas Brown's syndrome will have normal or near normal elevation in abduction.

O   **How can the ptosis that may be seen in double elevator palsy be determined to be a true ptosis or pseudoptosis?**

Have the patient fixate with the involved eye. If a pseudoptosis exists, it will disappear.

O   **What are the two types of double elevator palsies?**

Restrictive (forced duction positive on attempted elevation) and paretic (forced duction negative).

O   **What are the treatments options in double elevator palsy?**

They are based on the results of forced duction testing. If negative, a Knapp procedure may be performed. If positive, the tight inferior rectus is recessed.

O   **A woman has von Hippel-Lindau (VHL) disease. What is the risk that her daughter will develop the disease?**

VHL is an autosomal dominant phacomatosis. First degree relatives have a 50% risk of inheriting this disease. Annual evaluation including neuro-ophthalmologic, neurologic and MRI of the brain, spinal cord, chest, and pelvis should be performed in subjects at risk of inheriting VHL.

O   **What is heterogeneity?**

Different genotypes producing clinically similar phenotypic disorders are described by the term heterogeneity.

O   **What is the rubella syndrome?**

The rubella syndrome occurs if the mother is infected during the first trimester of pregnancy and may result in nuclear or lamellar congenital cataracts, corneal opacity, pigmentary retinopathy, hearing defects, and cardiac defects.

O   **What postoperative complication can occur if not all lens material is removed during cataract extraction in an infant with rubella syndrome?**

The rubella virus is present in the lens up to three years after birth. Incomplete removal of the lens will result in a viral-induced iridocyclitis.

O   **What are the features of congenital toxoplasmosis?**

Intracranial calcifications, chorioretinitis, seizures, hydrocephalus, microcephaly, hepatosplenomegaly, jaundice, anemia, and fever.

O   **What is the most common manifestation of congenital toxoplasmosis?**

Chorioretinitis.

O   **What is the incidence of congenital toxoplasmosis in offspring of women with toxoplasmosis during the first trimester?**

10 to 15% will demonstrate serological evidence of intrauterine disease, however these children have the most severe manifestations of the syndrome.

O   **What is the most common intrauterine infection?**

Congenital cytomegalovirus infection, which occurs in 0.5 to 2.5% of all newborns. Most infected children will develop normally, but 10 to 20% have congenital abnormalities.

O   **What are the manifestations of congenital cytomegalovirus infection?**

Hepatosplenomegaly, jaundice, petechiae, thrombocytopenia, microcephaly, cerebral calcification, optic atrophy and chorioretinitis.

❍   **What are the ocular manifestations of congenital cytomegalovirus infection?**

Chorioretinitis, microphthalmos, cataracts, keratitis, and optic atrophy.

❍   **What is Hutchinson's triad, and what disorder is associated with this?**

Interstitial keratitis, sensorineural deafness and malformed incisors in a child suggest congenital syphilis.

❍   **At what gestational age does exposure to syphilis produce congenital syphilis in fetuses?**

Congenital syphilis occurs in fetuses exposed to *Treponema pallidum* only after the 16th gestational week. Syphilis infections acquired earlier than this frequently result in fetal death.

❍   **What are the ocular manifestations of congenital syphilis?**

Interstitial keratitis, chorioretinitis, optic atrophy, uveitis.

❍   **At what age does interstitial keratitis from congenital syphilis occur?**

It occurs in up to 40% of untreated children and most commonly occurs in children 5-20 years of age.

❍   **How often is the interstitial keratitis of congenital syphilis bilateral?**

It is bilateral in 80% and is usually accompanied by iridocyclitis and iris atrophy.

❍   **Describe the features of congenital syphilitic chriorioretinis.**

It usually results in peripheral areas of pigment mottling, but in severe cases can result in extensive pigmentary changes resembling retinitis pigmentosa which is sometimes referred to as pseudoretinitis pigmentosa.

❍   **What is nanophthalmos?**

It is a rare disease characterized by a small eye, high hypermetropia, weak but thick sclera, and a tendency to angle closure glaucoma.

❍   **Why should eye surgery in a nanophthalmic eye be avoided where possible?**

Any surgery, but especially intraocular surgery and even laser trabeculoplasty may be complicated by severe uveal effusion.

❍   **What are the ocular manifestations of Treacher-Collins syndrome?**

Coloboma of the outer third of the lower lid and antimongoloid slant of the palpebral fissures. The mode of inheritance is autosomal dominant with complete penetrance but variable expressivity.

O   **What are the other facial abnormalities seen in Treacher-Collins syndrome?**

Malformations of the face include malar hypoplasia, often with absence of the zygomatic arch, absence of the nasofrontal angle giving a bird or fish-like profile, hypoplasia of the lower jaw with macrostomia and abnormal dention. The external ear is malformed, and there are often accessory auricular appendages and blind fistulae between the angles of the mouth and ears.

O   **What is Goldenhar's syndrome?**

This is characterized by epibulbar dermoids or lipodermoids, preauricular appendages, and vertebral anomalies. Cardiac or pulmonary abnormalities are common. Other ocular findings may include microphthalmos, ocular colobomata and coloboma of the eyelid, usually the middle third of the upper eyelid.

O   **What histologic feature is seen in all types of rhabdomyosarcoma?**

Cytoplasmic cross-striations.

O   **What is the most common type of rhabdomyosarcoma?**

Embryonal rhabdomyosarcoma.

O   **Which type of rhabdomyosarcoma has the best prognosis?**

Pleomorphic or differentiated type.

O   **Which type of rhabdomyosarcoma has the worst prognosis?**

Alveolar rhabdomyosarcoma.

O   **What does optimal management of rhabdomyosarcoma consist of?**

Biopsy, followed by radiotherapy and chemotherapy.

O   **What is the most common malignant solid tumor in children?**

Neuroblastoma.

O   **How often does neuroblastoma metastasize to the orbit?**

40% of cases, which typically presents with abrupt onset of proptosis accompanied by lid ecchymosis.

O   **What are the features of intracranial metastasis of neuroblastoma?**

Opsoclonus, ocular flutter, acute cerebellar ataxia.

○   **A child has a congenital facial palsy and inability to abduct her eyes. Vertical eye movements are normal, as are the pupils, the vision the optic nerves and fundus. What is your diagnosis?**

Möbius syndrome.

○   **A child is unable to elevate her left eye, which is complete when the eye is adducted and lessens considerable with abduction. Forced duction testing is positive on attempted passive elevation of the eye in adduction. What is your diagnosis?**

Brown's syndrome, which is a developmental anomaly of the superior oblique tendon, whose anterior portion is congenitally short.

○   **How will a child with a right IV nerve palsy prefer to hold his head?**

The child will prefer to rotate and tilt his head to the left.

○   **Following closed head trauma, a child prefers to depress his chin to achieve binocularity. What is the probable cause?**

Bilateral IV nerve palsy.

○   **What other condition must be considered in an acquired IV nerve palsy in a child without a history of head trauma?**

Posterior fossa tumor.

○   **How long does it takes for the anterior ciliary arteries to re-establish anterior segment perfusion after removing a rectus muscle during strabismus surgery?**

Vessels do not re-establish perfusion to the anterior segment.

○   **Which recti muscles provide more perfusion to the anterior segment, the horizontal or the vertical recti muscles?**

The vessels supplying the vertical recti are the most important in anterior segment perfusion, and one vertical muscle should remain intact during multiple muscle surgery to avoid anterior segment ischemia.

○   **What systemic disorders are associated with blue sclera?**

1.   Osteogenesis imperfecta.
2.   Hypophosphatasia.
3.   Syndromes: Marfan's, Ehler-Danlos, Crouzon's, Turner's, Albright's hereditary osteodystrophy, Hallermann-Streiff, Bloch-Sulzberger.

O   **A 10-year-old patient with a head tilt to the left since birth and a comitant LHT of 5 prism diopters undergoes patching of the right eye for several hours. What will be the result of patching in this patient?**

Patching has no effect on congenital torticollis.

O   **What will palpation of the neck in the patient above likely reveal?**

Palpation will likely reveal a firm, thickened sternocleidomastoid on the left side from fibrosis. There is marked resistance to passive straightening of the head.

O   **Which side may a patient with a right superior rectus palsy tilt his head?**

With paralyses of the vertical rectus muscles, the direction of the head tilt is inconsistent and are of little diagnostic significance. The head may be tilted toward either the paretic or the sound side in vertical rectus palsies.

O   **Which side will a patient with left inferior oblique palsy prefer to tilt his head?**

With inferior oblique paralysis, the head is tilted toward the paretic side; in this case, toward the left side.

O   **In Turner's syndrome, is the incidence of color deficiency increased, decreased or the same as in the normal male population?**

It is the same.

O   **What is the hereditary pattern of familial retinoblastoma?**

Although the hereditary pattern is that of an autosomal dominant mutation clinically, the mutation is recessive at the cellular level, specifically at the human chromosome 13q14 region.

O   **What is pleiotropism?**

Pleiotropism refers to multiple abnormalities produced by a single mutant gene.

O   **What is prism adaptation and how is it used?**

In prism adaptation, the patient is given press-on base-out prism for any residual esotropia that remains after prescribing the full hyperopic correction. The patient then returns in 2 weeks and if the esotropia has increased, a larger prism is then given. This process continues until the deviation remains stable. The surgeon then operates on the full "prism adapted" angle.

O   **What is cyclic esotropia?**

Cyclic esotropia is a rare motility disorder that is often acquired. Typically, it is a large-angle esodeviation that alternates with orthophoria on a 48 hour cycle. Other cycle frequencies have also been reported.

○ **What is congenital exotropia?**

A divergent strabismus that develops prior to six months of age and documented before one year of age.

○ **What are the characteristics of congenital exotropia?**

The characteristics of congenital exotropia are similar to congenital esotropia. The angle of deviation is large and other motility disorders such as inferior oblique overaction and dissociated vertical deviation commonly occurs. As in congenital esotropia, the treatment is surgical.

○ **Describe the characteristics of intermittent exotropia.**

Intermittent exotropia is a divergent strabismus that may be latent or manifest. The tropic stage may be seen when the patient is tired, ill or if fusion is interrupted, such as when one eye is covered.

○ **What is the natural course of intermittent exotropia?**

The long-term course of intermittent exotropia is unknown as most patients with the disorder generally undergo treatment at sometime in their lives. Most authorities believe that, left untreated, the disorder will worsen.

○ **How can intermittent exotropia be categorized?**

Intermittent exotropia may be characterized according to the size of the deviation at distance as compared to the size of the deviation at near. A common method of categorization has been:

Divergence excess: distance deviation greater than near.
Convergence insufficiency: near deviation greater than distance.
Basic: distance deviation same as near.
Pseudodivergence excess: near deviation is less than distance until the patient is measured at near through +3.00 D lenses when the near deviation increases to equal the distance.

○ **What is another way of categorizing the forms of intermittent exotropia based upon the distance and near deviations?**

By evaluating the AC/A ratio. Those patients with a near deviation less than the distance deviation are said to have a high AC/A ratio, those with a near deviation greater than the distance have a low AC/A and those where the deviation at near equals the distance have a normal AC/A.

○ **What are the typical characteristics of intermittent exotropia as it worsens?**

Intermittent exotropia may be considered as possibly evolving through four phases

Phase I.   Exophoria at distance, orthophoria at near.
Phase II.   Intermittent exotropia at distance, orthophoria or Intermittent exotropia at near.
Phase III.   Exotropia at distance, exophoria or intermittent exotropia at near.
Phase IV.   Exotropia at distance and near.

As the condition worsens, the deviation is seen more frequently. It may be seen when the patient is not tired or ill. In a young child, suppression may occur that allows the strabismus to be manifest constantly. The patient may be diplopic or infer it by closing one eye.

❍ What is lateral incomitance?

Lateral incomitance is a decrease in the deviation when it is measured in extreme right or left gaze. Several authors have stressed the importance of reducing the amount of surgery in laterally incomitant exotropia to avoid an overcorrection. Other authors believe that lateral incomitance occurs secondary to measurement artifact.

❍ What are the indications for treatment of intermittent exotropia?

In a younger child, if the condition is progressing from Phase II to Phase III, treatment is indicated to try to prevent the development of a suppression scotoma. If the child closes or covers one eye for viewing, the exodeviation is too large for the fusional convergence mechanisms to control and diplopia occurs. Treatment is indicated in this situation to correct the annoying symptom. In Phase III, with constant exotropia at distant fixation but an exophoria or intermittent exotropia at near, a suppression scotoma is present at distance fixation. At near, some degree of binocular function is usually present. Treatment should be offered at this stage in order to try and maintain whatever binocular function is present at near, and perhaps regain what has been lost at distance.

❍ What are some non-surgical methods that may be used to treat intermittent exotropia?

Orthoptic exercises, prism glasses, weak cycloplegics, occlusion therapy and overminus correcting lenses.

❍ What is the purpose of occlusion therapy in the treatment of intermittent exotropia?

Part time occlusion is used to eliminate the need for suppression in a young child with intermittent exotropia. When the deviation occurs while the child is not occluded, he/she will then be capable of experiencing diplopia and may attempt to control the deviation. It is generally used to delay surgery in young children until they are more visually mature.

❍ How may the classification system for intermittent exotropia be used when deciding upon the type of surgery to perform?

A surgeon may choose to weaken the apparently overacting or strengthen the apparently underacting muscles. Surgery based upon the classification system described earlier would be:

Divergence excess: bilateral lateral rectus recession.
Convergence insufficiency: bilateral medial rectus resection.
Basic type: unilateral lateral rectus recession combined with a
                                             unilateral medial rectus resection.

Many surgeons prefer to perform symmetric surgery and therefore use a bilateral lateral rectus recession regardless of the "type" of intermittent exotropia

O   **What is the desired early alignment status for a patient undergoing a bilateral lateral rectus recession for the treatment of intermittent exotropia?**

A small initial overcorrection with an esotropia of 5-10 pd in the first postoperative week.

O   **What are A and V patterns?**

An A pattern is a horizontal deviation that becomes more convergent (or less divergent) in upgaze and less convergent (more divergent) in downgaze. A V pattern is a horizontal deviation that becomes more convergent (less divergent) in downgaze and less convergent (more divergent) in downgaze. An A-Pattern is said to exist if divergence increases in down gaze by 10 or more prism diopters. A V-Pattern signifies an increase in divergence of 15 or more prism diopters in up-gaze.

O   **What is typically seen in patients with large A or V patterns?**

Oblique dysfunction. Large A patterns are typically seen in patients with superior oblique overaction. Large V patterns are commonly seen in patients with inferior oblique overaction or superior oblique underaction.

O   **How may A and V patterns be surgically treated when oblique dysfunction does not exist?**

Moving or offsetting the horizontal rectus muscle insertion up or down weakens the action of that muscle when the eye is moved in the direction of the offsetting. It follows that moving the medial rectus toward the apex of an A and V pattern is appropriate for correcting the incomitant deviation. Conversely, moving the lateral rectus muscle toward the open end of the A or V is also appropriate for correcting the incomitant deviation. This is true regardless of whether recession or resection is performed.

O   **How may A and V patterns be treated when associated with oblique dysfunction?**

By weakening or strengthening the involved oblique muscles.

O   **What type of A or V pattern should be treated cautiously when associated with oblique dysfunction?**

A pattern intermittent exotropia. Because these patients may be bifoveal fixators, performing a superior oblique tenotomy in these patients may lead to torsional diplopia, which may produce a head tilt if an asymmetric result occurs.

○   **How may complete oculomotor nerve palsy be surgically treated?**

Because the superior and inferior rectus will be paretic, they can not be transposed. Treatment may involve a significant weakening of the lateral rectus and transposition of the superior oblique tendon to an area adjacent to the medial rectus.

○   **How can superior oblique function be evaluated in the presence of a third nerve palsy?**

With attempted adduction and depression, the globe may be seen to incyclorotate.

○   **What are the results of the three step test in a superior oblique palsy?**

A hypertropia that is worse on gaze to the contralateral side and worse on head tilt to the ipsilateral side.

○   **How may newly acquired fourth nerve palsy be differentiated from a longstanding palsy that has only recently decompensated?**

Patients with longstanding fourth nerve palsy will display large vertical fusional amplitudes. Examination of old photographs in a person with a longstanding palsy will often demonstrate an abnormal head posture. Patients with congenital palsies will often have facial asymmetry manifest as midfacial hemihypoplasia on the dependent side opposite the affected superior oblique.

○   **What findings on clinical examination may help to detect the presence of bilateral fourth nerve palsy?**

Hypertropias that alternate on side gaze.
Hypertropias that alternate on head tilt testing.
A V pattern esotropia.
A large degree of cyclotorsion, often more than 10 degrees.

○   **What surgical procedures may be used to treat a unilateral superior oblique palsy?**

The involved superior oblique tendon may be tucked or the antagonist inferior oblique may be weakened. For large deviations, both may also be performed at the same time or either procedure may be combined with an ipsilateral superior rectus or contralateral inferior rectus recession. Knapp's classification is used by some surgeons to determine which muscle(s) to operate.

○   **How may a bilateral fourth nerve palsy with torsional diplopia be surgical treated?**

With the use of a bilateral Harada-Ito procedure where the anterior half of the superior oblique tendon is advanced to an area superior to the border of the lateral rectus.

○   **How may recently acquired sixth nerve palsy be managed?**

With observation and occlusion to eliminate diplopia (alternate occlusion in a child in the amblyogenic age group) or oculinum injection into the antagonist medial rectus to provide immediate alignment and/or prevent contracture of the medial rectus.

O   **What are surgical treatment options for a patient with a sixth nerve palsy?**

The ipsilateral medial rectus may be recessed in combination with a resection of the involved lateral rectus. In cases of a complete palsy, a transposition procedure may be performed. Transposition procedures include a Jensen, Hummelsheim or full tendon transfer of the superior and inferior rectus muscle to an area adjacent to the lateral rectus. The medial rectus may be recessed in conjunction with a transposition procedure but it carries the risk of anterior segment ischemia. Therefore, some surgeons will inject botulin toxin into the medial rectus along with a transposition procedure.

O   **Describe some problems associated with strabismus surgery.**

In addition to the well-known propensity of strabismus surgery to trigger the oculocardiac reflex, there is also an increased incidence of malignant hyperthermia in patients with conditions such as strabismus or ptosis. This observation is consistent with the impression that people susceptible to malignant hyperthermia often have localized areas of skeletal muscle weakness or other musculo-skeletal abnormalities. Other aspects of strabismus surgery of interest to include succinylcholine-induced interference with the forced duction test (FDT) and an increased incidence of postoperative nausea and vomiting.

O   **Describe the oculocardiac reflex.**

The oculocardiac reflex is a trigeminal-vagal reflex, leading to bradycardia, hypotension and premature ventricular contractions. The afferent pathway is by way of the ciliary ganglion to the ophthalmic division of the trigeminal nerve, and through the gasserian ganglion to the main sensory nucleus in the 4th ventricle. The efferent pathway is the vagus nerve. This reflex is triggered by pressure on the globe and by traction on the extraocular muscles as well as on the conjunctiva or on the orbital structures. Moreover, the reflex may also be elicited by performance of a retrobulbar block, by ocular trauma, and by direct pressure on tissue remaining in the orbital apex after enucleation. The incidence is augmented by anxiety, light general anesthesia, hypoxia, and hypercarbia.

O   **How do we treat the oculocardiac reflex, once established?**

There is consensus that continuous monitoring of the electrocardiogram (ECG) is important during all types of eye surgery to detect potentially dangerous cardiac rhythm disturbances. If a cardiac dysrhythmia appears, initially the surgeon should stop operative manipulation. Next, the patient's anesthetic depth and ventilatory status are evaluated. Commonly, heart rate and rhythm will return to baseline within 20 seconds after institution of these measures. Moreover, with repeated manipulation, bradycardia is less likely to recur, probably secondary to fatigue of the reflex arc at the level of the cardio-inhibitory center. However, if the initial cardiac dysrhythmia is especially serious or if the reflex tenaciously recurs, atropine should be administered intravenously.

RETINA AND VITREOUS

❍ **How do anatomists define the macula?**

That portion of the posterior retina with xanthophyllic pigment and two or more layers of ganglion cells.

❍ **How large is the macula?**

5-6 mm (5000-6000 microns).

❍ **What is the name for the small, slightly concave portion of the posterior retina that is devoid of capillaries and occupied almost exclusively by cones?**

Foveal avascular zone.

❍ **How large is the fovea?**

1.5 mm, 1500 microns, 1 disk diameter (DD), 5 degrees.

❍ **What area is defined by the lack of a ganglion cell and inner nuclear layer?**

Foveola: approx. 350 microns, approx. equal to the foveal avascular zone (FAZ).

❍ **What is the name for the depression in the center of the foveola?**

Umbo, clivus, light reflex.

❍ **What is the deepest portion of the retina supplied by branches of the central retinal artery?**

The inner portion of the inner nuclear layer.

❍ **What is the exception to the role of retinal blood supply of the choriocapillaris?**

Choriocapillaris normally supplies the outer portions of the retina up to the outer part of the inner nuclear layer—a cilioretinal artery can sometimes supply an area of inner retina.

❍ **What makes up the outer portion of the blood-retina border?**

Tight junctions between adjacent RPE cells (zonulae occludentes).

❍ **What makes up the inner portion of the blood-retina border?**

Retinal capillary endothelial cells.

❍   **What is the chromatophore for all four classes of human visual pigments (rhodopsin, red, blue, and green), and how is it oriented to the plane of the lipid bilayer?**

11-*cis*-retinaldehyde is oriented parallel to the plane of the lipid bilayer and, therefore, perpendicular to the path of photons.

❍   **When are old rod disks and cones shed?**

Rod disks are shed at dawn and cone disks are shed at dusk.

❍   **Why is the neuroretina usually devoid of water?**

The RPE has a high capacity for water transport.

❍   **What syndrome can be associated with congenital hypertrophy of the RPE?**

Gardner Syndrome (intestinal polyposis).

❍   **What are the parts of the ciliary body?**

The ciliary body has two parts, which are pars plicata ciliaris and pars plana ciliaris. The pars plicata is a circumficial zone about two and a half millimeters in the anterior posterior dimension, extending posteriorly from the iris root and contains 70 to 80 ciliary processes. The pars plana ciliaris is about three millimeters wide nasally and four and a half millimeters temporally, and extends from the pars plicata anteriorly to the ora serrata posteriorly. The posterior part of the pars plana is covered with vitreous base.

❍   **What artery is the origin for both the choroid and the central retinal artery?**

Ophthalmic artery.

❍   **How is pars plana vitrectomy performed?**

There are three incisions made in pars plana, for which one is used for infusion of fluid to maintain intraocular pressure. The second port is used for illumination with fiber optics. The third opening is used to allow a vitrectomy instrument to be used in the vitreous cavity. Other instruments (such as laser probes, intraocular scissors, etc.) are interchangeable through one of these openings.

❍   **What is open sky vitrectomy?**

It includes making a large incision in the cornea and removing the lens. The later techniques were pioneered by Schepens and Constable. For these operations, a long focal length microscope was used.

❍   **When is open sky vitrectomy performed?**

Open-sky vitrectomy is an operation used for desperate cases of detached retina. One of the best indications for this procedure is grade V retinopathy of prematurity, which has total fixed retinal detachment. For these patients, this procedure has been more effective than closed vitrectomy technique.

❍ **What is the best predictor of metastatic potential for retinoblastoma histopathologically?**

Optic nerve invasion.

❍ **Where are the attachment sites between the vitreous gel and the surrounding structures?**

The anterior surface of the vitreous gel is attached to the posterior lens capsule along a circular zone called the ligament of Wieger. This is a firm attachment in young individuals and weakly attached or completely absent in the elderly. The most important attachment site of vitreous gel is the vitreous base, which is a circumferential zone where the vitreous is attached to the adjacent epithelium of the pars plana and to the peripheral retina. The central vitreous is also attached alone the peripheral margin of the optic nerve head, to the retina in the posterior pole, and some retinal veins in the midperiphery. The vitreous gel is also adherent to the retina in other abnormal areas such as sites of lattice degeneration, cystic retinal tufts, and certain chorioretinal scars.

❍ **What wavelengths of light pass through the vitreous gel?**

The vitreous body is a clear gel that allows the transmission of about 90% of light wavelengths between 300 to 1400 nm.

❍ **What is the most common cause of cotton wool spots?**

Diabetic retinopathy.

❍ **What forms the external limiting membrane of the retina?**

It is formed by tight junctions between the photoreceptor inner segments and the lateral margins of Müller's cells.

❍ **Which of the following retinal proteins is/are involved in the phototransduction cascade: S antigen, interphotoreceptor retinoid binding protein (IRBP) and peripherin?**

Retinal S antigen.

❍ **What is a highly characteristic histologic finding in the iris pigment epithelium of diabetics?**

Lacy vacuolization of the iris pigment epithelium.

❍ **What organ is the most common site of metastasis for uveal melanomas?**

Liver.

○ **What type of collagen is vitreous composed of?**

Type II collagen, which is specific for vitreous.

○ **What is the most abundant component of the vitreous body?**

Water is the major component of the vitreous body. It comprises 98% of its volume.

○ **What is the optical function of the vitreous?**

It acts as an ultraviolet filter. There is decreased transmission at 350 to 300 nm wavelength and zero thereafter as well as decreased infrared transmission at 800 nm wavelength and zero after 1600 nm.

○ **How often do patients with acute posterior vitreous detachment and vitreous hemorrhage have retinal breaks?**

70% will have peripheral retinal breaks.

○ **How far is the ora serrata from the limbus?**

6 mm.

○ **Where do we make the incision for pars plana vitrectomy?**

An incision that is made three to four millimeters posterior to the limbus goes to the anterior part of the pars plana and avoids the vitreous base and the pars plicata. The blood vessels for pars plana are radially oriented and the circumficial incision rarely causes any bleeding into the eye.

○ **Is the insertion of the superior rectus muscle anterior or posterior to the ora serrata?**

Posterior.

○ **How far is the equator from the limbus?**

16 mm.

○ **How often is there no family history of retinitis pigmentosa in a patient with the disease?**

40% of patients with retinitis pigmentosa will have no family history of the disease.

○ **What is the probability that the next child of a patient with a history of bilateral retinoblastoma will develop the disease?**

50%.

❍ **In what other tumor besides retinoblastoma may Flexner-Wintersteiner and Homer Wright rosettes be seen?**

Medulloepithelioma.

❍ **What are Elschnig spots?**

They are choroidal infarcts seen in severe hypertensive retinopathy.

❍ **What is Terson's syndrome?**

Retinal and vitreous hemorrhage associated with posttraumatic subarachnoid and subdural hemorrhage.

❍ **What is the most common cause of spontaneous vitreous hemorrhage in adults?**

Diabetic retinopathy.

❍ **A 60-year-old patient has an acute, spontaneous vitreous hemorrhage that prevents visualization of the fundus. What diagnostic test should next be requested for in this case?**

Ultrasonography to rule out the possibility of retinal detachment or a neoplasm.

❍ **What is Cloquet's canal?**

It is the embryological remnant of the hyaloid vascular system.

❍ **What can be observed in essentially normal eyes that are remnants of the fetal vasculature?**

Mittendorf's dot, vascular loops, Bergmeister's papilla.

❍ **At what time during embryonic development does the primary vitreous first form?**

During the 3rd through 9th weeks.

❍ **What is the source of the secondary vitreous?**

Vitreous fibrils are formed by the inner retina while the Müller cells produce hyaluronic acid.

❍ **By which month is Cloquet's canal formed?**

5th month.

❍ **The tertiary vitreous forms what ocular structures?**

Zonular fibers.

○   **What is the most common presentation of PHPV?**

Leukocoria.

○   **What are the most common characteristics of PHPV?**

Unilateral in 90% of cases, normal full term infants, microphthalmia, shallow anterior chamber, natural course leads to blindness.

○   **What is the hallmark of hereditary vitreoretinopathies?**

Vitreous liquefaction resulting in an optically empty vitreous cavity.

○   **What are the most common fundus abnormalities that are seen in hereditary vitreoretinopathies?**

Equatorial and perivascular (radial) lattice, retinoschisis, chorioretinal atrophy, optic atrophy.

○   **What are the 2 hereditary vitreoretinopathies most commonly *not* associated with systemic abnormalities?**

Wagner's Disease and Jansen's Disease.

○   **What differentiates Wagner's and Jansen's Disease?**

Jansen's Disease has a high incidence of retinal detachment. Wagner's Disease is not associated with retinal detachment.

○   **What disease is associated with heredity vitreoretinopathies and systemic abnormalities?**

Stickler's Syndrome.

○   **What systemic abnormalities are generally found in Stickler's Syndrome?**

1. Hyperextensibility and enlargement of joints.
2. Arthritis and spondyloepiphyseal dysplasia.
3. Orofacial findings include mid-facial flattening, cleft palette, and the Pierre-Robin malformation complex (micrognathia, cleft palette, and glossoptosis).

○   **Why is it important to recognize Stickler's Syndrome?**

Because of the high incidence of retinal detachment which are normally very difficult to repair.

○   **What is the most common inheritance pattern in Stickler's Syndrome?**

Autosomal dominant.

○   **What are the findings in ocular ischemic syndrome?**

Stenosis of the carotid artery can lead to ocular ischemia, ipsilateral absence of arcus senilis, iris neovascularization and midperipheral retinal hemorrhages.

○   **What composes asteroid hyalosis?**

Calcium soaps.

○   **What is the ratio of pericytes to retinal vascular endothelial cells in normal retinal blood vessels?**

1 to 1 ratio.

○   **What type of configuration can choroidal melanomas assume on B-scan ultrasound?**

Collar button configuration.

○   **What are the criteria for diabetic clinically significant macular edema (CSME)?**

Retinal thickening within 500 microns of the center of the fovea.

Hard exudates at or within 500 microns of the center of the fovea if associated with thickening of adjacent retina.

Retinal thickening 1 disc diameter in size or larger if within 1 disc diameter from the center of the fovea.

○   **When should IDDM, NIDDM and pregnant patients have there first eye exam?**

IDDM - within 5 years of diagnosis.
NIDDM - at time of diagnosis.
Pregnant - early in 1st trimester.

○   **What are the retinal findings of preproliferative diabetic retinopathy?**

Cotton wool spots, dark blot hemorrhages, vascular changes (beading, looping, sausage-like), and intraretinal microvascular anomalies (IRMA).

○   **What was the conclusion of the Sorbinil Retinopathy Trial?**

Sorbinil, an aldose reductase inhibitor, was ineffective at preventing progression of diabetic retinopathy when given at a dosage of 250 mg daily.

○   **What did the Diabetes Control and Complications Trial demonstrate?**

Aggressive efforts to normalize blood sugars with insulin pumps may initially worsen the retinopathy in some patients during the first few months of treatment. Ultimately, strict control of blood sugar with intensive insulin therapy:

1. Reduced the risk of development of retinopathy in patients without retinopathy by 76%.
2. Reduced by 47% the risk of development of severe nonproliferative and proliferative retinopathy in patients with mild to moderate nonproliferative retinopathy, and slowed the progression of retinopathy in patients with mild to moderate nonproliferative retinopathy by 54%.

❍   What patients can the results of the Diabetes Control and Complications Trial be applied to?

Type I IDDM patients only.

❍   What group of patients can show a worsening of diabetic retinopathy with intensive control?

Patients with mild or moderate NPDR at the time of change to intensive control.

❍   How did the Diabetic Retinopathy Study (DRS) define Severe Visual Loss (SVL)?

VA less than 5/200 on two consecutive follow-up visits 4 months apart

❍   What are the high-risk characteristics for severe visual loss in proliferative diabetic retinopathy (PDR) which indicate treatment using laser photocoagulation?

Neovascularization of the disc (NVD) more than one-quarter disc in area
Vitreous or preretinal hemorrhage associated with:
1. NVD of any size or
2. Neovascularization elsewhere (NVE) more than one-half disc in area.

❍   What effect did the DRS demonstrate concerning severe visual loss in eyes treated with PRP?

A 50% or greater reduction in the rate of severe visual loss over a five year period.

❍   What treatment did the DRS recommend for high-risk PDR?

PRP - 1200 or more 500 micron burns separated by 1/2 burn width.

❍   How did the Early Treatment diabetic Retinopathy Study (ETDRS) define Moderate Visual Loss (MVL)?

Doubling of the visual angle, a drop of 15 letters on the ETDRS vision charts, or a drop of three or more lines of Snellen acuity.

❍   **What were the conclusions of the Early Treatment Diabetic Retinopathy Study (ETDRS)?**

Focal laser coagulation should be considered for all eyes with CSME because treatment reduces the risk of visual loss by 50%.

Panretinal photocoagulation (PRP) should be considered in patients who are at high risk of developing proliferative diabetic retinopathy (PDR) while mild to moderate nonproliferative diabetic retinopathy (NPDR) can be observed.

Systemic aspirin (650 mg/day) does not prevent the development of PDR, nor does it increase the risk of visual loss or vitreous hemorrhage.

❍   **Describe Severe NPDR as defined by the ETDRS.**

Severe NPDR was defined by the ETDRS as any one of the following: intraretinal heme and microaneurysms in 4 quadrants; venous beading in 2 quadrants; IRMA in 1 quadrant. Remember the 4:2:1 rule for severe NPDR.

❍   **How did the ETDRS define very severe NPDR?**

Any two of the preceding qualifications for severe NPDR will make the diagnosis very severe NPDR.

❍   **What did the ETDRS show concerning the optimal timing of PRP?**

Consider PRP when NPDR is severe - do not delay using PRP when a patient has high-risk PDR.

❍   **What groups of patients are predisposed to poor visual acuity even after photocoagulation?**

Those with diffuse macular edema, macular ischemia, hard exudates in the fovea, or marked CME.

❍   **What is the risk of developing high-risk PDR within one year for patients with very severe NPDR?**

Very severe NPDR - 45% risk of developing high-risk PDR within one year.

❍   **What systemic conditions may lead to a worsening of diabetic retinopathy?**

Hypertension, severe carotid vascular disease, and pregnancy.

❍   **Is photocoagulation recommended if high-risk PDR develops during pregnancy?**

Yes.

❍   **Which should be treated first, CSME or high-risk PDR?**

CSME.

○ **Describe the technique for focal laser photocoagulation.**

Focal - a 50-100 micron spot size, 0.1 second or less duration, attempt to whiten or darken all leaking microaneurysms between 500 and 3000 microns from the center of the macula.

○ **Describe the technique for grid laser photocoagulation.**

Grid - a 50-100 micron spot size, 0.1 second or less duration, spots at least 1 burn width apart applied to area of diffuse leakage >500 microns form the center of the macula and >500 microns from the optic disc.

○ **Which should be done first - focal laser or cataract extraction?**

Focal laser.

○ **What type of lasers may be more successful for PRP in patients with vitreous heme?**

Krypton red or diode lasers.

○ **When should NVI be treated with PRP?**

If there is contiguous NVI of the pupil and midstromal iris or any NVE.

○ **What are potential adverse effects of panretinal photocoagulation of diabetic retinopathy?**

1. Angle closure glaucoma from choroidal effusion.
2. Decreased night vision.
3. Central scotoma from worsening diabetic macular edema.
4. Retinal detachment from regression and contracture of neovascular fronds.

○ **What are the different types of central retinal vein occlusions?**

Nonischemic CRVO.
Ischemic CRVO.
Papillophlebitis.

○ **What is the probability that the next child of a patient with unilateral retinoblastoma but without a family history of the disease will develop retinoblastoma?**

6%.

○ **What is the most common primary intraocular malignancy?**

Uveal malignant melanomas.

❍   **Where is the most frequent primary site of choroidal metastatic tumors?**

1. Women: breast.
2. Men: lung.
3. Other causes include kidney, GI tract, prostate (rarely).

❍   **What are the layers of Bruch's membrane?**

The layers are, from internal to external:

1. The inner basal lamina of the RPE.
2. The inner collagenous zone.
3. Band of elastic fibers.
4. Outer collagenous zone.
5. Basal lamina of the choriocapillaris.

❍   **What are Roth spots and what can cause them?**

They are white spots in the middle of an intraretinal hemorrhage, which are thought to represent a fibrin thrombus occluding a ruptured blood vessel. They can be caused by:
1. infectious endocarditis
2. leukemia
3. anemia
4. hyperviscosity syndromes, eg. Multiple myeloma, Waldenstrom macroglobulinemia.

❍   **What are some of the causes of a bull's eye maculopathy?**

1. Drugs (chloroquine, chlorpromazine, thioridazine, tamoxifen).
2. Cone dystrophy.
3. Stargardt's disease.
4. Inverse (central) retinitis pigmentosa.
5. Batten's disease.

❍   **What are the risk factors for the development of choroidal neovascularization in age-related macular degeneration?**

1. Cigarette smoking.
2. Elevated serum cholesterol.
3. Large, bilateral, soft drusen.
4. Pigment irregularities in the macula.

❍   **What factors decrease the risk of choroidal neovascularization in age-related macular degeneration?**

1. Exogenous estrogen use in postmenopausal women.
2. Increased serum carotenoid levels.

❍   **How can retinoblastoma present clinically?**

1. Leukocoria.

2. Strabismus.
3. Secondary glaucoma.
4. Pseudouveitis (hypopyon, hyphema, red eye, pain) in older children.
5. Proptosis.
6. Orbital inflammation.

❍   **What are the most common organs involved with hematogenous spread of retinoblastoma?**

Bones, lymph nodes and liver.

❍   **What is the chance of a healthy patient having a child with retinoblastoma if he has a parent with bilateral retinoblastoma?**

6%.

❍   **What is the fundus appearance of retinoblastoma?**

Endophytic tumors project into vitreous, while exophytic tumors present as retinal detachment.

❍   **What laboratory investigations would you request for in evaluating a patient with retinoblastoma?**

Ultrasonography for presence of tumor, dimensions, calcifications. CT scan to detect calcifications and MRI scan to evaluate the optic nerve evaluation and look for pinealoblastoma with gadolinium enhancement.

❍   **What is the treatment for retinoblastoma?**

1. Enucleation.
2. Radiotherapy if good vision is present.
3. Photocoagulation for tumors <3mm diameter or <2 mm thickness.
4. Cryotherapy for tumors <3.5 mm or <2 mm thickness.
5. Systemic chemotherapy for orbital recurrences and metastatic disease (skull, orbit, long bones, viscera, spinal cord, lymph nodes).

Note: photocoagulation and cryotherapy are contraindicated if vitreous seeding is present.

❍   **What are retinal capillary hemangiomas called?**

Von Hippel's disease.

❍   **How many patients with Von Hippel's disease are associated with systemic lesions (Von Hippel-Lindau's syndrome)?**

Twenty five percent have systemic lesions such as:

1. Hemangioblastomas of the cerebellum, brainstem and spinal cord.
2. Cysts of the kidneys, pancreas, lungs, ovaries, and epididymis.
3. Phaeochromocytoma and hypernephroma.

❍   **What is its mode of inheritance?**

Autosomal dominant.

❍   **What is the differential diagnosis of Von Hippel's disease?**

1. Wyburn-Mason syndrome (racemose hemangiomatosis).
2. Coat's disease (aneurysmal dilatation of blood vessels with prominent subretinal exudates).

❍   **How would you workup patients with Von Hippel's disease and their relatives?**

1. Physical examination.
2. Urinalysis.
3. 24-Hour urine collection for levels of vanillylmandelic acid (VMA).
4. Renal ultrasonography.
5. Abdominal CT scan.
6. Brain CT or MRI scan.

❍   **What is the treatment of Von Hippel Lindau's disease?**

1. Photocoagulation or cryotherapy if it is affecting or threatening vision.
2. Genetic counseling.
3. Refer for medical treatment of the systemic lesions of Von Hippel-Lindau's syndrome.

❍   **What is Wyburn-Mason syndrome?**

1. It is a phacomatoses consisting of
2. Large, dilated, tortuous vessels forming AV communications in the retina,
3. Racemose hemangiomas in the midbrain causing seizures and hemiparesis, and
4. Hemangiomas in the ipsilateral pterygoid fossa, mandible and maxilla.
Note: Massive hemorrhage can result with ipsilateral dental or facial surgery.

❍   **What are the causes of peripheral retinal neovascularization?**

1. Diabetes mellitus.
2. Vein occlusion.
3. Sickle cell anemia.
4. Retinal vasculitis (sarcoidosis, collagen vascular disease, radiation retinopathy, pars planitis).
5. Retinopathy of prematurity.
6. Familial exudative vitreoretinopathy.
7. Eales disease.

❍   **Which form of sickle cell disease is associated with the most severe form of retinopathy?**

SC (sickle cell C) and Stahl (sickle cell thalassemia).

❍ **Which forms of sickle cell disease are associated with milder forms of retinopathy?**

SS (sickle cell anemia) and AS (sickle cell trait)(mildest form).

❍ **What are the critical signs of sickle cell retinopathy?**

Peripheral neovascularization (sea fans), sclerosed peripheral vessels, and a dull gray peripheral fundus resulting from ischemia.

❍ **What other ocular findings may occur in sickle cell retinopathy?**

Asymptomatic lesions include:

1. Black sunburst chorioretinal atrophy.
2. Salmon patch hemorrhages.
3. Venous tortuosity and silver-wiring of retinal arterioles.
4. Refractile deposits.
5. Angioid streaks.

Symptomatic lesions include vitreous hemorrhage, tractional retinal detachment, CRAO and BRVO.

❍ **How would you manage sickle cell retinopathy?**

1. Photocoagulation to areas of capillary nonperfusion.
2. Pars plana vitrectomy for tractional retinal detachment or vitreous hemorrhage.

❍ **Why would you not use acetazolamide to treat an acute attack of glaucoma in a patient with sickle cell disease?**

Sickling of RBCs may result.

❍ **What is the cause of retinal and optic disc colobomas?**

Incomplete closure of the fetal fissure.

❍ **What other ocular features may be associated with retinal colobomas?**

1. Posterior embryotoxon.
2. Non-rhegmatogenous retinal detachment.
3. Strabismus.
4. Nystagmus.
5. Posterior lenticonus.

❍ **What is the mode of inheritance of choroideremia?**

X-linked recessive.

❍ **What are the ERG findings in choroideremia?**

It may be normal in the early stages, but the scotopic ERG will eventually become non-recordable and the photopic ERG severely diminished by the end of the first decade.

❍ What biochemical abnormality is present in patients with choroideremia?

None.

❍ What metabolic error is present in gyrate atrophy?

Inborn error of the mitochondrial enzyme ornithine aminotransferase, leading to increased levels of ornithine in CSF, aqueous, serum and urine.

❍ How is gyrate atrophy treated?

Pyridoxine and arginine-restricted diet.

❍ What are two potentially lethal diseases may be associated with tyrosinase-negative oculocutaneous albinism?

1. Chédiak-Higashi syndrome: increased susceptibility to recurrent infections.
2. Hermansky-Pudlak syndrome: increased susceptibility to bleeding and bruising from a platelet defect.

❍ What is the mode of inheritance of Stargardt's disease?

It is autosomally recessive.

❍ What systemic diseases may be associated with congenital hypertrophy of the retinal pigment epithelium?

Gardner's syndrome and familial adenomatous polyposis (FAP). At least 4 lesions in each eye are generally considered necessary to suggest the possibility of either FAP or Gardner's syndrome.

❍ What should all patients with either FAP or Gardner's syndrome undergo early in adult life?

Prophylactic total colectomy because virtually all patients will develop colorectal carcinoma by age 50 years.

❍ What systemic diseases may be associated with angioid streaks?

1. Paget's disease.
2. Pseudoxanthoma elasticum.
3. Ehlers-Danlos syndrome.
4. Hemoglobinopathies (homozygous sickle cell disease, thalassemias).
5. Acromegaly.
6. Calcinosis.
7. Senile elastosis.

○   **What posterior segment features may be caused by Ehlers-Danlos syndrome?**

High myopia and retinal detachment from giant tears.

○   **What gastrointestinal problem may occur in patients with pseudoxanthoma elasticum?**

GI bleed can occur within the first decade of life and which may be life threatening.

○   **When does the retina become vascularized in an infant?**

The nasal retina is usually vascularized by 36 weeks gestation, while the temporal retina is usually completely vascularized by term.

○   **Which infants are at risk for developing retinopathy of prematurity (ROP)?**

Infants born less than 36 weeks of age, weighing less than 2000 g and who have received supplemental oxygen.

○   **What is threshold disease in ROP?**

Threshold disease includes:

1. Stage 3 ROP.
2. Zone 1 or 2 involved.
3. 5 or more continuous clock hours or 8 cumulative clock hours of retina involved.
4. Plus disease present.

○   **When should neonates at risk for ROP be screened?**

Initially, they should be screened between postconceptual ages of 32 and 36 weeks after birth then every 2 weeks until 36 weeks if the fundi are normal and weekly if there is evidence of zone 1 or 2 disease present.

○   **How often does ROP in infant eyes spontaneous regress?**

85%.

○   **What is a retinal detachment?**

It is a separation of the sensory retina from the RPE by subretinal fluid.

○   **What is the significance of pigment cells (tobacco dust) in the retrolental space of a patient complaining of sudden onset of floaters and flashing lights?**

It suggests the possibility of a retinal tear. The cells represent macrophages containing RPE cells.

○   **What potential complication can occur in areas of "white-without-pressure"?**

Giant tears can occur along the posterior border of "white-without-pressure."

❍   **Do snail-track degenerations have the same complications as lattice degeneration?**

Yes. Large round holes can form in areas of snail-track degeneration, and there is a high risk of retinal detachment.

❍   **What is retinoschisis?**

It is a splitting of the neurosensory retina into two layers.

❍   **Where does the splitting occur in degenerative retinoschisis?**

Degenerative retinoschisis can either be typical (split at outer plexiform layer) or reticular (split at nerve fiber layer).

❍   **What group does degenerative retinoschisis occur more frequently in, myopes or hypermetropes?**

Hypermetropes (70%).

❍   **What are the clinical features of juvenile X-linked retinoschisis?**

It is a bilateral, vitreoretinal degeneration in children characterized by tiny cystoid spaces in a bicycle wheel pattern in the macula eventually resulting in an atrophic macular scar and associated with retinoschisis in up to 50% of cases. Retinal detachment and vitreous hemorrhage can also occur in up to 40% of cases.

❍   **What does the inner wall of the schisis in juvenile X-linked retinoschisis consist of?**

Retinal nerve fiber layer and the inner limiting membrane.

❍   **What is a characteristic ERG finding found in juvenile X-linked retinoschisis?**

The b-wave is disproportionately decreased as compared to the a-wave.

❍   **What type of visual field defects do retinoschisis and retinal detachments produce?**

A retinal detachment produces a relative scotoma while a retinoschisis produces an absolute scotoma.

❍   **What other features can help you distinguish between a retinoschisis and a retinal detachment?**

It is unusual to find "tobacco dust" and or hemorrhage in a retinoschisis, while it is a common finding in rhegmatogenous retinal detachment. Second, the retinoschisis has a smooth surface and usually appears to be a dome shaped structure in contrast to rhegmatogenous retinal detachment, which is often corrugated with an irregular surface. Finally, a long term rhegmatogenous retinal detachment may appear smooth and thin, very similar to retinoschisis, however a long-standing rhegmatogenous retinal detachment can have atrophy of the underlying retinal pigment epithelium with demarcation lines and macrocyst. In a retinoschisis, the underlying retinal pigment epithelium appears normal.

O **How can retinoschisis produce a retinal detachment?**

For a retinoschisis to cause a retinal detachment there should be an outer wall hole present. There are two possible scenarios. In the first case, only outer wall hole(s) of schisis cavity is/are present. This results in the content of the schisis cavity to slowly detach the retina. In the second type of retinal detachment secondary to retinoschisis, there is a hole in both the inner and the outer walls of the cavity.

O **How are retinal detachments classified?**

There are three main classes of retinal detachment including rhegmatogenous retinal detachment, tractional retinal detachment and exudative retinal detachment.

O **What is a tractional retinal detachment?**

Tractional retinal detachment is caused by vitreous membranes produced by penetrating injuries or proliferative retinopathy, which can cause traction on neurosensory retina and pull it away from the retina pigment epithelium layer.

O **Describe the appearance of the retina in tractional retinal detachment.**

The retina has a smooth surface and is immobilized. The detachment is concave toward the anterior segment of the eye and rarely extends to the ora serrata.

O **How are tractional retinal detachments repaired?**

Treatment may require both vitrectomies to release the traction on the detached retina and a scleral buckle procedure to seal the break.

O **When does exudative retinal detachment occur?**

Exudative retinal detachment is seen when there is damage done to the retinal blood vessels or the retinal pigment epithelium. This allows the passage of fluid into the subretinal space. The most common causes of this exudative retinal detachment are neoplasia and inflammatory disease. This can present as a "shifting fluid" in appearance, which responds to the force of gravity, detaching the area of the retina in which it accumulates.

O **What are signs of long-standing rhegmatogenous retinal detachments?**

1. Pigment demarkation (high-water marks).
2. Secondary intraretinal cysts.
3. Retinal thinning.
4. Subretinal fibrosis.

O **What is the most common cause of rhegmatogenous retinal detachment?**

The most common cause of rhegmatogenous retinal detachment is lattice degeneration which is found in 8-10% of the general population, however, only a small number of affected individuals develop retinal detachment. It is estimated that 20-40% of all rhegmatogenous detachments has lattices degeneration as the underlying cause.

○ **What is the most common cause of failure to repair a rhegmatogenous retinal detachment?**

Proliferative vitreoretinopathy (PVR).

○ **How do we classify PVR?**

PVR is classified according to its location, type, and extent of retinal contraction. If the PVR is posterior to the equator, it is considered as posterior PVR, and if it is anterior to the equator, it is considered as anterior PVR. Anterior and posterior PVR can be further classified based on the extent of the proliferation or retinal contraction.

○ **What is the treatment for a retinal giant tear?**

A giant retinal tear is a retinal tear greater than 90 degrees in circumferential extent. Following the vitrectomy the retinal flap can be unfolded with air, silicone oil, or perflurocarbon. After reattachment of the retina, long acting tamponade gas or silicone oil is used to reattach the retina with the extensive laser photocoagulation therapy around the retinal tear to stabilize the retina. Using these recent techniques the patient can be in supine position during the surgery, unlike the earlier techniques which require the prone position to permit the unfolding of the giant tear.

○ **What are potential complications of drainage of subretinal fluid?**

1. Postoperative endophthalmitis.
2. Retinal incarceration.
3. Vitreous prolapse.
4. Choroidal hemorrhage.
5. Iatrogenic retinal breaks.
6. Fishmouthing of U-tears.

○ **What are causes of early failure of retinal detachment surgery?**

1. Failure to find all retinal breaks.
2. Buckle failure due to inadequate size, height and positioning.
3. Fishmouthing of the retinal tear.
4. Missed iatrogenic breaks during drainage of subretinal fluid.

○ **What are the causes of a re-detachment following initially successful retinal detachment surgery?**

1. Proliferative vitreoretinopathy.
2. Insufficient cryotherapy.
3. Inadequate buckle.

4. New retinal break formation.

○ What are the indications for vitrectomy?

1. Non-resolving vitreous opacities, eg. Bleeding, inflammation, neoplastic.
2. Proliferative retinopathy.
3. Complicated retinal detachments, including giant tears.
4. Macular epiretinal membranes.
5. Dislocated crystalline lens or lens fragments after cataract surgery.
6. Diagnostic vitrectomy for uveitis.
7. Aphakic cystoid macular edema in which vitreous is incarcerated in the wound.

○ What are the intraoperative complications of vitrectomy?

1. Iatrogenic retinal detachment or retinal breaks.
2. Severe hemorrhage.
3. Cataract formation.
4. Pressure induced optic nerve damage.

○ What are the postoperative complications of vitrectomy?

1. Endophthalmitis.
2. Retinal detachment.
3. Recurrent vitreous hemorrhage.
4. Phthisis bulbi.
5. Sympathetic ophthalmia.
6. Glaucoma.
7. Anterior segment neovascularization.
8. Flat anterior chamber.
9. Cataract.
10. Fibrin formation.
11. Inflammation.
12. Recurrent corneal erosions.

○ How can you perform closed vitrectomy in the presence of a corneal opacity?

Under severe cases of corneal opacification one can use a temporary keratoprosthetic device during the surgery and a donor cornea must be available which can be used after the vitrectomy is done.

○ What did the Diabetic Retinopathy Vitrectomy Study (DRVS) evaluate?

The benefit of early (1-6 months) versus late (at 1 year) vitrectomy for eyes with severe vitreous heme and visual loss of 5/200 or worse.

○ What did the DRVS show concerning vitrectomy in patients with vitreous hemorrhage?

Benefit of early vitrectomy was clearly demonstrated in IDDM patients. No such advantage was found in NIDDM patients.

○ **What did the DRVS show concerning vitrectomy in eyes with very severe PDR?**

There was an advantage for early vitrectomy compared to conventional treatment in eyes with very severe PDR.

○ **What can cause a traumatic retinal break?**

Retinal breaks can result following perforating eye injuries by direct retinal perforation, contusion, and vitreous traction, which is produced by fibrocellular proliferation.

○ **When is pneumatic retinopexy used?**

It is used to treat uncomplicated retinal detachments with a small retinal break or a group of breaks over an area of less than two clock hours located in the upper two-thirds of the retina. Air, sulfur hexafluoride (SF6) and perfluoropropane (C3F8) are most commonly used.

○ **Which of the gases used in fluid-gas exchange lasts the longest inside the eye?**

Perfluoropropane (C3F8) lasts 55-65 days, while sulfur hexafluoride (SF6) and perfluoroethane (C2F6) last 10-14 days and 30-35 days respectively.

○ **What are the indications for treatment of macular holes with vitrectomy and fluid-gas exchange?**

Full thickness macular holes less than one-year-old and associated with a visual acuity worse than 20/60.

○ **When is an inferior iridectomy performed when using silicone oil as a permanent tamponade?**

Inferior iridectomy is placed in an aphakic eye when silicone oil is used to fill the vitreous cavity. This is to minimize the anterior segment complications by preventing the prolapse of silicone oil into the anterior chamber.

○ **What are the most common causes of spontaneous vitreous hemorrhage in adults?**

1. Diabetic retinopathy (39-54%).
2. Retinal break without detachment (12-17%).
3. Posterior vitreous detachment (7.5-12%).
4. Rhegmatogenous retinal detachment (7-10%).
5. Retinal neovascularization from BRVO and CRVO (3.5-10%).

○ **What are the main methods used in intraocular surgery to create a chorioretinal scar?**

1. Photocoagulation.
2. Cryotherapy.
3. Diathermy.

○   What is the mechanism of action of photocoagulation?

The light energy is absorbed by an opaque tissue and is converted into heat that produces thermal damage. The chorioretinal adhesion is made during photocoagulation by different wavelengths of light, which produces burns in the retina and pigment epithelium. Photocoagulation should be used in the area that the retina is in contact with the pigment epithelium.

○   What potential complications may result from peripheral retinal photocoagulation?

1. Cystoid macular edema.
2. Choroidal detachment.
3. Secondary angle closure glaucoma resulting from forward rotation of the ciliary body from a choroidal detachment.
4. Rhegmatogenous retinal detachment from secondary tear formation.
5. Exudative retinal detachment.
6. Inadvertent treatment of the fovea.
7. Perforation of the retina.

○   What is the mechanism of action of diathermy?

The diathermy probe conducts the radiofrequency energy to the ocular tissue. The energy is then converted to heat as it penetrates the tissue, and produces a burn within the ocular tissue.

○   What is the disadvantage of using diathermy to create a chorioretinal scar?

The main disadvantage of diathermy is that it causes shrinkage and weakening of the sclera. It also requires scleral dissection for best results.

○   What is cryotherapy?

Cryotherapy is a common method used to create a chorioretinal adhesion during intraocular surgery. Cryotherapy causes dissolution of cellular membrane by freezing. When the temperature is rapidly lowered during cryotherapy, intracellular ice crystal form, which can cause mechanical damage. During the thawing, water and electrolytes separate, which results in a change in the PH with rupture of the cell membrane. The longer the cryoprobe is used on the sclera, the stronger the adhesion is between the retina and the retina pigment epithelium.

○   What are causes of choroidal folds?

1. Hypermetropia.
2. Ocular hypotony.

3. Choroidal tumors.
4. Posterior scleritis.
5. Orbital disease, eg. Thyroid ophthalmopathy.

❍ What is retinal telangiectasia?

It is defined by an exudative retinal detachment associated with telangiectatic vascular anomalies. It is found predominantly in males, usually unilateral and not hereditary.

❍ What are the types of retinal telangiectasias?

1. Coat's disease (children).
2. Leber's miliary aneurysms (adults).
3. Idiopathic juxtafoveolar telangiectasis (adults).

❍ What are causes of leukocoria in children?

1. Retinoblastoma.
2. Coat's disease.
3. Persistent hyperplastic primary vitreous (PHPV).
4. Cataract.
5. Toxocariasis.
6. Cicatricial ROP.
7. Incontinentia pigmenti (Bloch-Sulzberger syndrome).
8. Retinal dysplasia.
9. Retinal astrocytoma.
10. Inflammatory cyclitic membranes.

❍ What is Coat's disease?

It is a severe form of unilateral retinal telangiectasia mainly occurring in boys and resulting in massive exudative retinal detachment. It typically presents in the first decade of life with visual loss, leukocoria, or strabismus.

❍ What are risk factors associated with retinal vein occlusion?

Systemic risk factors: age, systemic hypertension, and diabetes mellitus, blood dyscrasias Ocular risk factors: glaucoma,hypermetropia, periphlebitis, and congenital anomalies of the central retinal vein.

❍ At what site in the retina do branch retinal vein occlusions occur in?

At AV crossings.

❍ At what site does a central retinal vein occlusion usually occur in?

At the prelaminar layer of the optic nerve head.

❍ What was the conclusion of the Branch Vein Occlusion Study regarding the use of argon macular grid laser for macular edema?

Sixty percent of eyes treated for macular edema with photocoagulation recovered 20/40 vision or better compared to 34% in nontreated eyes.

O   **Is the chronic cystoid macular edema resulting from nonischemic CRVO responsive to conventional laser photocoagulation?**

No.

O   **What is the risk of developing neovascularization in an eye with 5 disk diameters or more of nonperfusion following a retinal vein occlusion?**

30-50% of eyes.

O   **What percentage of eyes with nonischemic CRVO will convert to ischemic CRVO?**

Fifteen percent of cases within 4 months and 34% of cases within 3 years.

O   **When does rubeosis iridis develop in eyes with ischemic CRVO?**

Rubeosis iridis usually develops within 2-4 months in approximately 50% of eyes.

O   **In what percentage of people is a cilioretinal artery present?**

It is present in up to 30% of individuals.

O   **What is Eales' disease?**

It is an idiopathic vasculitis in young boys or men with associated positive reaction to PPD, epistaxis, constipation and occasionally with potentially fatal cerebral vasculitis.

O   **What are lacquer cracks?**

Lacquer cracks are large breaks in Bruch's membrane found in highly myopic eyes.

O   **What is a Fuch's spot?**

It is pigmentary proliferation following absorption of macular hemorrhage from choroidal neovascularization in highly myopic eyes.

O   **What does visual loss in acute retinal necrosis (ARN) syndrome usually result from?**

Visual loss in ARN can result from optic neuritis, which may occur early in the disease, and proliferative vitreoretinopathy and retinal detachment.

O   **What viruses have been implicated in ARN syndrome?**

Herpes simplex and varicella zoster.

❍   **What is the appropriate treatment for ARN syndrome?**

Intravenous acyclovir for 5 to 10 days, followed by oral acyclovir.

❍   **What are causes of bull's eye maculopathy?**

1. Chloroquine toxicity.
2. Cone dystrophy.
3. Bardet-Biedl syndrome.
4. Batten's disease.
5. Inverse retinitis pigmentosa.
6. Benign concentric annular macular dystrophy.
7. Fenestrated sheen dystrophy.
8. Stargardt's disease.

❍   **What are angioid streaks?**

They are cracks in Bruch's membrane radiating from the optic disc with secondary changes in the choriocapillaris and RPE.

❍   **What ocular complications can occur from angioid streaks?**

1. Foveal involvement.
2. Choroidal neovascularization.
3. Choroidal rupture from trauma.

❍   **What systemic diseases are associated with angioid streaks?**

1. Ehlers-Danlos syndrome.
2. Pseudoxanthoma elasticum.
3. Paget disease.
4. Sickle cell diseases and thalassemias.

❍   **What systemic diseases may be associated with lattice degeneration?**

1. Marfan's syndrome.
2. Stickler's syndrome.
3. Ehlers-Danlos syndrome.

❍   **What are the main indications for prophylactic treatment of lattice degeneration?**

1. Retinal detachment in the opposite eye
2. Highly myopic eye with extensive lattice degeneration
3. Family history of retinal detachment
4. Systemic diseases associated with lattice degeneration

❍   **What clinical features are suggestive of a malignant change of a choroidal nevus into a melanoma?**

1. Evidence of growth.
2. Presence of symptoms.
3. Lipofuscin pigment on the surface.
4. Dilated vessels within the tumor.
5. Posterior margin of the lesion is within 3 mm of the optic disc.
6. Subretinal fluid.
7. Cystoid changes of overlying retina.

❍   **What is Leber's congenital amaurosis?**

It is an autosomal recessive congenital blindness presenting at birth or within the first few years of life.

❍   **What are the ERG findings in Leber's congenital amaurosis?**

The ERG is nonrecordable, even if the fundus appears normal.

❍   **What is the oculodigital syndrome, which commonly occur in children with Leber's congenital amaurosis?**

Constant rubbing of the eyes by the child in an effort to stimulate the retina causes enophthalmos as a result of resorption of orbital fat.

❍   **What is the volume of the vitreous?**

4 mL.

❍   **What is the wave in the ERG?**

It is the initial negative or downward deflection, which arises from the photoreceptors.

❍   **What is the b wave in the ERG?**

It is the positive or upward deflection generated by Müller cells representing processes occurring in the bipolar cell region.

❍   **What are causes of selective or predominant decrease in the amplitude of the b-wave?**

1. Siderosis.
2. Congenital stationary night blindness.
3. Central renial artery or vein occlusion.
4. Quinine or methanol toxicity.
5. Juvenile X-linked retinoschisis.

❍   **What is the implicit time?**

It is the time between the flash of light and the peak of the b-wave.

❍   **Is the ERG useful in the diagnosis of disorders affecting the ganglion cell layer or the optic nerve such as glaucomatous optic neuropathy?**

No. The ERG is a function of the first two neurons in the retina and thus will not be useful in diseases affecting the third neuron and its fibers, such as glaucomatous optic neuropathy or optic neuritis.

❍   **How can rod responses to the ERG be isolated?**

A fully dark adapted eye is stimulated with a flash of very dim light or with blue light.

❍   **What ERG techniques are used to isolate cone responses?**

1. Stimulation of a fully light-adapted eye with a bright flash of light or red light.
2. Flicker light stimulus of 30-40 Mhz to which rods cannot respond.

❍   **What does the electro-oculogram (EOG) measure?**

The EOG measures the standing action potential between the electrically negative cornea and the electrically positive back of the eye. It reflects the activity of the RPE and the photoreceptors.

❍   **Will a patient with optic atrophy resulting from demyelinating optic neuritis have a recordable EOG?**

Yes. Widespread disease of the RPE is needed to affect the EOG response significantly. Eyes with lesions proximal to the photoreceptors will have a normal EOG.

❍   **What is the mode of inheritance of Best's disease?**

Autosomal dominant.

❍   **What electrophysiologic findings are present in Best's disease?**

The EOG is subnormal (decreased light peak:dark trough ratio), while the ERG is normal.

❍   **Is the EOG abnormal in adult onset foveomacular dystrophy?**

No.

❍   **What are the stages of Best's disease?**

Stage 1:   Previtelliform (normal fundus, abnormal EOG).
Stage 2:   Vitelliform (egg-yolk stage).
Stage 3:   Pseudohypopyon.
Stage 4:   Vitelliruptive (scrambled egg).
Stage 5:   Macular scar.

❍   **Give two complications that may be produced by choroidal nevi.**

Malignant transformation and choroidal neovascular membranes.

O   **What is the classic triad of clinical findings in retinitis pigmentosa?**

1. Retinal bone-spicule-like pigmentation.
2. Arteriolar attenuation.
3. Waxy disc pallor.

O   **What are the ERG and EOG findings found in retinitis pigmentosa?**

The ERG is abnormal with reduced amplitude of photopic and scotopic b-waves and a delayed implicit time. The EOG shows an absence of the light rise.

O   **What other ocular findings may be associated with retinitis pigmentosa?**

1. Posterior subcapsular cataracts.
2. Myopia.
3. Optic disc drusen.
4. Keratoconus.
5. Open angle glaucoma.
6. Intermediate uveitis.
7. Posterior vitreous detachment.

O   **What is the name of the syndrome characterized by retinitis pigmentosa and sensorineural hearing loss?**

Usher Syndrome.

O   **What is Refsum's disease?**

It is an accumulation of phytanic acid, resulting in pigmentary retinopathy, cataracts, hypertrophic peripheral neuropathy, and cerebellar ataxia, deafness, ichthyosis, arrhythmias and elevated CSF protein.

O   **What mucopolysaccharidoses are associated with pigmentary retinopathy?**

Hurler, Hunter, Scheie, and Sanfilippo.

O   **What contributes to the outermost layer of Bruch's membrane?**

Choriocapillaris.

O   **I can't smell, see or hear. My skin is scaly. My heart doesn't work well and I can't keep my balance. What disease do I have?**

Refsum disease.

O   **What is Oguchi's disease?**

It is a recessive form of stationary night blindness characterized by a 2-12 hour delay in attaining normal dark-adapted rod thresholds and associated with Mizuo's phenomenon.

❍   **What is Mizuo's phenomenon?**

It is a change in fundus color from a golden brown fundus in the light-adapted state to a normal color in the dark-adapted state. It is found in Oguchi's disease.

❍   **What is fundus albipunctatus?**

It is a recessive form of stationary night blindness characterized by a multitude of tiny yellow-white spots, which extend from the posterior pole to the periphery and sparing the macula.

❍   **Are the visual fields and visual acuities adversely affected in fundus albipunctatus?**

No. They remain normal.

❍   **What are the ERG findings in cone dystrophy?**

The photopic response will be subnormal or non-recordable, while the scotopic response will be normal.

❍   **What is the mode of inheritance of Stargardt's macular dystrophy and fundus flavimaculatus?**

Usually autosomal recessive, although autosomal dominant cases have been reported.

❍   **What fluorescein angiographic finding may be seen in Stargardt's macular dystrophy and fundus flavimaculatus?**

Absence of the normal background fluorescence-giving rise to a "dark choroid" may be found 85% of patients.

❍   **What is North Carolina macular dystrophy?**

It is an autosomal dominant retinal dystrophy characterized by drusen-like deposits in the retinal periphery and the macula, later progressing to confluence of the macular lesions and atrophic or exudative maculopathy in young adults.

❍   **What is familial dominant drusen?**

It is an autosomal dominant retinal disease characterized by large drusen located at the macula and around the optic nerve. The prognosis is good, although some patients may develop macular degeneration.

❍   **What is Stickler's syndrome?**

It is an autosomal dominant vitreoretinal degeneration characterized by high myopia, an empty vitreous cavity, large areas of lattice degeneration with RPE hyperplasia, retinal detachment in 30% from multiple breaks and gian tears, presenile cataracts in 50% of cases. Ectopia lentis and glaucoma develops in 10% of cases.

○   **What is a characteristic retinal lesion found in sphingolipidoses such as Tay-Sachs disease (Gm2 gangliosidosis type 1) and Neiman-Pick disease?**

Cherry-red spot in the macula.

○   **What drugs can cause crystalline deposits to be deposited in the macula?**

Tamoxifen, canthaxanthin, and methoxyflurane.

○   **What layer of Bruch's membrane do Müller cells contribute to?**

None.

○   **What mucopolysaccharidoses are associated with progressive rod-cone dystrophy?**

Hurler's, Scheie's, Hunter's and Sanfilippo's but not in Morquio's and Maroteaux-Lamy's.

○   **A 24-month-old girl with no signs of external injuries and no history of medical problems is seen in the emergency room with bilateral subhyaloid hemorrhages on fundus examination. What is the most likely cause of her fundus abnormalities?**

Child abuses, especially shaken baby syndrome.

○   **At what CD4 lymphocyte count level does CMV retinitis become more common?**

CMV retinitis becomes more common when CD4 lymphocyte countsdrop to 50 cells/mm^3 or less.

○   **How often does iris neovascularization and neovascular glaucoma occur following a central retinal artery occlusion?**

Approximately 5%.

○   **What explains the decreased choroidal fluorescence of the fovea on fluorescein angiography?**

The foveal RPE cells contain larger, more abundant melanosomes than the RPE cells in the periphery.

○   **What is Wyburn-Mason syndrome?**

This is a phacomatoses consisting of AV malformations in the retina and midbrain.

❍   **How many patients with classic choroidal neovascularization, who received verteporfin in the Treatment of Age-Related Macular Degeneration with Photodynamic Therapy study, lost fewer than 3 lines of vision after two years compared to those receiving placebo?**

After 2 years, 59.1% of patients lost fewer than 3 lines of vision compared with 31.3% of those receiving placebo.

❍   **How does verteporfin work in photodynamic therapy for CNVin age-related macular degeneration (AMD)?**

Verteporfin is a photosensitizing drug that is administered intravenously and selectively accumulates in neovascular tissue of AMD by attaching to low-density lipoproteins. Because cells in CNV are actively dividing and growing, they need higher levels of lipoprotein compared with normal cells. Therefore, high concentrations are absorbed rapidly in these areas. When activated by laser light, free radicals and singlet oxygen is produced, which damages cell components.

❍   **How is the laser treatment delivered to activate verteporfin after it is administered to the patient?**

The laser treatment is administered 15 minutes after verteporfin infusion intravenously at a predetermined spot size through the slit lamp and contact lens at 689 nm targeted by a low intensity helium-neon beam for 83 seconds, with 50 J/cm^2 delivered to the lesion.

❍   **How often do patients need to be retreated according to the Treatment of Age-Related Macular Degeneration with Photodynamic Therapy study (TAP)?**

Patients need to be retreated at 3-month intervals. The TAP study found that patients required an average of 3.4 treatments over one year and 5.5 treatments over 2 years.

❍   **What precautions should be taken during photodynamic therapy with verteporfin?**

Following infusion of verteporfin, care should be taken to avoid exposure of skin and eyes to direct sunlight or bright indoor lights for 5 days with dark sunglasses and long-sleeved shirts and pants. In the event of extravasation during infusion, the area should be thoroughly protected from direct light until the swelling and discoloration have faded to avoid a severe burn.

❍   **Are UV sunscreens effective in protecting against photosensitivity reactions following verteporfin infusion?**

No, because photoactivation of the residual drug in the skin can be caused by visible light.

❍   **Why should patients receiving photodynamic therapy be encouraged to expose their skin to ambient indoor light rather than stay in the dark?**

This helps inactivate the drug through a process called photobleaching.

❍   **What is a characteristic fundus finding in acute macular neuroretinopathy?**

A cloverleaf or wedge shaped pattern of dark red lesions in the macula is the characteristic fundis finding in AMN. It is a rare cause of mild visual loss and paracentral scotomas in young adults.

❍   **A child is diagnosed with Leber's congenital amaurosis. What is the chance that succeeding children will also have this condition?**

There is a 1 in 4 chance that succeeding children will have Leber's congenital amaurosis because it is transmitted in an autosomal recessive fashion.

❍   **What is the most common form of congenital defect in color vision?**

Deuteranomalous trichromatopsia, which affects 5 percent of the male population.

❍   **What is the incidence of lattice degeneration in the general population?**

7 to 8 percent.

❍   **What is the long-term risk of retinal detachment in patients with lattice degeneration?**

1%.

❍   **What is the incidence of progressive retinal detachment from atrophic retinal holes in phakic eyes with lattice degeneration?**

2%.

❍   **When should patients with lattice degeneration be prophylactically treated?**

Prophylactic treatment is indicated only if:
1. Retinal traction tears that are symptomatic are present, unless the patient is aphakic.
2. There is a history of retinal detachment in the other eye.
3. There is a strong family history of retinal detachment.

❍   **How much carotid artery stenosis is required to cause ocular ischemic syndrome?**

90% or greater ipsilateral obstruction.

❍   **A patient with history of vitreous surgery and intraocular gas placement of the right eye two days ago presents with painful, blind right eye. What is the most likely diagnosis?**

Elevated intraocular pressure is a serious complication of intraocular gases, which can lead to central retinal artery occlusion and blindness.

❍   **A patient is seen one day after vitrectomy with intravitreal gas bubble. What findings should alert you to improper head position?**

A feathery posterior subcapsular lens opacity indicates lens damage by prolonged contact with the gas bubble. The patient should be instructed to maintain facedown position to avoid contact between the gas bubble and the lens. If proper head positioned is maintained, the feathery opacity usually disappears within one to two days after contact between the lens and the gas bubble.

❍   **What is the most accurate way of measuring intraocular pressure for a patient with intravitreal gas bubble?**

The most accurate method of measuring intraocular pressure for a patient with intraocular gas bubble is by applanation tonometry. Indentation (Schiötz) tonometry can give a falsely low reading presumably because of the compressibility of the gas.

❍   **What are the common causes of lens opacity during the vitrectomy?**

Direct contact between the lens and the surgical instruments and the composition of the irrigating solution seem to be important factors in maintaining lens clarity.

❍   **What is the 5 year mortality rate of patients with ocular ischemic syndrome?**

Approximately 40%, mainly due to complications of cardiovascular disease.

❍   **What is the most common opportunistic ocular infection in acquired immunodeficiency syndrome (AIDS)?**

Cytomegalovirus (CMV) retinitis.

❍   **In a patient with CMV retinitis and rhegmatogenous retinal detachment, where is the most common location for retinal breaks?**

The most likely position for retinal breaks is within or adjacent to the area of retinal necrosis.

❍   **What is the most common treatment technique for a rhegmatogenous retinal detachment in an eye with CMV retinitis?**

Closed vitrectomy techniques with an intraocular tamponade (silicone oil), with or without scleral buckle.

❍   **What is the role of vitrectomy in management of proliferative diabetic retinopathy?**

There are two main objective of vitrectomy for proliferative diabetic retinopathy. First, it is used to remove media opacities such as vitreous hemorrhage or cataract. The second objective is to relieve vitreous traction causing detachment or distortion of the macula.

❍   **What was the recommendation of the Diabetic Retinopathy Vitrectomy Study group (DRVS) for type I versus type II diabetes?**

The DRVS was designed to evaluate the risks and benefits of performing early pars plana vitrectomy in eyes with advanced proliferative diabetic retinopathy. In patients with Type I diabetes, early vitrectomy (after one month) offered a greater chance of visual recovery, however, in type II and mixed type diabetes no significant difference was noted between the early versus late (after one year) vitrectomy.

○   **How are intraocular gases sterilized?**

To ensure sterility of the gases, they all are passed through 0.22 micrometer Millipore filter to remove the bacteria and fungi before injection.

○   **What are the harmful effects of intraocular gases?**

Their harmful effects are due to the physical properties such as volume expansion causing increased intraocular pressure, and prolonged contact with corneal endothelium or posterior lens surface. The prolonged contact with corneal endothelium can cause corneal damage and prolonged contact with posterior surface of the lens can cause cataract. The most serious complication of using an expanding gas is central retinal artery occlusion and blindness. This can be secondary to elevation of intraocular pressure after using intraocular gases.

○   **When is silicone oil used during vitrectomy surgery?**

Silicone oil can be used to provide a long-term or permanent internal tamponade in some cases of severe retinal detachment including giant tears and retinal detachment complicated by proliferative vitreoretinopathy.

○   **What is the specific gravity of silicone oil?**

0.975, which is slightly less than fluid in the vitreous cavity.

○   **Can you mix intraocular blood with silicone oil?**

Intraocular blood does not mix with silicone oil and it remains outside the bubble.

○   **What are the commercially available silicone oil viscosities?**

Silicone oils of 1,000 to 5,000 centistokes are used for vitreous surgery. The viscosity of silicone oil is related to the length of the polymer chains that make the oil. The average molecular weight of the silicone oil molecules of 1,000 centistokes is about 25,000, and the average molecular weight of silicone oil with a viscosity of 5,000 centistokes is about 50,000. In the United States, commercially available silicone oil is 5000 centistokes.

○   **What are the most common complications of silicone oil?**

Most complications of silicone oil are due to its entering the anterior chamber or causing pupillary block with secondary shallowing of the anterior chamber. These complications include band keratopathy, generalized corneal decompensation, iritis, chronic inflammation glaucoma, hypotony, cataract, and retinal damage.

❍ **What proportion of patients with an acute symptomatic PVD have a retinal tear?**

10%.

❍ **What proportion of patients with an acute symptomatic PVD and associated vitreous hemorrhage have a retinal tear?**

75%.

❍ **What is usually present in the history of a majority of patients with superonasal retinal dialyses?**

Head or eye trauma.

❍ **What is the prevalence of lattice degeneration in the adult U.S. population?**

10%.

❍ **What is the prevalence of lattice degeneration in patients with rhegmatogenous retinal detachment?**

25-30%.

❍ **In what percentage of patients with rhegmatogenous retinal detachment will a retinal break not be found?**

3%, usually in aphakic or pseudophakic eyes.

❍ **Does cobblestone degeneration increase the risk of developing a rhegmatogenous retinal detachment?**

No.

❍ **What are the important histologic features of lattice degeneration?**

1. Discontinuity of the internal limiting membrane.
2. Pocket of overlying liquified vitreous.
3. Vitreoretinal condensation and adherence at the margin of the lesion.
4. Sclerotic vessels.
5. Variable degrees of retinal atrophy.

❍ **What is the most important prognostic factor for visual recovery following retinal detachment surgery?**

The presence and duration of macular detachment.

❍ **What conditions require retinal detachment repair with vitrectomy techniques instead of conventional scleral buckling?**

Retinal detachment with accompanying vitreous hemorrhage and retinal detachment associated with advanced proliferative vitreoretinopathy.

O   **What is the most feared problem following retinal detachment surgery?**

Preretinal membrane formation.

O   **What color and wavelength of light is absorbed by fluorescein?**

Blue – 490 nm.

O   **What color and wavelength of light is emitted by stimulated fluorescein?**

Yellow-green – 530 nm.

O   **What color filter is used on the camera used for taking pictures in FAs?**

Yellow-green.

O   **What are the two broad categories of hypofluorescence?**

Blockage and nonperfusion.

O   **What are the five broad categories of hyperfluorescence?**

Leakage, staining, pooling, transmission, and autofluorescence.

O   **When does the hyperfluorescence of a window defect peak?**

At the peak of choroidal fluorescence.

O   **How does one differentiate leakage and pooling?**

The borders of leakage become increasingly blurred, while the borders of pooling remain distinct.

O   **How long does skin discoloration last after injection of fluorescein? Urine discoloration?**

Skin - 6-12 hours, Urine - 24-36 hours.

O   **Nausea, vomiting, or vaso-vagal reaction occur in what percentage of FA patients?**

10%.

O   **What percentage of FA patients experience anaphylactoid and anaphylactic reactions?**

Anaphylactoid - 1%, Anaphylactic - 1:100,000.

❍   **At what wavelength does fluorescence peak for ICG?**

835 nm.

❍   **What three things are necessary for retinal neovascularization?**

Angiogenic stimulus, source of endothelial cells, intact posterior cortical vitreous (usually).

❍   **What is necessary for choroidal neovascularization to occur?**

A defect in the outer aspect of Bruchs' membrane.

❍   **What are the signs of potential CNV?**

Subretinal or sub-RPE fluid or blood, subretinal or intraretinal lipid, subretinal gray-white lesion, CME, sea fan pattern of subretinal small vessels.

❍   **What is the difference between classic and occult CNV during FA?**

Classic hyperfluoresces very early and has distinct boundaries, while occult hyperfluoresces later, may be associated with RPE detachment and may have indistinct borders.

❍   **How longs does it take the cones and rods to reach their threshold in dark adaptation?**

Cones - 5-10 minutes, Rods - 30 minutes.

❍   **What is the range of human retinal light sensitivity?**

10-11 log units.

❍   **What is the range of human color vision?**

Between 400-700 nm.

❍   **What is protan color deficiency? Deutan? Tritan?**

Protan - lack or deficiency of red sensing cones.
Deutan - lack or deficiency of green sensing cones.
Tritan - lack of blue sensing cones.

❍   **In what way are the Farnsworth panels more useful than pseudoisochromic plates?**

Farnsworth panels discriminate well between acquired and congenital defects, while pseudoisochromic plates do not.

❍   **A Tritan deficiency almost always signifies what type of disease?**

Acquired.

O   **We normally are most sensitive to contrast at what spacial frequency?**

2-5 cycles/degree.

O   **In what group of patients is central serous retinopathy (CSR) most common?**

Men between 30 and 50.

O   **What is most likely defective in patients with CSR?**

RPE barrier or pumping functions.

O   **Describe the fluorescein pattern in CSR.**

A small area of hyperfluorescence that increases in size and intensity - 10% have "smokestack."

O   **What must be ruled out in older patients with CSR?**

Choroidal neovascular (CNV) membranes.

O   **What is the usual natural history of CSR?**

Between 80-90% will spontaneously resolve in 1-6 months and 40-50% will have at least one recurrence.

O   **What did a 1974 study of photocoagulation of CSR show?**

Median resolution of CSCR was 5 weeks in the treated vs. 23 week in the non-treated group. No difference in final VA was shown.

O   **Describe the current treatment guidelines for CSR.**

Hold off on laser for 3-4 months unless:

1. Recurrent episode.
2. Persistent VA decrease from CSR in fellow eye.
3. Development of chronic signs.
4. Occupational needs.

O   **What is a rare complication of laser treatment for CSCR?**

CNV - follow-up in 3-4 weeks for this reason.

O   **What is the purpose behind sending patients home with an Amsler Grid?**

Testing for metamorphopsia and scotoma, which may be early symptoms of CNV.

O   **Why are most ophthalmologists hesitant to treat POHS with photocoagulation?**

Because CNV from POHS does not uniformly progress to severe visual loss and up to 10% may spontaneously resolve (also submacular surgery is promising)

❍ **What is intermediate myopia?**

Abnormally long axial lengths, but only minimal changes in the posterior pole. Usually with spherical equivalents between -5.00 and -8.00 and axial lengths between 25.5 and 32.5 mm.

❍ **What is pathologic myopia?**

Changes in the retina associated with very abnormal elongation of the eye, usually with axial lengths >32.5mm and spherical equivalents >-8.00 diopters.

❍ **What are Fuch's spots?**

Area of RPE hyperplasia found in pathologic myopia presumably developing in response to a small area of CNV that does not progress to disciform scarring.

❍ **What is the most serious complication of pathologic myopia?**

CNV.

❍ **How do epiretinal membranes (ERM) develop?**

A dehiscence of the internal limiting membrane allows retinal glial cells (myofibroblasts and fibroblasts) to proliferate along the retinal surface. Contraction of these membranes causes cellophane maculopathy or macular pucker. Detachment of the posterior vitreous is present in almost all eyes.

❍ **What is an indication for surgery for ERM?**

Visual acuity of 20/60 or worse.

❍ **What is the difference between vitreomacular traction syndrome (VMTS) and ERM?**

In vitreomacular traction syndrome the posterior vitreous separation is incomplete at the macula.

❍ **What may happen to the macula in VMTS?**

The macula may become shallowly detached.

❍ **What can angiography show in VMTS?**

Angiography may show leakage from vessels in the macular region and from the optic disc.

❍ **What is thought to cause idiopathic macular holes?**

Tangential vitreomacular traction.

○ **What percent of stage 1 macular holes will undergo spontaneous resolution?**

Approximately 50%.

○ **What is the incidence of bilaterality of idiopathic macular holes?**

Between 25% and 30%.

○ **What is considered protection from developing macular holes?**

Complete posterior vitreous separation.

○ **What can occur in the retina after a sudden rise in intra-abdominal pressure?**

Valsalva retinopathy - the rise in intraocular venous pressure may be sufficient to rupture small capillaries in the macula.

○ **Where is the hemorrhage located in valsalva retinopathy?**

Under the internal limiting membrane.

○ **What is in the differential diagnosis of valsalva retinopathy?**

PVD and macroaneurysm.

○ **What is the prognosis for valsalva retinopathy?**

Excellent - most recover completely in 2-3 months.

○ **Where is the pathology usually centered in Purtscher's retinopathy?**

Surrounding the optic disc.

○ **What is the pathophysiology of Purtscher's retinopathy?**

Injury activates complement, which causes granulocyte aggregation and leukoembolization. Complement-mediated leukostasis and obstruction may follow local retinal vascular injury.

○ **What may cause Purtscher's-like retinopathy?**

Acute pancreatitis, collagen vascular diseases, and childbirth.

○ **How are the fundus findings caused by fat embolism different from Purtscher's?**

Heme is found in the paramacular area and cotton wool spots are generally found more peripherally.

❍ **The syndrome of intraocular hemorrhages associated with abrupt intracranial hemorrhage is known as what?**

Terson Syndrome.

❍ **What is the suspected cause of Terson Syndrome?**

The acute intracranial hemorrhage may cause an abrupt rise in intraocular venous pressure resulting in a rupture of peripapillary and retinal vessels.

❍ **What percentage of patients with subarachnoid hemorrhage will have associated intraocular hemorrhage, and what percent will have vitreous hemorrhage?**

Approximately 33% will have associated intraocular hemorrhage and 6% will have vitreous hemorrhage.

❍ **Describe the five stages of hypertensive retinopathy with the Modified Scheie Classification.**

Grade 0 - No changes.
Grade 1 - Barely detectable arterial narrowing.
Grade 2 - Obvious art. narrowing with focal irregularities.
Grade 3 - Grade 2 + retinal heme and/or exudate.
Grade 4 - Grade 3 + disc swelling.

❍ **What intraocular findings other than arterial narrowing are associated with hypertension?**

Intraretinal heme, BRAO, BRVO, CRVO, arterial macroaneurysms.

❍ **In what type of patient do we normally see hypertensive choroidopathy?**

Young patients experiencing acute hypertension, such as in preeclampsia, eclampsia, pheochromocytoma, or accelerated hypertension.

❍ **What are Elschnig spots?**

Hyperpigmented patches with a surrounding zone of hypopigmentation found over zones of choroidal nonperfusion.

❍ **What are Siegrest streaks?**

Linear configurations of hyperpigmentation that develop over choroidal arteries in patients with uncontrolled hypertension.

❍ **Describe the FA of a patient with hypertensive choroidopathy.**

Early choroidal hypoperfusion and late leakage.

❍   **What syndrome is AR, carried on chromosome 16 and characterized by obesity, polydactyly, hypogonadism, mental retardation and pigmentary retinopathy?**

Bardet-Biedl syndrome.

❍   **A defective myosin gene would affect cells that contain what structure? Why is this important?**

Ciliated cells would be affected. Photoreceptors are modified ciliated cells and cilia are end organs for otologic function-- both are affected in Usher Syndrome and a defective myosin gene has been identified in some Usher Syndrome patients.

❍   **What disease has AR inheritance of juvenile-onset renal failure and retinal pigmentary degeneration?**

Juvenile nephronophthisis or renal-retinal dysplasia.

❍   **What diseases share ichthyosis and pigmentary retinopathy?**

Refsum disease and Sjögren-Larsson syndrome.

❍   **What retinal finding associated with pseudoxanthoma elasticum is more consistent than angioid streaks?**

A *peau d'orange* fundus.

❍   **What should you be suspicious of in any patient over 50 with rapidly progressive retinal dysfunction?**

Underlying malignancy.

❍   **What is the presumed mechanism for retinal degeneration associated with cancer?**

Immunologic.

❍   **Describe the fundus of a true albino.**

Foveal hypoplasia with no foveal light reflex or yellow macular pigment.

❍   **Histologically, what is the difference between oculocutaneous albinism and ocular albinism?**

Oculocutaneous albinism is characterized by a reduction in the amount of primary melanin found in each melanosome, while ocular albinism has an absolute decrease in the number of melanosomes.

❍   **What is the inheritance pattern of oculocutaneous albinism? Ocular albinism?**

Oculocutaneous albinism is AR, while ocular albinism is X-linked.

❍ **Name and describe the two potentially lethal forms of albinism.**

Chediak-Higashi syndrome is oculocutaneous albinism combined with severe susceptibility to infection. Hermansky-Pudlak syndrome patients easily bruise and bleed secondary to a platelet defect.

❍ **What therapy can prevent or treat the retinal degeneration associated with abetalipoproteinemia?**

Vitamin A and E.

❍ **What is the storage abnormality in mucopolysaccharidosis patients that have retinal dystrophies?**

Heparin sulfate.

❍ **Which of the phenothiazines is associated with severe retinopathy if used in abnormally high doses?**

Thioridazine.

❍ **How common is cobblestone degeneration in patients over the age of 20?**

Cobblestone degeneration is found in 22% of the population >20yo.

❍ **Cobblestone degeneration is actually a discrete area of ischemic atrophy. What is absent histologically from the affected areas?**

Choriocapillaris, RPE and outer retina are absent. The remaining inner retina is firmly attached to Bruch's-- this is why retinal detachments don't usually spread through areas of cobblestone.

❍ **Why is it that acute operculated holes are rarely treated prophylactically, while acute symptomatic flap tears are almost always treated?**

The operculated hole is not under residual vitreoretinal traction, while the flap tear remains under traction and carries a high risk of detachment.

❍ **What is Shafer's sign?**

Small clumps of pigmented cells, called tobacco dust, seen in the vitreous or AC. This sign can be helpful in diagnosing the type of retinal detachment when no hole can be found.

❍ **What cells are responsible for PVR?**

RPE and glial cells.

○   **Why is there no Grade C-4 in the classification of RD with PVR?**

Grade C-4 RD with PVR would mean full-thickness retinal fold in 4 quadrants, and this, of course, is the definition of Grade D RD with PVR.

○   **What type of lens must be used to diagnose Class D-2 RD with PVR?**

A +20 D condensing lens, because the anterior end of the funnel must be completely visible within the field of view of this lens.

○   **What is the current rate of anatomic success after retinal detachment repair?**

About 90% of eyes will be anatomical success after retinal detachment repair.

○   **Why is a macula on detachment a more urgent case than a macula off detachment?**

If the macula is spared 87% of eyes will attain 20/50 or better, while only 37% will reach that level of acuity if the macula is detached. A macular detachment should be repaired within the first week because studies have shown a decline in post-op VA in eyes repaired >1 week out.

○   **How soon should a patient with an exudative retinal detachment be scheduled for surgery?**

They should not be scheduled for surgery because the treatment of exudative detachments is aimed at treating the underlying condition (usually neoplasm or inflammatory disease).

○   **Describe a typical choroidal metastasis (i.e., appearance, associated signs and symptoms). What is the most common symptom of a patient who presents with this disorder?**

Typically, it is seen in the posterior pole, secondary to the relative greater blood flow (i.e., via short posterior ciliary arteries). It presents as a yellowish-whitish mass, often associated with serous retinal detachments. Blurred vision is found as the presenting complaint 80% of the time.

○   **Compare and contrast the A-scan findings of a metastatic tumor v. choroidal melanoma.**

A-scan of a metastasic tumor usually shows a high internal reflectivity (i.e., more heterogenous in character), where A-scan of a choroidal melanoma shows a low internal reflectivity (i.e., more homogenous in character).

○   **What are the most common quadrants for retinal break following trauma?**

1. Inferotemporal, which is noted to be the least protected (i.e., less bony structure) area of the globe.
2. Superonasal (due to the coup contrecoup effect).

❍   **What's the most common quadrant for a spontaneous (i.e., non-traumatic) retinal break? How does age affect this risk?**

1. Less than 20 years of age: superotemporal quadrant, followed by inferotemporal, followed by superonasal, followed by inferonasal.
2. 20-40 years of age: superotemporal quadrant, followed by inferotemporal and superonasal (equal), followed by inferonasal.
3. Over 40 years of age: superotemporal quadrant, followed by superonasal, followed by inferotemporal, followed by inferonasal.

❍   **What is the histopathology of a retinal cavernous hemangioma?**

It is a tumor rising from the inner half of the retina, with multiple endothelial lined thin-wall aneurysms, separated by thin, fibrous septa. There is no evidence of intraretinal or subretinal exudates.

❍   **What must you rule out when a patient presents with posterior scleritis?**

1. Syphilis.
2. Wegener's granulomatosis.
3. Inflammatory bowel disease.
4. Rheumatoid arthritis.
5. Relapsing polychondritis.
6. Systemic lupus erythematosus.
7. Sarcoid.

❍   **Name the four stages of macular hole formation, according to the Gass system.**

Stage I is a foveal detachment, with loss of foveal pigment (i.e., yellow spot). Stage II is a full-thickness macular hole, less than 400 microns. Stage III is a full-thickness macular hole, greater than 400 microns. Stage IV is a full-thickness retinal hole greater than 400 microns, with detached vitreous. Typically, Stages II-IV are repaired operatively. Stage I holes are observed. A macular cyst can be a precursor to a macular hole.

❍   **What is the rare retinal disorder that affects patients at about age 40 and often displays bilateral subfoveal neovascular membranes?**

Sorby's macular dystrophy. The gene for Sorby's dystrophy codes for a tissue inhibitor of metalloproteinase, which is involved in the extracellular matrix remodeling (i.e., therefore the increased risk for CNVM).

❍   **What is the differential diagnosis of intraretinal crystals?**

Crystals can be from Tamoxifen, canthaxanthine, cystinosis, primary hyperoxaluria, Bietti's crystalline dystrophy, idiopathic juxtafoveal telangiectasia Type II, diabetic macular edema, talc retinopathy and methoxyflurane toxicity.

❍   **What are some risk factors associated with retinal detachment?**

Family history or previous history of retinal detachment in a companion eye of a patient, lattice degeneration, meridional folds, vitreoretinal tufts, enclosed ora bays and peripheral retinal excavations. Cobblestone degeneration, RPE hypertrophy and hyperplasia are not risk factors.

O   **With regard to intraocular foreign bodies, which substances are more reactive, or more significant, than others are are?**

Aluminum, zinc, glass, stone and plastic are especially well tolerated. Copper (containing more than 85%) causes chalcosis and iron causes siderosis. Cooper and iron are the main metals that cause extensive damage with ERG changes, initially producing a large A-wave and a normal B-wave. As the siderosis progresses, the B-wave amplitude will diminish and eventually become extinguished. ERG's are useful for following these patients with intraocular foreign body. Vegetable matter is an organic foreign body that can cause a severe inflammatory response, and an increased risk for endophthalmitis. The copper from chalcosis can produce a KF (Kaiser-Flescher) ring.

O   **After extracapsular cataract extraction, a patient presents to the Retina clinic two weeks later. The vision is noted to be decreased to approximately 20/70. The anterior segment of the eye looks to be within normal limits, with a well-centered PC IOL, with minimal cell and flare. The interesting point of the case is that the surgery was approximately two hours in duration. Your fundus exam shows a yellowish-white lesion deep in the retina, adjacent to the fovea, as well as a paracentral scotoma. What is the most likely diagnosis?**

Phototoxicity from the ophthalmic operating microscope is the most likely diagnosis. This typically presents with a yellowish-white lesion deep to the retina. The lesion involves a zone of mottled retinal pigment epithelium, and transmits hyperfluorescence on angiography. Phototoxicity has been reported in some cases, as small as 10 minutes duration. Filtering light sources, shields and macular protectors may be useful in these cases.

O   **A 75-year-old age related macular degeneration patient comes in your office, stating that she heard that large doses of different vitamins would help her AMD (and has been taking them). She complains of decreased visual acuity. On your exam, she is noted to be 20/70 OU, with significant cystoid macular edema OU. Which vitamin is most likely the cause of these findings?**

Nicotinic acid, which can cause cystoid macular edema. Discontinuation of this vitamin in large doses may help resolve the cystoid macular edema. In addition, the anti-oxidant in the treatment of AMD is still considered controversial.

O   **A patient with parafoveal telangiectasia Type II should have which blood test performed?**

The patient should be screened for diabetes. A glucose tolerance test should be performed, as a population of these patients has abnormal glucose tolerance tests.

O   **What wavelengths should be used when treating a melanin-containing lesion?**

As melanin absorbs most wavelengths well, the choice of wavelengths is less critical. Argon green is useful for most purposes.

❍ **What wavelengths should be considered when treating a blood-containing lesion?**

Krypton 568 nm or organic dye 570-575 nm is maximally absorbed by blood with minimal scatter.

❍ **What is the least significant parameter in retinal photocoagulation?**

Adjusting exposure time generally has less impact than adjusting spot size or power.

❍ **What needs to be taken into account when using a Rodenstock or Volk lens for retinal photocoagulation?**

The spot size will be magnified.

❍ **How can laser photocoagulation be used to distinguish a rhegmatogenous retinal detachment from retinoschisis?**

A reaction will be visible in the outer layer of schisis, but not on the bare RPE of a retinal detachment.

❍ **What type of detachment related to acquired retinoschisis is more likely to progress?**

Detachments secondary to inner and outer layer breaks are more likely to progress, while detachments involving outer breaks alone more often remain localized.

❍ **What factors would suggest that a retinal break might require prophylactic treatment?**

Lack of chronicity, presence of symptoms, myopia, aphakia or pseudophakia, superior location, family history of retinal detachment, or history of detachment in the fellow eye.

❍ **Photocoagulation is the preferred treatment for which parasitic disease?**

DUSN.

❍ **When is photocoagulation of retinoblastoma appropriate?**

When the tumors are small, confined to the sensory retina, few in number and remote from the disc and macula. Direct treatment is contraindicated secondary to poor absorption.

❍ **When is it appropriate to consider the use of laser photocoagulation in the treatment of choroidal melanoma?**

In tumors less than 3 mm thick and greater than 3 mm from the foveola and risk of liberating tumor cells.

O   **What is the role of laser photocoagulation in the treatment of capillary hemangiomas associated with Von-Hippel/Von-Hippel-Lindau?**

Direct treatment with large spot size and low intensity burns applied to the surface of the lesion should be undertaken when they are discovered, since small lesions are more easily treated.

O   **How and when should the lesions of Coat's disease be treated with laser photocoagulation?**

Lesions threatening the macula and not associated with a large exudative retinal detachment may be treated directly with 200-500 micron spots of moderate power and wavelengths absorbed by hemoglobin, such as argon green or yellow dye laser.

O   **When should arterial macroaneurysm be treated?**

Aneurysms that threaten the macula may be treated directly with argon laser using large spot size. Lesions that have ruptured and bled acutely rarely rebleed, and treatment may be associated with arteriolar occlusion.

O   **When is photocoagulation required for cavernous hemangiomas?**

Photocoagulation is rarely required, but has been advocated for recurrent vitreous hemorrhage.

O   **What groups were studied by the Macular Photocoagulation Study Group?**

The MPS studied classic CNV in age-related macular degeneration, presumed ocular histoplasmosis and idiopathic causes.

O   **How were "extrafoveal CNV" and "juxtafoveal CNV" defined in the MPS?**

The foveal edge of CNV and blockage by pigment or blood is located 200-2500 microns from the center of the FAZ in extrafoveal CNV. The foveal edge of juxtafoveal CNV and blockage by pigment or blood is located 1-199 microns from the center of the FAZ.

O   **What was the laser technique used in the MPS for treatment of extrafoveal CNV?**

CNV, contiguous blockage and 100 microns beyond were covered.

O   **What was the laser technique used in the MPS for treatment of juxtafoveal CNV?**

On the non-foveal side, cover CNV, contiguous blockage and 100 microns beyond. On the foveal side, cover CNV and (if greater than 100 microns from the center of the FAZ and contiguous blood is also present) contiguous blood up to 100 microns beyond.

❍   **What were the results of the Macular Photocoagulation Study for POHS?**

A treatment benefit was demonstrated using argon blue-green to treat extrafoveal CNV and krypton red to treat juxtafoveal CNV. The recurrence rate was higher in juxtafoveal CNV.

❍   **What were the conclusions of the Age-Related Eye disease Study (AREDS)?**

1. People at high risk for developing advanced AMD reduced their risk by 25 percent when treated with antioxidants plus zinc and also reduced the risk of central visual loss by 19 percent.

2. The risk of developing advanced AMD in people at high risk was reduced by 21 percent by zinc alone and reduced the risk of central visual loss by 11 percent.

3. The risk of developing advanced AMD in people at high risk was reduced by 17 percent by antioxidants alone and reduced the risk of central visual loss by 10 percent.

❍   **What were the specific daily amounts of antioxidants and zinc used in the AREDS study?**

500 mg of vitamin C
400 international units of vitamin E
15 mg of beta-carotene
80 mg of zinc as zinc oxide
2 mg of copper as cupric oxide.

UVEITIS

○ **Which uveitic disease has the best prognosis with regards to cataract surgery?**

Fuch's heterochromic iridocyclitis, where posterior synechiae do not commonly form and formation of pupillary membranes are unlikely.

○ **"River blindness," a major cause of blindness worldwide, characterized by uveitis, chorioretinal changes and optic atrophy is caused by what organism?**

Microfilariae of Onchocerca volvulus cause this disease also known as onchocerciasis.

○ **What is the primary host of *Onchocerca*?**

Black fly larvae.

○ **What is the treatment for ocular cysticercosis?**

Surgical removal of the cysticerci; medical treatment or photocoagulation can lead to an intense inflammatory reaction from the dead organism.

○ **What are the major active components of the slow reacting substance of anaphylaxis (SRS-A)?**

Leukotrienes C_4 and D_4.

○ **Do NSAIDs inhibit lipoxygenase?**

No, but nordihydroguaiaretic acid (NDGA) does.

○ **What are Koeppe and Busacca nodules?**

They are iris granulomas. Koeppe nodules are found at the pupillary margin, while Busacca are found on the iris stroma.

○ **What uveitic disease is the HLA-A29 phenotype strongly associated with?**

Birdshot retinochoroidopathy is strongly associated with the HLA-A29 phenotype, which is present in up to 96% of patients with this disease. People who are HLA-A29 positive have a 50 to 224 times greater chance of developing birdshot retinochoroidopathy that those with other HLA phenotypes.

○ **What are the complications of birdshot retinochoroidopathy?**

Cystoid maculopathy, choroidal neovascularization, retinal atrophy, optic atrophy, and cataract.

O   **What is keratoderma blenorrhagica?**

They are blister like lesions in the feet and are associated with Reiter's syndrome.

O   **What is the mechanism of action of alkylating immunosuppressive agents?**

They interact with the 7-nitrogen guanine of DNA and cause strand breakage and cross-linking of DNA strands.

O   **What type of hypersensitivity reaction is present in ocular cicatricial pemphigoid?**

Type II hypersensitivity.

O   **What are the three most common causes of anterior uveitis?**

Idiopathic iridocyclitis (12%), HLA-B27-associated iridocyclitis (3%) and JRA (2.8%).

O   **What are the presenting symptoms of patients with acute posterior multifocal placoid pigment epitheliopathy (AMPPE)?**

Patients with AMPPE complain of mildly impaired visual acuity in one eye followed a few days later by involvement of the other eye. Half of all patients will report a prodromal flu-like illness, which may be associated with erythema nodosum.

O   **What is the appearance of the active lesions of AMPPE with fluorescein angiography?**

The active lesions appear hypofluorescent during the early phases of the fluorescein angiogram.

O   **Do most patients with AMPPE generally require treatment?**

No. The disease resolves spontaneously in a few weeks in the vast majority and the visual acuity usually returns to normal or near normal.

O   **A man working in a pig farm accidentally stabs himself in the eye when a pig kicks his hand holding a knife. On examination in the operating room, you see a laceration extending from the cornea to the sclera with uvea and vitreous prolapsing through the wound. There does not appear to be an exit wound. Is this an ocular penetrating injury or a perforating injury?**

This is an ocular penetrating injury. Had the knife created an exit wound at the opposite end, it would be called an ocular perforating injury.

O   **What is the risk of sympathetic ophthalmia in this patient?**

The incidence of sympathetic ophthalmia is thought to be 1.9/1000 nonsurgical penetrating injuries and 1/10,000 surgical cases.

❍ **When should enucleation be performed in this patient to prevent sympathetic ophthalmia?**

Enucleation should be performed within 2 weeks of the injury if there is no hope of restoring vision in that eye. If sympathetic ophthalmia occurs in the opposite eye, removing the blind, injured eye within 2 weeks of the onset of SO may reduce the severity of the disease.

❍ **What is the main difference between sympathetic ophthalmia and Vogt-Koyanagi-Harada's (VKH) syndrome histopathologically?**

Sympathetic ophthalmia shows sparing of the choriocapillaris, while VKH shows inflammation affecting all layers of the choroid.

❍ **What are spondyloarthropathies?**

They are a group of diseases that affect the spine and entheses (insertions of tendons and ligaments).

❍ **Name the HLA-B27-associated spondyloarthropathies where uveitis can occur.**

1. Ankylosing spondylitis.
2. Reiter's syndrome.
3. Psoriatic arthritis.
4. Inflammatory bowel disease (Crohn's disease, Ulcerative colitis).

❍ **Why should all young men with acute, unilateral iritis undergo X-rays of the sacroiliac joints irrespective of the presence or absence of low back symptoms?**

Radiographs may show the presence of sacroiliitis before the patient becomes symptomatic. Early appropriate therapy may prevent the more severe structural changes to the spine.

❍ **What percentage of males who are HLA-B27 positive will develop ankylosing spondylitis?**

20%.

❍ **What are the major symptoms of Reiter's syndrome?**

1. Arthritis of more than a month's duration typically affecting knees and ankles.
2. Urethritis.
3. Ocular inflammation (papillary conjunctivitis, acute nongranulomatous iridocyclitis, keratitis).

❍ **What are some minor symptoms of Reiter's syndrome?**

Achilles tendonitis, plantar fasciitis, sacroillitis, painless oral ulcers, keratoderma blenorrhagica involving palms and soles, circinate balanitis, prostatitis, diarrhea.

○   **What are the diagnostic criteria for Reiter's syndrome?**

1. Complete: Three major symptoms.
2. Probable: two major and two minor symptoms.
3. Possible: two major and one minor symptoms.

○   **How often are patients with Reiter's syndrome HLA-B27 positive and have an associated sacroiliitis?**

About 70% are HLA-B27 positive, and about 60% may have an associated sacroiliitis.

○   **What other diseases producing oral ulcers, iridocyclitis, and large joint arthritis must be ruled out when making the diagnosis of Reiter's syndrome?**

Behçet's disease and sarcoidosis. Reiter's disease is not associated with retinal vasculitis, which can occur with these two diseases.

○   **What HLA phenotypes have been associated with ocular Behçet's disease in other countries?**

HLA-B5, HLA-B51.

○   **What are the major symptoms of Behçet's disease?**

1. Uveitis (66%)
2. Painful oral ulcers (100%)
3. Genital ulcers (84%)
4. Skin lesions (erythema nodosum, cutaneous vasculitis) (66%)

○   **What are the Japanese diagnostic criteria for Behçet's disease?**

1. Complete: 4 major symptoms (oral ulcers, uveitis, genital ulcers, and skin lesions).
2. Incomplete: 3 major symptoms or uveitis + one major symptom.
3. Suspect: 2 nonocular major symptoms.
4. Possible: One major symptom.

○   **What are the ocular manifestations of Behçet's disease?**

1. Acute recurrent iridocyclitis.
2. Retinitis.
3. Retinal vasculitis.
4. Retina edema and exudation.
5. Vitritis.

○   **How can you test for cutaneous hypersensitivity in patients with Behçet's disease?**

Scratching the skin with a needle will cause a pustule to form ("prick" or pathergy test), while stroking the skin can cause the appearance of lines (dermatographism).

○ **What is the differential diagnosis of Behçet's disease?**

Reiter's syndrome can produce acute anterior uveitis, oral ulcers, urethritis, sacroiliitis and arthritis. The uveitis is recurrent and unilateral and is not associated with retinal vasculitis. Sarcoidosis produces chronic uveitis with retinal vasculitis, oral ulcers, and large joint arthralgias. It is associated with hilar lymphadenopathy, systemic anergy, and elevated serum angiotensin converting enzyme (ACE) and lysozyme levels.

○ **In what forms of juvenile rheumatoid arthritis (JRA) is uveitis likely to occur?**

Uveitis affects about 20% of children with the pauciarticular (≤4 joints affected within a 6 month period) form of JRA, which accounts for 50% of all JRA cases. Uveitis occurs in about 5% of the polyarticular form (≥5 joints affected), which accounts for 40% of all JRA cases, and is extremely rare in the acute toxic form (Still's disease).

○ **What are risk factors for developing uveitis in the pauciarticular form of JRA?**

Early onset JRA, positive ANA and HLA-DR5.

○ **How often should children with JRA be screened for eye disease?**

Children with the pauciarticular form should be screened by an ophthalmologist at least every 3 months, while children with the polyarticular form should be seen at least every 6 months. Patients with Still's disease can be seen at least once a year.

○ **Are JRA patients who develop uveitis usually symptomatic?**

No. They are usually asymptomatic even with 4+cells in the anterior chamber, and the uveitis is frequently detected only on slit lamp examination. The eyes are usually uninjected even in the presence of severe uveitis, which is chronic, nongranulomatous and bilateral in 70% of cases.

○ **A 75-year-old patient presents with a chronic vitritis that was initially responsive to corticosteroids but has now become resistant. What is the most likely diagnosis?**

This patient may have intraocular lymphoma. It is a non-Hodgkin's large cell lymphoma occurring usually in the elderly that can originate in the brain or the eye. It may masquerade as a chronic posterior uveitis and vitritis that may initially seem to respond to corticosteroids and then become resistant.

○ **How is intraocular lymphoma diagnosed?**

Vitreous biopsy is required to confirm the diagnosis, while CT scan or MRI scan may confirm CNS involvement. Radiation therapy and systemic chemotherapy are the mainstays of treatment. The prognosis is generally poor.

○ **What is Vogt-Koyanagi syndrome?**

It is characterized by chronic, granulomatous anterior uveitis and skin changes (alopecia, poliosis, and vitiligo).

○   **What is Harada's syndrome?**

This is characterized by posterior segment involvement (multifocal choroiditis and exudative retinal detachment) associated with neurologic features (meningeal and auditory symptoms, encephalopathy, CSF lymphocytosis).

○   **What is the most common cause of poor visual acuity in patients with intermediate uveitis?**

Cystoid macular edema.

○   **What systemic disorders can be associated with intermediate uveitis with long-term followup?**

Multiple sclerosis and sarcoidosis.

○   **What percentage of MS patients will show peripheral retinophlebitis with vitreous snowballs?**

10%.

○   **What is the description of the keratic precipitates produced by Fuch's heterochromic iridocyclitis?**

Diffusely scattered, stellate keratic precipitates

○   **What percentage of patients with Fuch's heterochromic iridocyclitis eventually develop glaucoma?**

25-50%.

○   **What can gonioscopy of an eye with Fuch's heterochromic iridocyclitis reveals?**

Fine vessels crossing the trabecular meshwork without synechiae.

○   **You are consulted by Pediatrics to see a newborn child with seizures, hydrocephalus and paralysis. On examination, you find bilateral chorioretinal scars. What is the most likely diagnosis?**

Congenital systemic toxoplasmosis.

○   **What may be found in skull radiographs of children born with congenital toxoplasmosis?**

Intracranial calcifications.

❍   **What are the critical ocular signs of active ocular toxoplasmosis?**

A unilateral yellowish-white retinal lesion, usually adjacent to an old chorioretinal scar, and associated with a hazy vitreous.

❍   **Which is the active form of *Toxoplasma gondii* responsible for the tissue destruction and inflammation?**

Tachyzoite. Sporocysts are oocysts excreted in cat feces while bradyzoites are the encysted form in tissues.

❍   **How is toxoplasmosis acquired?**

1. Eating undercooked meat-containing bradyzoites.
2. Ingestion of sporocysts from contamination of hands or eating dirt containing sporocysts.
3. Transplacental spread to the fetus in a pregnant woman with acquired systemic toxoplasmosis.

❍   **What should you request from the laboratory when obtaining a serum antitoxoplasma antibody titer in the workup of a patient with possible ocular toxoplasmosis?**

Ask the laboratory to do a 1:1 dilution.

❍   **What are the main indications for treatment of active ocular toxoplasmosis?**

An active lesion threatening the macula, optic nerve or a major blood vessel.
Severe vitritis.
AIDS.

❍   **What drugs can be used in the treatment of toxoplasmosis?**

Pyrimethamine with folinic acid, sulfadiazine, clindamycin, and trimethoprim-sulfamethoxazole.

❍   **What is the main side effect of pyrimethamine?**

Bone marrow depression, which is why folinic acid is given concurrently to counteract against. CBC and platelet counts should be checked at least weekly, and the dosage of pyrimethamine should be reduced and folinic acid increased if the platelet count goes below 100,000.

❍   **What should patients taking pyrimethamine and folinic acid be instructed not to take?**

Multivitamin preparations containing folic acid.

❍   **What will result if systemic corticosteroids alone or regional corticosteroids are given to a patient with active ocular toxoplasmosis?**

Acute necrotizing retinitis.

O   **What are the critical signs of presumed ocular histoplasmosis (POHS)?**

Atrophic "histo" spots in the posterior pole and mid-periphery.
Peripapillary atrophy.
Choroidal neovascularization (late sign).
Quiet vitreous.

O   **What is the visual prognosis of POHS patients who develop choroidal neovascular membranes involving the macula according to the Macular Photocoagulation Study Group?**

Twenty-two percent of laser treated eyes will develop a six-line loss of vision compared with 50% of untreated eyes within 2 years.

O   **What types of choroidal neovascular membranes should be treated with focal laser photocoagulation?**

Juxtafoveal (within 1-200 microns of the center of the foveal avascular zone) and extrafoveal (within 200 and 2500 microns from the foveal avascular zone) membranes

O   **How often are the VDRL and the FTA-Abs titers positive in a patient with syphilis?**

Seventy-six percent of primary syphilis patients are VDRL positive while 86% are FTA-Abs reactive. All secondary syphilitics are VDRL and FTA-Abs positive. In latent and neurosyphilis, the VDRL is positive in 70% while the FTA-Abs is positive in 97%.

O   **What are the most common ocular manifestations of syphilis?**

Chronic granulomatous or nongranulomatous iridocyclitis, multifocal chorioretinitis, neuroretinitis, choroiditis, scleritis, and interstitial keratitis.

O   **What are some neuro-ophthalmic manifestations of ocular syphilis?**

1. Argyll-Robertson pupils.
2. Retrobulbar neuritis, papillitis.
3. III nerve and VI nerve palsies.
4. Visual field defects from syphilitic brain lesions.

O   **What is the treatment for ocular syphilis?**

IV penicillin for 10 days followed by intramuscular penicillin for 3 weeks using the same therapeutic regimen for neurosyphilis. Penicillin-sensitive patients can be treated with oral tetracycline or erythromycin for 30 days. The VDRL declines to undetectable levels after effective therapy, while the FTA-ABS and MHA-TP are detectable throughout life.

O   **What are the clinical features of tuberculous uveitis?**

Tuberculous uveitis can present as acute, recurrent, or chronic granulomatous iritis and fulminating, granulomatous, caseating tubercles in the iris and choroid. Retinal periphlebitis and choroidal neovascularization may be present. With specific therapy, the lesions quiet down and may disappear entirely.

❍   **What does histopathology of tuberculous lesions demonstrate?**

Caseating granulomas with Langerhans' giant cells.

❍   **How do you test for tuberculosis in a patient suspected of having tuberculous uveitis?**

The diagnosis is made by chest X-ray and by skin testing using the PPD-T (5TU). If the skin reaction to 5TU is negative, the PPD 2 (250TU) should be used. Any reaction suggests that the uveitis can be due to tuberculosis.

❍   **How is isoniazid (INH) used as a therapeutic test for tuberculous uveitis?**

300 mg is given daily for 3 weeks while keeping other therapy constant and observing the eye at weekly intervals for improvement. If tuberculous uveitis is strongly suspected, other anti-tuberculous agents such as rifampin and ethambutol are added to the regimen.

❍   **How often should monitoring for isoniazid-induced liver toxicity be performed?**

Monthly monitoring for liver toxicity is recommended by the FDA, and INH should be discontinued at least temporarily if values exceed 3 times the upper limit of normal.

❍   **How can peripheral neuritis produced by INH be prevented?**

Administer pyridoxine 25 mg/day.

❍   **What ocular side effect should be watched out for when using ethambutol to treat tuberculosis?**

Ethambutol can produce an optic neuropathy.

❍   **Which species is the most common cause of toxocariasis in humans, *T. canis* or *T. catis*?**

Toxocara canis, which is a roundworm parasite of dogs.

❍   **Do antihelminthics have a role in treating ocular toxocariasis?**

No, because the larva incites inflammation and granuloma formation only after its death. Oral and periocular corticosteroids are the treatment of choice when vitritis, retinal edema or exudative retinal detachments are present. Vitreoretinal surgery can be performed in the presence of severe endophthalmitis to clear the media and control the inflammation.

❍   **How is toxocara usually acquired?**

Oral ingestion of soils containing feces or larvae, usually by young children.

❍   **Is ocular toxocariasis associated with visceral larval migrans (VLM)?**

No. VLM is a systemic illness, usually in young children, caused by *T. canis* and presents with fever, hepatosplenomegaly, cough, and a pruritic skin rash. Peripheral eosinophilia and leukocytosis are also present. It is not associated with ocular disease.

❍   **What are the most common ocular lesions found in toxocariasis?**

Chronic endophthalmitis, posterior pole granuloma, peripheral granuloma.

❍   **Does a positive anti-Toxocara antibody titer rule out retinoblastoma?**

No. Any positive titer should be interpreted in conjunction with the clinical findings and is consistent but not necessarily diagnostic of toxocariasis.

❍   **Do anti-helminthic agents play any role in treating ocular toxocariasis?**

No, because the death of the larva causes the inflammation and granuloma formation.

❍   **What are the ocular manifestations of Lyme disease?**

Conjunctivitis, uveitis, episcleritis, stromal keratitis and orbital myositis.

❍   **What is the vector for Lyme disease?**

The tick *Ixodes* sp. transmits the spirochete *Borrelia burgdorferi* though its bite.

❍   **What is the differential diagnosis of posterior scleritis?**

1. Choroidal tumor.
2. Uveal effusion syndrome.
3. Harada's disease.
4. Orbital inflammatory disease.

❍   **How do you distinguish between the retinal vasculitis of acute retinal necrosis (ARN) versus the retinal vasculitis produced by sarcoidosis?**

Diseases such as ARN and polyarteritis nodosa produce an arteriolitis, whereas other diseases such as sarcoidosis and syphilis often affect the retinal venules.

❍   **What is Heerfordt's syndrome?**

It is seen in sarcoidosis and consists of:

1. Anterior uveitis.
2. Facial palsy.
3. Parotid enlargement.

❍   **Which form of inflammatory bowel disease does iritis more commonly occur in?**

Iritis occurs in over 10% of patients with ulcerative colitis, while less than 3% with Crohn's disease will develop iritis.

❍   **What are Dalen-Fuchs nodules?**

They are epithelioid cell accumulations between Bruch's membrane and the retinal pigment epithelium and are classically found in some patients with sympathetic ophthalmia and Vogt-Koyanagi-Harada syndrome.

❍   **What HLA phenotype is associated with intermediate uveitis?**

None.

❍   **What is the differential diagnosis of intermediate uveitis?**

Lyme disease, Fuch's heterochromic iridocyclitis, toxocariasis, JRA, and toxoplasmosis should be considered. In younger children, retinoblastoma must also be in the differential diagnosis.

❍   **What is the main indication for treatment of intermediate uveitis?**

Cystoid macular edema with reduction in vision.

❍   **What is the treatment for intermediate uveitis?**

Periocular corticosteroids are the mainstay of treatment. Oral NSAIDs reduce the frequency and severity of attacks. Oral corticosteroids are used for patients resistant to periocular steroids. If that fails, pars plana cryotherapy using a freeze-refreeze technique to areas of active exudation, vitrectomy or systemic immunosuppression with azathioprine, methotrexate, cyclosporin or cyclophosphamide can be used.

❍   **A 55-year-old patient presents with retinal vasculitis, vitritis, chronic diarrhea and arthritis. Intestinal biopsy reveals PAS-positive material. What is the most likely diagnosis?**

Whipple's disease.

❍   **What cell is the main target for HIV?**

T-helper lymphocytes.

❍   **What are the treatment options available for CMV retinitis?**

1. Oral valganciclovir
2. Ganciclovir implant
3. IV ganciclovir

4. IV or intravitreal foscarnet or cidofovir for patients whose retinitis is resistant to ganciclovir

O   **What types of conjunctivitis can chronic use of atropine eye drops produce?**

Follicular conjunctivitis.

O   **What is the mechanism of action of methotrexate?**

Methotrexate is a folate analog and inhibits dihydrofolate reductase, which is required in nucleotide synthesis.

O   **What is the most common cause of endogenous fungal endophthalmitis?**

Candida species.

O   **In what clinical setting is Candida endophthalmitis usually seen?**

This is usually seen in hospital inpatients receiving hyperalimentation or indwelling catheters, IV drug users and immunocompromised patients.

O   **What are the ocular manifestations of Candida endophthalmitis?**

This infection presents with fluffy, yellow-white, multifocal choroidal lesions and vitreous "puffballs" when the fungus breaks through the retina and into the vitreous.

O   **How often does acute retinal necrosis present unilaterally?**

It is unilateral in two-thirds of cases.

O   **What is the mechanism of action of NSAIDs?**

It inhibits the cyclooxygenase enzyme that is essential in the production of prostaglandins.

O   **List the mydriatic/cycloplegic agents in order of increasing duration of effect.**

1. Tropicamide.
2. Cyclopentolate.
3. Homatropine.
4. Scopolamine.
5. Atropine.

O   **What is the most common organism found in posttraumatic endophthalmitis where soil contamination might be a factor?**

Bacillus cereus.

O   **How many times more common is sarcoidosis in African Americans compared to white Americans?**

It is 10-15 times as common in African Americans as in white Americans.

○   **Give three noninvasive ways of diagnosing sarcoidosis.**

Serum angiotensin converting enzyme (ACE) levels, chest X-ray (hilar adenopathy in 80% of ocular sarcoidosis) and gallium scanning (looking for lacrimal gland, parotid gland or pulmonary involvement).

○   **How often does uveitis develop in patients with systemic sarcoidosis during the silent stage of the disease?**

80% of patients.

○   **What will biopsy of sarcoid lesions reveal?**

Noncaseating granulomas.

○   **What is the safest drug to use to treat toxoplasmosis in a pregnant woman?**

Clindamycin.

○   **In which uveitis syndromes have lymphocytes taken from patients with these diseases been shown to develop an in vitro response to retinal S-antigen?**

Lymphocytes taken from patients with sympathetic ophthalmia, Vogt-Koyanagi-Harada (VKH) syndrome, and birdshot retinochoroidopathy all develop an *in vitro* response to retinal S-antigen.

○   **What can multiple evanescent white dot syndromes (MEWDS) show with visual field testing?**

Enlarged blind spot.

○   **What percentage of patients with sarcoidosis will show an elevated serum angiotensin converting enzyme level?**

60% in all sarcoid patients, 90% with active disease, and 40% with inactive disease.

○   **Which will show greater calcium levels when testing for sarcoidosis, serum calcium or urine calcium levels?**

Urine calcium levels are more often raised than serum levels in sarcoidosis.

○   **What is the most potent corticosteroid?**

Dexamethasone.

○   **What parasite believed to be associated with diffuse, unilateral, subacute neuroretinitis (DUSN)?**

Bayliascaris, which is a raccoon ascarid, worm.

O   **What does flare in the anterior chamber represent?**

Flare represents breakdown of the blood-aqueous barrier and should not be used to guide treatment of uveitis.

O   **What type of hypersensitivity reaction is present in scleritis?**

Type III (immune complex) hypersensitivity.

O   **What organism is thought to be responsible for Lyme disease, and how is it transmitted?**

Borrelia burgdorferi, which is transmitted by tick bites.

O   **What is the significance of elevated fetal IgM levels?**

It indicates the presence of an intrauterine infection since IgM cannot cross the placental barrier from the mother to the fetus.

O   **At what stage does uveitis usually occur in Lyme disease?**

Stage II disease.

O   **What HLA phenotype has been associated with presumed ocular histoplasmosis with macular involvement?**

HLA B-7.

O   **What ear problems can be associated with VKH syndrome?**

Tinnitus, vertigo, and deafness.

O   **What is the most common ocular manifestation of HIV infection?**

Cotton wool spots from infarction of the retinal fiber layer, which may result from Deposition of immune complexes in the retinal capillaries.

O   **What is the incidence of CMV retinitis in patients with AIDS in adults?**

CMV retinitis occurs in a third of adults with AIDS.

O   **What are the characteristics of CMV retinitis?**

It is bilateral in 30 to 50% of cases and characterized by areas of retinal whitening and hemorrhages. It typically begins in the posterior pole along major blood vessels. Without treatment, it slowly progresses to blindness.

O   **What is the cause of visual loss in serpiginous choroidopathy?**

Visual loss occurs with involvement of the macula by the active lesion or by choroidal neovascularization developing from the edge of chorioretinal atrophy and involving the fovea.

❍   **A 26-year-old woman complains of photopsias and blurring of vision in one eye. Her visual acuity is 20/40 in the involved eye, and the fundus exam reveals small, subtle, gray-white lesions at the level of the outer retina and RPE which show early hyperfluorescence in a wreath-like pattern and late staining on fluorescein angiography. What is the probable diagnosis?**

Multiple evanescent white dot syndrome.

❍   **What is the treatment for multiple evanescent white dot syndromes?**

No treatment is necessary. The white dots disappear within weeks of onset, and the visual symptoms gradually resolve.

❍   **What immune cell possesses cytotoxic activity against tumors and virally infected cells without any previous exposure to antigen?**

Natural killer cells.

❍   **What types of hypersensitivity reaction are Wessely rings?**

Type III (immune complex) hypersensitivity.

❍   **What percentage of patients with ankylosing spondylitis are HLA-B27 positive?**

90-100%.

❍   **What percentage of Americans are HLA-B27 positive?**

5 to 14%.

❍   **In what diseases can Dalen-Fuchs nodules are found in?**

Sympathetic ophthalmia, VKH syndrome, tuberculous choroiditis, and sarcoidosis.

❍   **What type of hypersensitivity reaction is myasthenia gravis?**

Type V, where antibodies react with cell surface receptors and either stimulate or depress cellular function.

❍   **How do nonsteroid antiinflammatory drugs reduce inflammation?**

NSAIDs block the cyclo-oxygenase pathway, which produces prostaglandins, prostacyclin and thromboxane.

❍   **What is the primary immunoglobulin found in tears?**

IgA.

○   **On what type of cells are Class II cell surface antigens found?**

They are found on B-cells, monocytes and some activated T-cells and are coded by the Dr, Dp and Dq regions of the HLA system.

○   **Do AIDS patients exhibit elevated or decreased immunoglobulin levels?**

They exhibit elevated immunoglobulins, especially IgG and IgA.

○   **What is the mechanism of immune suppression by cyclosporine?**

Cyclosporine suppresses interleukin-2 production, preventing activated T cells from dividing and proliferating.

○   **What are the most common infectious organisms causing chronic postoperative endophthalmitis after intraocular surgery?**

S. epidermidis produces chronic postoperative endophthalmitis within 6 weeks after surgery, while *Candida* endophthalmitis occurs within 1- to 3 months and *P. acnes* within 3 months to 2 years after surgery.

○   **How sensitive are serologic tests for Lyme disease?**

Lyme antibody titers and ELISA for IgG and IgM are positive in only 40 to 60% of cases.

○   **Is rheumatoid factor found in patients with juvenile rheumatoid arthritis?**

No, rheumatoid factor is typically absent in this disease.

○   **What is phacoanaphylactic endophthalmitis?**

It is a unilateral, chronic endophthalmitis with granulomatous inflammationaround a ruptured lens. The latent period is up to 2 weeks after lens injury and occurs in up to 46% of cases of sympathetic ophthalmia. Treatment includes steroids, antibiotics, and removal of the lens.

○   **Why is phacoanaphylactic endophthalmitis rarely associated with cataract surgery?**

Bacteria probably act as an adjuvant in phacoanaphylactic endophthalmitis.

○   **What is the appearance of keratic precipitates found in Fuch's heterochromic iridocyclitis?**

They are small, non-pigmented stellate KPs which tend to be uniformly distributed over the endothelium.

❍ **What percentage of normal subjects experience an elevation of IOP in response to topical steroid therapy within 2 to 3 weeks of therapy?**

33%.

❍ **What are the ocular manifestations of Crohn's disease?**

1. Uveitis.
2. Scleritis and episcleritis.
3. Retrobulbar neuritis.
4. Extraocular muscle paresis.
5. Keratoconjunctivitis sicca.
6. Subepithelial keratopathy.
7. Recurrent blepharitis and conjunctivitis.

❍ **What type of uveitis does Cryptococcus produce and what is the treatment?**

Cryptococcus is a fungal opportunist occurring in immunocompromised patients. Ocular infection occurs after cerebral infection and produces a chorioretinitis. Treatment is with amphotericin B.

❍ **A young child with high fever, rash, lymphadenopathy, erythema of the soles and palms, and stomatitis develops bilateral eye redness. On examination, iritis is present in both eyes. What is the probable diagnosis, and what cardiac and neurologic complications are they at risk for?**

This child has Kawasaki's disease. Ocular manifestations include bilateral conjunctivitis and iritis. Patients may also develop myocarditis and coronary arteritis as well as meningitis.

❍ **A 40-year-old woman with arthralgia, fatigue, and weight loss develops a mild, nongranulomatous iritis. Her fundus reveals retinal vasculitis with associated intraretinal hemorrhages, cotton wool spots, and retinal edema. Laboratory tests reveal an elevated white count with eosinophilia, negative rheumatoid factor and ANA, elevated ESR, decreased complement, elevated circulating immune complexes, positive anti-neutrophilic cytoplasmic antibody (ANCA) and a positive hepatitis B surface antigen. What is the probable diagnosis?**

Polyarteritis nodosa (PAN).

❍ **How often is hepatitis B surface antigen positive in patients with classic PAN?**

10% to 50%.

❍ **What is the treatment for herpes simplex associated iridocyclitis in a patient with a herpetic ulcer?**

Topical cycloplegics such as homatropine and scopolamine are used to control the uveitis and topical antivirals are given for the ulcer. If the uveitis is severe, a short course of systemic prednisone 30-40 mg PO each morning for 10 days may be given. Trials using oral acyclovir 200 mg 5 times daily for infectious ulcers suggest efficacy, while clinical trials using the same dose of oral acyclovir on stromal keratitis and iritis showed no effect.

○   **Which uveitic syndrome has an increased frequency of HLA-BW22J, a unique Japanese antigen?**

VKH syndrome.

○   **How often is HLA-Bw54 positive in patients with Posner-Schlossman syndrome (glaucomatocyclitic crisis)?**

It is positive in up to 40% of patients.

○   **What viral disease has been associated with glaucomatocyclitic crisis in some cases using PCR on aqueous samples taken in these patients?**

HSV.

○   **What is the treatment for glaucomatocyclitic crisis?**

Treatment consists of cycloplegia, topical steroids, topical beta-blockers, topical alpha agonists, and topical and systemic carbonic anhydrase inhibitors.

○   **What is the uveitis of herpes zoster ophthalmicus due to?**

It is a vasculitis due to live virus invasion, which may result in hypopyon, hyphema, and glaucoma, sector iris atrophy, chorioretinal exudates, vascular sheathing and exudates, and serous retinal detachment.

○   **What is the therapy for acute herpes zoster ophthalmicus?**

Acyclovir 800 mg PO 5 times daily for 10 days, preferably started within 72 hours of onset of the disease. Famciclovir 750 mg PO tid for 7-14 days and valacyclovir 1 g PO tid for 7 days has a greater effect on postherpetic neuralgia.

○   **What are the clinical findings of acute retinal necrosis (ARN)?**

ARN usually occurs in otherwise healthy patients and is characterized by multiple, focal areas of retinal necrosis in the peripheral retina outside of the temporal arcades, which rapidly progress circumferentially, marked vitritis and iritis, and occlusive vasculopathy. Bilateral involvement can occur sequentially or simultaneously in one third of patients.

○   **When does the second eye most often become involved after the onset of acute retinal necrosis in the first eye?**

Six weeks.

○   **What is the treatment for acute retinal necrosis?**

Acyclovir 5-10 mg/kg or 500 mg/m^2 IV q8h for 5-7 days, then oral acyclovir 400-600 mg 5 times daily for up to 6 weeks from the onset of infection. Famciclovir or valacyclovir may be useful in cases that do not respond to acyclovir.

❍ **What HLA phenotype is associated with serpiginous choroiditis?**

HLA-B7.

❍ **What are the clinical characteristics of serpiginous choroiditis?**

It generally affects young, healthy adults with no systemic findings and is usually unilateral, although the other eye may be involved years later. Vitritis occurs in 30%. It is characterized by a cream-colored lesion moving in a snake-like spread from the disk area and lasting for 18 months. Focal phlebitis and APMPPE-like lesions may be present. Vision is lost if the macula is involved. There is no treatment other than laser photocoagulation for choroidal neovascular membranes.

OCULAR PHARMACOLOGY AND THERAPEUTICS

○ **Why do eyedrops have the potential to achieve high serum levels rapidly?**

The first-pass effect (metabolism of a significant fraction of absorbed drug as it crosses the gut wall and passes through the liver) doesn't apply for topical ophthalmic drugs absorbed through the nasal mucosa.

○ **Should patients with glaucoma receive atropine?**

Atropine premedication in the dose range used clinically (0.4 to 0.6 mg IM) however, has no effect on IOP in open-angle glaucoma. When 0.4 mg of atropine is given to a 70-kg person, the eye absorbs only 0.0001 mg. In closed-angle glaucoma, however, atropine may be contraindicated unless a topical miotic agent is instilled into the conjunctiva to guarantee a small pupil. Scopolamine has a greater mydriatic effect than atropine and it is best avoided in patients with known or suspected narrow-angle glaucoma.

○ **Does a dose of atropine; such as used in the reversal of muscle relaxants, affect intraocular pressure?**

Reversal doses of atropine, when given in conjunction with neostigmine do not significantly alter intraocular pressure and this combination may be safely used, even in patients with glaucoma.

○ **What are the effects of anesthetic medications on IOP?**

Inhalation anesthetics cause dose-related decreases in IOP. Postulated etiologies include depression of a central nervous system (CNS) control center in the diencephalon, reduction of aqueous humor production, enhancement of aqueous outflow, or relaxation of the extraocular muscles. Moreover, virtually all CNS depressants, including barbiturates, neuroleptics, opioids, tranquilizers and hypnotics (such as etomidate and propofol), lower IOP in both normal and glaucomatous eyes. It is interesting that etomidate, despite its tendency to produce pain on intravenous injection and skeletal muscle movement, is associated with a significant reduction in IOP. However, etomidate-induced myoclonus may be hazardous in the setting of a ruptured globe. Ketamine's effect on IOP remains controversial. Administered intravenously or intramuscularly, ketamine initially was thought to increase IOP significantly, as measured by indentation tonometry. However, ketamine is not a good drug for ophthalmologic surgery, regardless of the effects on IOP. The nystagmus caused by this drug makes measurement of IOP difficult and may result in inaccurate results.

○ **By what mechanism(s) does epinephrine reduce IOP?**

By reducing outflow resistance through trabecular outflow channels and by increasing uveoscleral outflow.

○   **How many milligrams of epinephrine are there in one drop of a 2% solution?**

Approximately one milligram (a substantial systemic dose).

○   **How is thymoxamine beneficial in the treatment of pigmentary glaucoma?**

As an alpha-blocker, thymoxamine constricts the pupil with no effect on the ciliary body. This flattens the iris, reducing iridozonular touch, without induced myopia or anterior rotation of the lens-iris diaphragm.

○   **What are the potential life-threatening adverse effects associated with systemic acetazolamide use?**

Bone marrow suppression, aplastic anemia, potassium depletion and arrhythmias, and metabolic acidosis.

○   **A glaucoma patient taking acetazolamide is scheduled for surgery. What are some things to remember about carbonic anhydrase inhibitors if general anesthesia is planned?**

Acetazolamide, a carbonic anhydrase inhibitor with renal tubular effects, should be considered contraindicated in patients with marked hepatic or renal dysfunction or in those with low sodium levels or abnormal potassium values. Severe electrolyte imbalances can trigger serious cardiac dysrhythmias during general anesthesia. Furthermore, people with chronic lung disease may be vulnerable to the development of severe acidosis with long-term acetazolamide therapy. Topically active carbonic anhydrase inhibitors have been developed and are now commercially available. Such topical agents might well be expected to be relatively free of clinically significant systemic effects.

○   **How does acetazolamide increase the risk of renal stones?**

By reducing urinary citrate excretion.

○   **Why is echothiophate of importance when planning surgery under general anesthesia?**

Echothiophate is an irreversible inhibitor of acetylcholinesterase and as such is useful in the chronic treatment of glaucoma. It constricts the pupil, increasing the outflow of aqueous humor. Systemically however, it decreases the efficacy of the enzyme pseudocholinesterase. Since this enzyme metabolizes succinylcholine, the combination of echothiophate and succinylcholine may result in prolonged neuromuscular blockade. Because of its extremely long half-life, it is advisable to have a patient discontinue the use of echothiophate at least two weeks prior to surgery.

○   **Is mannitol contraindicated in diabetic patients?**

No. Unlike glycerol, mannitol is not metabolized and poses no hyperglycemic threat to diabetics.

○   **What iris characteristics increase the risk of latanoprost-induced color changes? Describe the nature of the color changes.**

Color changes occur most commonly in eyes with mixed-iris color: brown peripupillary pigment fading to gray-green or blue peripherally (this phenomenon is not seen in uniformly brown or blue eyes). Color changes start at the pupil and spread peripherally, and appear to be permanent.

○   **By what mechanism does ethacrynic acid reduce IOP?**

It reduces trabecular outflow resistance, presumably by altering trabecular endothelial cell cytoskeletal structures.

○   **What factors limit ocular penetration of systemically administered medications?**

The blood-aqueous barrier at the level of the anterior uveal vessels, the inner blood-retinal barrier at the retinal capillary level, and the outer blood-retinal barrier at the RPE level.

○   **What are the most common side effects associated with systemic ganciclovir therapy?**

Myelosuppression is most common. Elevated liver enzymes, skin rash, GI and CNS toxicity may also occur. In children, carcinogenicity and reproductive toxicity are also issues of concern.

○   **What is the initial treatment regimen for HSV retinitis (acute retinal necrosis)?**

Oral and IV acyclovir. If no response and the lesions are sight threatening, add foscarnet and/or ganciclovir.

○   **A patient with traumatic hyphema is treated with aminocaproic acid to prevent secondary hemorrhage. What side effects should you monitor for?**

Nausea and vomiting (25% of patients), and dizziness and hypotension (20% of patients).

○   **An elderly woman with macular degeneration reports high-dose vitamin supplementation in an effort to slow the progression of her disease. What are your concerns?**

High zinc levels can cause copper deficiency anemia and decreased HDL. High vitamin E levels can lead to fatigue, muscle weakness and decreased thyroid function.

○   **What regimen is appropriate for endophthalmitis prophylaxis in the setting of a ruptured globe?**

No single regimen is best, but ceftazidime and vancomycin offer good coverage against gram positive, gram negative and anaerobic organisms.

○   **A 12-year-old girl presents with a two-day history of preseptal cellulitis. What germs are you worried about and what antibiotic coverage is appropriate?**

Common bugs include Staph and Strep species, as well as H. flu and some anaerobes. Amoxicillin-clavulonic acid or a second-generation cephalosporin would be adequate coverage.

○   **A 28-year-old male presents with conjunctivitis and urethritis. Inclusion bodies are seen on conjunctival smear. The diagnosis of chlamydial inclusion conjunctivitis is made. What treatment is appropriate?**

Systemic (oral) administration of tetracycline to the patient and his partner(s).

○   **What adverse reactions to chloramphenicol led to its disuse despite its broad spectrum of activity?**

Aplastic anemia, optic atrophy, peripheral neuritis, and gray syndrome (vomiting, cyanosis, gray stools, ashen skin color, tachypnea, vasomotor collapse, and a 40% mortality rate).

○   **What is the mechanism of action of the fluoroquinolones?**

They are bactericidal via inhibition of DNA gyrase.

○   **What is the mechanism of action of rifampin? What are its side effects?**

Rifampin inhibits bacterial RNA synthesis with no effect on mammalian nucleic acid synthesis. Adverse reactions are rare (4% or less) and include nausea, vomiting, fever, rash, and hepatitis. Rifampin causes orange discoloration of bodily secretions, and has been reported to stain soft contact lenses.

○   **Does oral acyclovir add to topical trifluorothymidine and steroids in the treatment of stromal HSV keratitis?**

No.

○   **How do the antiviral agents' trifluorothymidine, idoxuridine, vidarabine and acyclovir work?**

All are nucleoside analogues targeting viral DNA polymerase.

○   **Antiallergy agents lodoxamide and cromolyn block histamine-mediated allergic responses in what way?**

They stabilize mast cells, preventing degranulation of histamine-filled intracellular granules. These agents possess no direct antihistaminergic activity at histamine receptors.

❍   **By what mechanism does mitomycin C work?**

As an alkylating agent, MMC inhibits DNA synthesis by cross-linking DNA strands.

❍   **Which non-steroidal anti-inflammatory agents do not prolong bleeding time?**

None. They all inhibit platelet aggregation by inhibiting production of thromboxane A2.

❍   **Why must topical NSAIDS be applied pre-operatively to prevent intra-operative miosis?**

They block synthesis of prostaglandins rather than blocking prostaglandin effect at the iris; so they must be administered ahead of time to be effective.

❍   **Which immunosuppressive agent is most effective in the setting of rheumatoid peripheral ulcerative keratitis? Ocular Wegener's granulomatosis? Polyarteritis nodosa?**

Cyclophosphamide is best for all these entities.

❍   **After your ROP screening exam, an infant has feeding intolerance. Explain why.**

Cyclopentolate achieves significant enough systemic levels to delay gastric emptying (via its anti-muscarinic action) in infants.

❍   **A hypertensive patient on systemic propranolol undergoes routine dilated funduscopic exam, and winds up in the ER later that night in hypertensive crisis. Why?**

Beta-blockers may enhance the vasopressor effect of phenylephrine by inhibiting vasodilation.

❍   **Chronic management of myasthenia gravis depends on direct-acting cholinergic agents--true or false?**

False. The agents of choice are indirect-acting cholinergics (cholinesterase inhibitors).

❍   **How long must a patient receive high-dose oral steroids before being at risk for developing posterior subcapsular cataracts?**

0% of patients treated for under one year, 42% of patients treated from 1-3 years, and 58% of patients treated over four years will develop PSC cataracts.

❍   **Rank the following steroids in terms of potency (lowest to highest): methylprednisolone, prednisone, dexamethasone, cortisone, and hydrocortisone.**

Cortisone, hydrocortisone, prednisone, methylprednisolone, dexamethasone.

❍   **How do the acetate and sodium phosphate salts of prednisolone differ pharmacologically?**

Prednisolone sodium phosphate is water-soluble (solution); ocular absorption is limited by duration of eye-solution contact. Prednisolone acetate is water insoluble (suspension; requires shaking) and absorption is two-phased: rapid delivery of the small solubilized fraction, then extended delivery as particles in cul-de-sac dissolve.

❍   **List the barriers to ocular penetration which topical ophthalmic preparations must overcome.**

Basal tear flow washes drug away; local irritation stimulates reflex tearing, washing drug away; tear film itself has hydrophobic (lipid layer) and hydrophilic (aqueous layer) components, as well as a mucinous layer with drug-binding potential; hydrophobic epithelium challenges water-soluble drugs; hydrophilic stroma challenges lipid-soluble drugs; the endothelium (hydrophobic) is too thin to form an effective barrier.

❍   **A 28-year-old woman is diagnosed with pigmentary glaucoma and betaxolol is prescribed. She mentions she's 2 months postpartum and breast-feeding. Is your management still appropriate?**

No. Betaxolol is secreted in breast milk in high enough concentration to cause systemic beta-blockade in the infant. Timolol achieves lower breast milk concentrations and is deemed safe by the American Academy of Pediatrics for breast-feeding mothers.

❍   **How are acetylcholine and carbachol different pharmacokinetically?**

Acetylcholine acts directly at post-synaptic receptors; carbachol also has indirect activity by inactivating acetylcholinesterase, thus increasing its potency.

❍   **Why must the anesthesiologist be informed, prior to general anesthesia, that a patient is taking echothiophate?**

Phospholine Iodide inhibits plasma pseudocholinesterase (as well as acetylcholinesterase), the enzyme responsible for metabolism of succinylcholine. Intraoperative administration of succinylcholine might lead to cardiovascular collapse and respiratory shutdown.

❍   **Which of the alpha-2 agonists (clonidine, apraclonidine, and brimonidine) is most likely to produce CNS side effects such as drowsiness and fatigue? Which is least likely?**

Clonidine is most likely, apraclonidine is least likely.

❍   **A 62-year-old woman with 2mm of left ptosis and unilateral glaucoma OS has uncontrolled IOP with timolol and dorzolamide. What might you consider as a third agent and why?**

Apraclonidine can cause 1.4 mm (average) lid retraction, presumably due to sympathetic stimulation of Mueller's muscle.

○ **Propine is generally not additive to beta-blockers, with one exception. Which agent and why?**

Propine's IOP-lowering effect is via stimulation of beta-2 receptors in the eye. Nonselective beta-blockers block this effect, but betaxolol relatively spares the beta-2 adrenergic receptors and is additive to propine.

○ **Which beta-blocker would you choose for a patient with several risk factors for myocardial infarction, including an unfavorable lipid profile?**

Carteolol--it elevates LDL to a lesser degree than timolol possibly due to its intrinsic sympathomimetic activity.

○ **The two most common adverse reactions reported with dorzolamide is?**

Transient ocular surface irritation (33%) and bitter taste (26%).

○ **What is the mechanism of action of 5-fluorouracil in modulating wound healing?**

Competitive inhibition of thymidylate synthetase during cell replication.

○ **How does the ocular side effect profile of mitomycin C (MMC) differ from that of 5-fluorouracil (5-FU)?**

MMC—little epitheliopathy, risk of endotheliopathy and ciliary body toxicity if introduced intraocularly. 5-FU—severe epitheliopathy, punctal stenosis, minimal risk of endotheliopathy.

○ **What aspect of intracellular acyclovir activation gives the drug exquisite specificity for HSV- or VZV-infected cells?**

Acyclovir is a prodrug, and is activated by a viral (rather than a cellular) enzyme; thus activity is only achieved in infected cells.

○ **What options are available for the CMV retinitis patient who is systemically intolerant to ganciclovir (GCV) therapy?**

GCV intraocular implant or periodic intravitreal GCV injections; systemic foscarnet; intravitreal or systemic cidofovir.

○ **An African immigrant from a region where river blindness is endemic presents with uveitis and the diagnosis of onchocerciasis is made. What is the treatment of choice, and what is its mechanism of action?**

Ivermectin, which paralyzes nematodes by enhancing signal transmission in peripheral, nerves of microfilaria but not in adult worms.

❍   **A neonate born to a woman with chlamydial infection develops conjunctivitis in both eyes. What antibiotic would you prescribe, by what route of administration, and what is its mechanism of action?**

Erythromycin is given orally to provide systemic prophylaxis against pneumonia, and it works by binding to the 50S subunit of the bacterial ribosome, preventing bacterial protein synthesis.

❍   **What is the mechanism of action of the aminoglycoside?**

They bind to the 30S subunit of the bacterial ribosome, preventing protein synthesis.

❍   **What is the spectrum of activity of the aminoglycoside class?**

Aerobic gram negatives and pseudomonas. Limited activity against gram positives. Little activity against anaerobes.

❍   **What is the clinical spectrum of activity of polymyxin B?**

Gram negative rods (except Proteus, Serratia, and Brucella). No gram positive organisms, gram negative cocci, or fungi.

❍   **What are the consequences of co-administration of intravitreal vancomycin with intravitreal dexamethasone? Vancomycin and ceftazidime?**

Co-administering vancomycin and dexamethasone results in decreased vancomycin levels. Co-administering vancomycin and ceftazidime may result in vancomycin precipitation.

❍   **A 22-year-old contact lens wearer presents with a red eye, pain, and a ring-shaped stromal infiltrate after swimming in a pond. You diagnose acanthamoeba infection. What are your medical management options?**

Propamidine (only available in United Kingdom); Neosporin (polymyxin B, neomycin, gramicidin); pentamidine (use transiently while waiting for a colleague in England to send you propamidine); miconazole/ketoconazole/clotrimazole; polyhexamethylene biguanides; sulindac.

❍   **Is flucytosine adequate monotherapy for intraocular fungal infections?**

No, due to widespread resistance in many fungal species; but it makes great co-therapy with amphotericin B.

❍   **In the treatment of Candida albicans endophthalmitis, is systemic treatment with amphotericin B adequate for vitreous coverage?**

No, intravitreal administration is required to achieve therapeutic vitreous levels.

❍   **What is the function of magnesium in BSS intraocular irrigating solution? What about calcium?**

Magnesium is a cofactor for many ATPases, and its presence allows normal biochemical reactions to occur. Calcium helps maintain the apical junctional complexes, which in turn maintain the corneal endothelial barrier (preventing corneal edema).

○   **During cataract surgery, you ask for BSS for hydrodissection, and instead the nurse hands you sterile water. What effect (if any) will this have on ocular tissues?**

The relatively hypertonic corneal endothelium will take on water to lessen the ionic concentration gradient, resulting in corneal edema. If the cells rupture, permanent corneal decompensation may occur.

○   **Povidone-iodine, a popular ophthalmic prep solution, is an iodophor. What does this mean?**

An iodophor is a complex of iodine and organic compounds. Free iodine (which has antimicrobial activity against most bacteria, fungi, viruses, protozoa and yeasts) is released slowly in low concentrations.

○   **What are two potentials ophthalmic uses for cyanoacrylate tissue adhesives?**

To glue nonadherent surfaces together (ie, an otherwise irreparable stellate corneal laceration), and to provide a temporary protective surface (ie, over nonhealing corneal ulcers).

○   **A 29-year-old man is treated for idiopathic anterior uveitis with topical prednisolone acetate, and presents during treatment with mild ptosis of the treated eye as well as 1 mm of anisocoria (the treated eye having the larger pupil). What's going on?**

These transient findings have been attributed to the steroid vehicle, and resolve with cessation of therapy.

○   **What percent of normal volunteers will manifest an IOP over 20mmHg after 6 weeks of topical steroid therapy? How many will be over 30mmHg? What are the risks factors predicting steroid responsivity?**

30% over 20 mmHg and 4% over 30 mmHg. POAG, diabetes, and myopia all are risk factors.

○   **What is the duration of mydriasis for each of the following agents: tropicamide, cyclopentolate, homatropine, scopolamine, and atropine?**

6-24 hrs, 24 hrs, 1-3 days, 3-7 days, and 7-10 days, respectively.

○   **Name as many clinical uses for mydriatic-cycloplegic agents as you can.**

Dilated funduscopic examination, cycloplegic refraction, preoperative dilation, anterior uveitis treatment, lysis of posterior synechiae, treatment of glaucomas associated with lens subluxation or aqueous misdirection, amblyopic fogging therapy, treatment of accommodative esotropia, diagnosis of Horner's syndrome, and as a provocative test for angle closure glaucoma.

O   **What is the mechanism of action of the local anesthetics?**

Blockade of sodium channels in peripheral nerves, preventing depolarization and nerve conduction.

O   **When dilating children in the peds clinic, why is proparacaine (or tetracaine) the first drop instilled?**

Comfort? No! Topical anesthetics induce corneal epithelial microdefects which enhance penetration of dilating drops, while decreasing reflex tearing prevents drug washout.

O   **A 62-year-old woman is undergoing IVFA to evaluate her ARMD. What is her likelihood of experiencing nausea? Does this likelihood change if we know she experienced nausea with a previous IVFA? What is her chance of cardiopulmonary arrest?**

Around 5% of patients experience nausea, and those who do stand a 50% chance of similar discomfort on subsequent IVFA tests. The risk of cardiopulmonary arrest is approximately 1 in 220,000.

O   **A 16-year-old male psychiatric patient presents with blurred vision after eating his cat raw, and is found to have active chorioretinitis with adjacent satellite scars. What is the probable diagnosis and appropriate treatment for the ocular disease?**

Toxoplasmosis chorioretinitis. Treatment includes sulfonamides, clindamycin, and steroids.

O   **What is the importance of nitrous oxide in eye surgery?**

Nitrous oxide is a substance that is 34 times less soluble in blood than is nitrogen. Therefore, it diffuses into an air bubble extremely fast. This can cause large increases in pressure by expanding that bubble. This is obviously hazardous when a bubble is present intra-ocularly. It can compromise retinal blood flow. At the end of surgery, during which nitrous was used, it diffuses out much faster as well, possibly causing the opposite, retinal detachment. In cases, where sulfur hexafluoride is used, nitrous oxide should be avoided for at least ten days. Sulfur hexafluoride has a very low water-solubility and is injected to restore pressure after vitreous surgery. It remains in the eye for several days. Combining this with nitrous oxide could lead to disastrous consequences.

OCULAR TRAUMA

○ **Demographically, who is most likely to suffer severe ocular trauma?**

Males between the ages of 15 and 40 are the most likely group to suffer this injury.

○ **When does severe ocular trauma commonly occur?**

Three main categories of activity constitute the most common settings of ocular trauma:
1. Industrial.
2. Recreational.
3. Victims of assault.

○ **What is the single most important preventative measure one can take to avoid severe ocular trauma?**

The use of impact-resistant protective eyewear.

○ **What are some common recreational activities associated with severe ocular trauma?**

Sports involving small high-speed projectiles (golf, racquetball, baseball, paintball war-games); basketball (elbows and fingers); many others if you think about it.

○ **Automobile airbags have saved many lives since their introduction. What types of ocular injuries have been reported as a result of their deployment?**

Traumatic hyphema, dislocated lenses, retinal tears, and globe rupture.

○ **The evaluation of a patient with ocular trauma requires all the elements of a comprehensive examination. Why is the exploration of the injury mechanism so critical to this evaluation?**

Patients with ocular trauma present with a wide variety of signs and symptoms, which reflect the frequent association of multiple levels of pathologic changes seen in these eyes. To begin to appreciate the depth and breadth of complex injuries, it is vital to document and analyze temporal aspects of the injury, the magnitude of force and directionality of the impact, the risk of particulate invasion of the globe or orbit, and the possible exposure to toxic chemicals or infectious agents.

○ **What common metallic substances are particularly biochemically toxic if internalized in the eye?**

Copper, iron, lead.

O   **What common variety of glass is radio-opaque, aiding in the detection of intraocular foreign bodies?**

Automobile windshield glass is leaded. Even minute particles are easily visible on CT scan.

O   **What potentially blinding disorder can result from a small retained intraocular iron foreign body?**

Siderosis retinae.

O   **What are important clinical signs that can aid in the diagnosis of ocular siderosis, prior to severe loss of vision?**

Pigment changes of the lens and cornea, as well as electroretinographic abnormalities may precede symptomatic visual loss.

O   **What is retinitis sclopetaria?**

A condition resulting from the effects of a missile passing through the orbit without direct globe contact. There is diffuse disruption of the outer retinal layers manifesting as hemorrhage and RPE disorganization.

O   **Describe the mechanism of an orbital floor blowout fracture.**

As a result of blunt force trauma to the globe, the antero-posterior diameter of the globe acutely shortens while the equatorial diameter elongates forcing orbital tissue against the floor of the orbit, out-fracturing it.

O   **What are clinical indications for surgery to reduce an orbital floor blowout fracture?**

Controversy exists about operative indications. Some facial and orbital surgeons feel the goal of repair is to restore normal orbital volume to prevent debilitating enophthalmos. Others are guided by the size of the floor defect, commonly identifying a >50% defect as an indication for repair. Most surgeons agree that extraocular muscle entrapment is an absolute indication for repair.

O   **What is the differential diagnosis of acute post-traumatic proptosis?**

One must consider retro-orbital hemorrhage, traumatic arterio-venous fistula (carotid-cavernous), and acute orbital volume reduction, as in the case of crush injury to the skull base and posterior orbit.

O   **What is emergency management of acute retro-orbital hemorrhage?**

Immediate assessment to ascertain whether neuro-vascular compromise of the eye exists (severe reduction of visual acuity and/or ocular motility, presence of an afferent pupillary defect). There is typically a marked increase in ocular pressure, which must be treated by an emergency canthotomy with cantholysis (lower and upper if indicated).

❍   **What is "Commotio Retinae"?**

This is a contrecoup injury manifesting as a disruption with opacification of the outer retinal layers. When seen in the macula, it is termed "Berlin's edema" which is a confusing term as studies have shown that intercellular fluid is not present.

❍   **What manner of injury can produce traumatic optic neuropathy?**

Shearing force injuries, such as those resultant from blunt force trauma to the globe, can cause disruption of the optic nerve at its attachment to the posterior eye wall. Clinically this can produce an optic nerve avulsion. Forces may transmit along the pyramidal orbit wall structures and concentrate at the optic canal, causing a form of "closed-tunnel" injury to the intracanalicular portion of the optic nerve. This can occur in the absence of a fracture of the optic canal. Orbital missiles or stab wounds to the orbit may also directly traumatize the optic nerve.

❍   **Describe the evolution of traumatic angle recession.**

Blunt force applied to the anterior globe produces a sudden rise in fluid pressure in the anterior segment. The fluid dissects a tract along anatomically susceptible planes, in the case the region between the longitudinal and circular musculature of the ciliary body.

❍   **Describe the management of traumatic hyphema.**

Controversy exists about the preferred mode of treatment. For small to moderate size hyphemas, many authors recommend a combination of a topical or systemic steroid with a cycloplegic and close observation for evidence of rebleeding, corneal staining or IOP rises. Parenteral aminocaproic acid can be used acutely to help reduce the incidence of rebleeding. Oral or topical carbonic anhydrase inhibitors should not be used in patients at risk for sickle cell trait or disease. Surgical intervention is indicated if corneal bloodstaining is evident, or the IOP is elevated in the face of a total hyphema. Aspirin should be avoided.

❍   **What is the significance of a vitreous base avulsion?**

Most authors agree that this is pathognomonic of blunt trauma to the globe, and has medicolegal implications.

❍   **Describe the typical configuration of choroidal rupture after blunt trauma.**

Choroidal ruptures often assume a concentric pattern centered around the optic nerve. This is presumably due to the relatively inelastic attachments of retinal and choroidal elements to the scleral ring and optic nerve.

❍   **What are cardinal signs of globe rupture?**

Hypotony, severely reduced visual acuity, vitreous hemorrhage, globe deformity.

O   What two areas are anatomically most susceptible to scleral rupture after blunt trauma?

The limbus and the area under rectus muscle insertions. Incisional corneal refractive surgery scars may emerge as a new risk factor for ocular rupture after blunt trauma.

O   Name two post-traumatic retinopathies caused by distant extraocular trauma.

Purtscher's retinopathy is characterized by diffuse retinal hemorrhages, cotton wool spots, and exudate most often as a complication of acute chest-compressing trauma. Shaken-baby retinopathy is characterized by diffuse, sometimes large preretinal, intraretinal, and occasionally subretinal hemorrhages, which correlate highly with the presence of intracranial bleeding.

O   What is the significance of angle recession after blunt ocular trauma?

Secondary glaucoma can result in some patients.

O   What is the differential diagnosis of pulsatile proptosis after blunt head/orbit trauma?

Traumatic aterio-venous fistula (often carotid-cavernous sinus), and transmitted meningeal arterial pulses with orbit roof fractures.

O   What major types of ocular dysmotility syndromes may result from orbit blowout fractures?

Acutely it may be difficult to differentiate between orbital edema and an entrapped or palsied extraocular muscle, as motility may be globally impaired due to both of these factors. A short course of parenteral corticosteroids may bring about a rapid decrease in edema to better evaluate the patient's motility. Extraocular muscle palsy may result from injury to the branches of motor nerves that innervate traumatized muscles. Forced duction testing can help differentiate between a palsied muscle and an entrapped muscle.

O   Name the elements of a tripod orbit fracture.

A triangular piece of lateral orbit bone results from forces that fracture across the lower orbital rim, the fronto-zygomatic bone, and the maxilla. Varying degrees of orbital floor deformity can be seen with this type of injury.

O   LeFort type facial fractures can damage what important structure adjacent to the orbit?

The lacrimal drainage system.

O   In the case of retained intraocular foreign bodies, why is it critical to determine the composition of the fragment.

Certain metals and alloys are extremely immunologically reactive and toxic to the retina. It is very helpful to know ahead of time if the fragment is magnetic, which would possibly aid in its extraction.

○   **Why is the rate of endophthalmitis lower than expected with retained metallic foreign bodies?**

Often times, the mechanism of injury involves a super-heated high-speed projectile, which renders it microbiologically sterile.

○   **What is the "at-risk" period for sympathetic ophthalmia to occur after penetrating ocular trauma?**

Patients have been diagnosed with SO in as little as ten weeks and as long as 50 years following penetrating ocular injury.

○   **What early symptoms can a patient with sympathetic ophthalmia manifest at the time of presentation?**

Subtle early symptoms include loss of accommodation in the sympathizing eye, mild photophobia, and blurring.

○   **A child presents to the emergency room with a history of being poked in the eye while riding a bicycle in the park. The child is in pain and very agitated. How should you proceed to examine this child for ocular injury?**

Because the likelihood of obtaining an unobstructed examination of the globe is small in a child who is frightened and in pain, one should proceed to an examination under general anesthesia to rule out serious ocular injury. Thorn injuries from plant matter are particularly serious types of injuries because the puncture sight may be obscured by conjunctival edema or blood. A careful dilated examination should follow to rule out penetrating trauma, as secondary endophthalmitis following exposure to pathogens associated with plant matter can be extremely aggressive.

○   **A patient presents to the emergency room after being hit in the eye with something. He was not wearing eye protection when he went to pick up his car from the repair garage. His vision is slightly blurred and he is photophobic. Slit lamp and indirect ophthalmoscopic examinations do not reveal any signs of an intraocular foreign body. What important diagnostic test should also be done?**

Gonioscopy should also be performed to rule out a penetrating injury with foreign body tucked into the angle of the anterior chamber.

○   **What are the medicolegal implications of diffuse bilateral retinal hemorrhages noted in an infant?**

One must first rule out conditions like severe anemia or myeloproliferative disorders before considering non-accidental trauma. Physicians are required in most states to report suspected cases of NAT.

○   **A homeless person returns to the emergency room complaining of increasing pain and swelling of the orbit which started three days after having brow and lid lacerations repaired following a stabbing attack. On examination, the lids are erythematous and tensely swollen. The globe is proptotic and unable to duct. CT scan shows a fusiform mass along the medial orbit wall, which clinically correlates with a small laceration of the medial upper lid, which is draining some pus. What may have happened, and what is your initial management going to be?**

This scenario is consistent with a penetrating stab wound deep into the orbit medially. There may be a retained radiolucent foreign body in the area that now has developed into an expanding subperiosteal abscess. This mass needs to be surgically drained in order to take pressure off of the globe to prevent a terminal insult to the optic nerve or central retinal vasculature. Cultures and gram stains should be obtained prior to starting parenteral broad-spectrum antibiotics.

BIBLIOGRAPHY

Age-Related Eye Disease Study Research Group: A randomized, placebo-controlled, clinical trial of high-dose supplementation with vitamins C and E, beta carotene, and zinc for age-related macular degeneration and vision loss: AREDS report no. 8. *Arch Ophthalmol.* 2001 Oct;119(10):1417-36.

Albert DM, Jakobiec FA. Clinical Practice Principles and Practice of Ophthalmology . Philadelphia: W. B. Saunders Company, 1994.

Apple DJ, Kincaid MC, Mammalis N, Olson RJ. Intraocular Lenses: Evolution, Designs, Complications and Pathology. Baltimore: Williams & Wilkins, 1989.

Apple DJ, Rabb MF. Ocular Pathology: Clinical Applications and Self-assessment. St. Louis: Mosby Year Book, Inc., 1991.

Arrffa, R. Graysonís Diseases of the Cornea 4ᵗʰ Ed, St. Louis: Mosby-Year Book, Inc., 1997.

American Academy of Ophthalmology. Basic and Clinical Science Course. Sections 1-12; 2000-2001.

Beck RW, Cleary PA, Trobe JD, et al: The effect of corticosteroids for acute optic neuritis on the subsequent development of multiple sclerosis. The Optic Neuritis Study Group. *N Engl J Med* 1993 Dec 9; 329(24): 1764-1769.

Beck RW, Arrington J, Murtagh FR, et al: Brain magnetic resonance imaging in acute optic neuritis. Experience of the Optic Neuritis Study Group. Arch Neurol 1993 Aug; 50(8): 841-846.

Beck RW, Trobe JD, Moke PS, et al: High- and low-risk profiles for the development of multiple sclerosis within 10 years after optic neuritis: experience of the optic neuritis treatment trial. *Arch Ophthalmol* 2003 Jul; 121(7): 944-949.Bohigian GM. Handbook of External Diseases of the Eye. Fort Worth: Alcon Laboratories, Inc., 1980.

The Branch Vein Occlusion Study Group. Argon laser photocoagulation for macular edema in branch vein occlusion. *American Journal of Ophthalmology.* 1984: 98: 271-282.

Cameron, John, Current Surgical Therapy, Mosby, 2004.

Casper DS, Chi TL, Trokel SL. Orbital Disease: Imaging and Analysis. New York: Thieme Medical Publishers, 1993.

The Central Vein Occlusion Study Group. Evaluation of grid pattern photocoagulation for macular edema in central vein occlusion: the Central Vein Occlusion Study Group M report. *Ophthalmology*. 1995; 102:1425-1433.

The Central Vein Occlusion Study Group. A randomized clinical trial of early panretinal photocoagulation for ischemic central vein occlusion: the Central Vein Occlusion Study Group N report. *Ophthalmology*. 1995; 102: 1434-1444.

Choplin NT, Lundy DC. Atlas of Glaucoma. London: Martin Dunitz Ltd, 1998.

The Diabetic Retinopathy Vitrectomy Study Research Group: Early vitrectomy for severe vitreous hemorrhage in diabetic retinopathy vitrectomy study report 2. Arch Ophthalmol. 1985; 103: 1644-52.

Endophthalmitis Vitrectomy Study Group, Results of the endophthalmitis vitrectomy study. Arch Ophthalmol. 1995; 113: 1479-1496.

Kanski JJ. Clinical Ophthalmology. Oxford: Butterworth-Heinemann Ltd, 5th Ed, 2003.

Michael A. Kass, Dale K. Heuer, Eve J. Higginbotham, et al. The Ocular Hypertension Treatment Study: A randomized trial determines that topical ocular hypotensive medication delays or prevents the onset of primary open-angle glaucoma. *Arch Ophthalmol*. 2002;120:701-713.

Krachmer JH, Mannis MJ, Holland EJ. Cornea. St. Louis: Mosby-Year Book, Inc., 1997.

Kline, Lanning, Neuro-*Ophthalmology*, Slack, 2003.

Kline LB. Optic Nerve Disorders. San Francisco:American Academy of Ophthalmology, 1996.

Kunimoto, Derek, *The Wills Eye Manual*, Lippincott Williams & Wilkins, 2004.

Kuppermann B.D., Flores-Aguilar M., Quiceno J.I., et. al. Combination Ganciclovir and Foscarnet in the Treatment of Clinically Resistant Cytomegalovirus Retinitis in Patients with Aquired Immunodeficiency Syndrome, Arch Ophthalmol. 1993; III: 1359-1366.

Loewenstein, John, *Ophthalmology*, McGraw-Hill, 2003.

Mae O. Gordon, Julia A. Beiser, James D. Brandt, et al. The Ocular Hypertension Treatment Study: baseline factors that predict the onset of primary open-angle glaucoma. *Arch Ophthalmol*. 2002;120:714-720.

Mannis, Mark, *Contact Lenses in Ophthalmology*, Springer, 2003.

Milder B, Rubin ML. The Fine Art of Prescribing Glasses Without Making a Spectacle of Yourself. Gainesville: Triad Publishing Company, 2nd Ed, 1991.

Nema, H, *Diagnostic Procedures in Ophthalmology*, 2003.

Opremcak EM. Uveitis: A Clinical Manual for Ocular Inflammation. New York: Springer-Verlag, 1995.

Pavan-Langston, D. Manual of Ocular Diagnosis and Therapy. Boston: Little, Brown and Company, 4th Ed, 1996.

Pepose JS, Holland GN, Wilhelmus KR. Ocular Infection and Immunity. St. Louis: Mosby-Year Book, Inc., 1995.

Rhee DJ, Pyfer MF. The Wills Eye Manual. Philadelphia: Lippincott Williams & Wilkins, 3rd Ed, 1999.

Rapuano, Christopher, *Year Book of Ophthalmology*, 2003.

Ryan SJ. Retina, 2nd Ed, St. Louis: Mosby-Year Book, Inc., 1994.

Sadun, A, Brandt JD. Optics for Ophthalmologists. New York: Springer-Verlag, 1987.

Schepens C, Neetens A., Ed. The vitreous and Vitreoretinal Interface. New York: Springer-Verlag, 1987.

Skuta GL. ProVision: Preferred Responses in Ophthalmology Series 2. San Francisco: American Academy of Ophthalmology, 1996.

Smolin G, Thoft RA. The Cornea. Boston: Little, Brown and Company, 3rd Ed, 1994.

Spalton, David, *Atlas of Ophthalmology*, Mosby, 2004.

Taylor D. Pediatric Ophthalmology. Boston: Blackwell Scientific Publications, 1990.

Uram, Martin, *Diagnostic Procedures in Ophthalmology*, Alpha Science, 2003.

Von Noorden, GK. Atlas of Strabismus. St. Louis: The C.V. Mosby Company, 4th Ed, 1983.

Weingeist TA. ProVision: Preferred Responses in Ophthalmology. San Francisco: American Academy of Ophthalmology, 1993.

Wilkinson CP, Rice TA. Retinal detachment. New York: Mosby, 1997.

Yanof, M, Ophthalmology, Mosby, 2003.

NOTES

NOTES

NOTES

NOTES

NOTES

NOTES

NOTES

NOTES

NOTES